ATHLETES' HEALTH
& Top Performance

Dr.med. German E. Clénin

National Library of Australia Cataloguing-in-Publication entry

Creator: Clénin, German E., author.

Title: Athletes' health and top performance/Dr German E. Clénin.

ISBN: 9781925497243 (paperback)

Subjects: Sports medicine–Popular works.
Sports sciences–Popular works.
Self-care, Health.
Athletes–Health and hygiene.

Dewey Number: 613.711

Published by **Dr German E. Clénin** and InHouse Publishing
www.inhousepublishing.com.au

Dedication

I dedicate this book to my wife Susanne, who keeps me grounded, has supported me very much during my professional career, and with whom I like to share my ideas and thoughts. Many hugs and lots of love to you, Susanne!

I also dedicate this book to my parents, who have done everything to enable an excellent education leading to my professional and personal development. Thanks a lot to both of you, Ma and Pa!

Table of Contents

Acknowledgements

I'm very thankful having had the great support of two friends and mates in sports: Rev. Graham Dempster (previously P.E. teacher) and Tim Bagshaw (MSc in Physiotherapy). They gave me a lot of valuable feedback and helped to make my English much smoother. Many thanks to PD Dr.med. André Leumann, Dr.med Mareike Cordes, Barbara Harisberger, and Ewa Haldemann who all made extremely valuable and constructive comments to the content of the book. Special thanks to Sabrina, Sarah, Nadine, Susanne, Rémy, and Marc-André for their support with illustrations, photos, drawings, and website. Thanks to Fran and Bob, Catherine and Andrew, Joël and Jonin for their support and great friendship. And last but not least: thanks to Ocean, Kaya, Caroline, and the whole team at InHouse Publishing – you were truly inspiring.

Foreword

As an athlete, I often push my very limits. This is essential to achieve top performance, but it is equally important not to go too far. Exactly this happened in spring, when I had a persistent cough. Following a good winter training season, I was looking forward to the start of competition season and was fully motivated to train intensively with my goals in mind. A cold turned into a cough, as it happens, but I saw no reason to adjust or alter my training.

The cough persisted and even a reduced training schedule did not lead to improvement. The warning shot and the decision to see a doctor came one night when the coughing became so severe that my chest started hurting. The next day, I immediately went to my sports medicine physician and, following a clinical examination and two x-rays, early stage pneumonia was diagnosed. Thanks to my quick action and the targeted therapy, I was able to minimise my training downtime and resume competition season within only a short time. I also found the Return to Play Plan recommended by the doctor very helpful, which made me understand that I really had to stop completely for a few days in order not to delay the healing process. Very soon, I was already able to commence with shorter training units in the extensive area of endurance.

This and similar situations are common in the career of an athlete. When can I resume training and when is a doctor's consultation a must?

The book at hand serves as an excellent and specific advisor across the entire range of sports. A variety of potential issues are presented in a well-structured manner and complemented with valuable tips of an experienced author. For me as an athlete, this book provides a great level of security, and this is one piece in the puzzle of success!

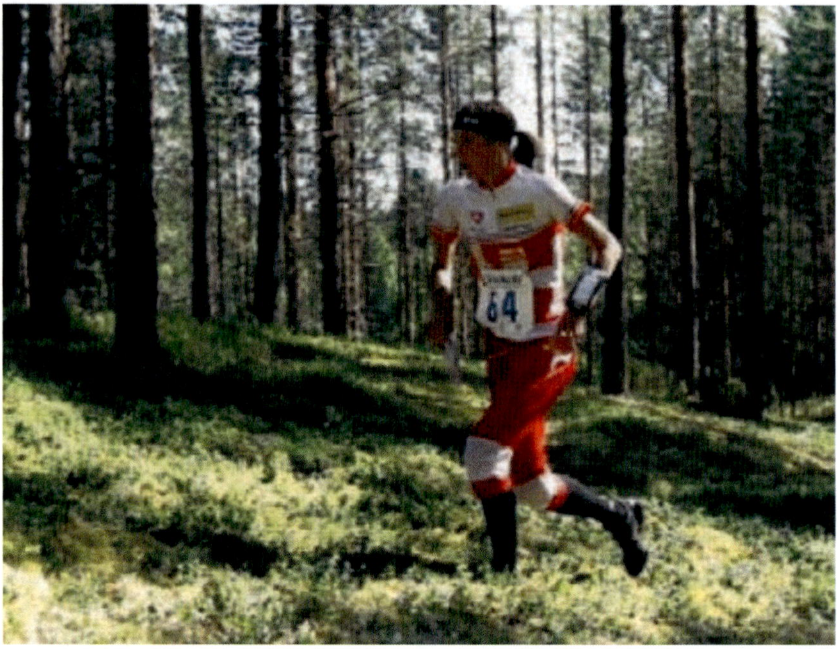

Simone Niggli-Luder
Orienteering World Champion (23-times)
World Cup Winner (8-times)
Swiss Sports Woman of the Year (3-times)

Introduction

Dear athletes, coaches, parents, and sport and health professionals,

Athletes' Health and Top Performance. What a promising title! I do have two thoughts to share:

1. There's a broad knowledge and deep understanding in the various disciplines around the physiology of performance: novel insights in sports sciences and sports medicine, recent findings in training and recovery strategies, evidence-based and approved practices in sports physiotherapy, and new concepts in sport nutrition and successful strategies in sports psychology. Even for health and sport professionals it is a challenge to keep abreast of it all and to stay up to date. An overview in the form of a handbook for athletes, coaches, parents, and often many more involved persons is the answer to this need.
2. Athletes are good patients as they want to get back into the action, the sooner, the better. 'Doc, when'll I be back?' is one of the very first questions I hear in my practice—that's a big advantage for any health professional in the field of elite sports. However, in the life of an athlete, there are often issues that need a closer look and some patience. The approach of, 'Just train harder, it will get better then,' is neither a long term nor an effective solution—especially as the proper healing of an injury or an illness is too important for high performance and the sustainability of a sports career. *Athletes' Health* is not at all just about the absence of illnesses and sport-injuries, but as the WHO definition says:

   > *'Health is a state of complete physical, mental and social well-being and not merely the absence of disease or infirmity.'*[1]

That's where we should all look for. No doubt, sport is a wonderful thing, whether it's your profession, your passion, or just a leisure activity. There are many positive effects related to sports activity. To be successful you need to give much of

---

[1] *Preamble to the Constitution of the World Health Organization (WHO) Geneva 23.3.2016 http://www.who.int/about/definition/en/print.html*

yourself, and a consistently high level of performance in sports is extremely demanding and challenging. We all agree that elite sport is therefore quite often on the edge (and occasionally even a bit beyond). This means that with an injury, whether it be an acute trauma or overuse, there is often a pressure situation—a time pressure to be back as soon as possible, with expectations of the media, the club, the coach, and, last but not least, your very own, enhancing this dilemma. It's essential in this situation to take one step back and to make a serious analysis of what the medical diagnosis is and what treatment and return to play plan we are talking about.

Knowing the athlete's side from both my own experience, and from my professional involvement in this field, I understand how not being allowed to perform feels. But an athlete's health is as essential in leading up to top performance as it is to allowing a long lasting, successful sports-career, not to mention life after sport.

So, I hope that this manual will be a help for a better understanding for all of us.

Sincerely,
Dr.med. German E. Clénin

Goals for This Manual About Athletes' Health

1. Breaking down recent and essential findings in sports medicine and sports sciences and presenting them to you in a written and understandable manner, supported by pictures and illustrations.
2. Empowering of athletes, coaches, and parents by directly bringing you applied knowledge and practical skills to support you in your everyday life as sportsmen and women.
3. Giving practical advice for good preventive measures, early self-treatment options, and recommendations when to see a doctor.

This manual can't replace a sports medicine physician's or sport physiotherapist's diagnosis and treatment, but it will make you more self-sufficient and hopefully allow you to feel safer in your daily work as an athlete and coach.

How Are the Topics Organised and Structured?

Topics are organised according to organ systems throughout the table of contents, with a focus on important sport relevant information. The structure follows this order:

Title: Disease XY – Additional Information

The first part is a neutral medical title. While the second part works as a catchy description and reminder. This second part is personal coloured by experience and possibly not always 100% objective. But I feel that makes it more interesting and, hopefully, is an added value for you. For example: Runner's knee – when the ilio-tibial band rubs and causes lateral knee pain.

Symptoms

Describes the classical symptoms, as you may observe them. Possibly with an illustration or a figure to assist recognition.

Figure 1: or Illustration 1:

Background

Gives background information to the illness or injury, as far as necessary.

Prevention and Treatment Table for *XY*

Prevention	What to do or not to do so that an illness, an overcharge, or an injury is NOT going to happen.
Treatment by Yourself	Showing good and easily applicable treatment options.
When is a Doctor Needed?	To make you feel safer in your decision-making when to see a doctor.
Return to Play/Sports	Gives an idea about the time frame. Some propositions how to start training again and for alternative training may be given.

What Does the Doctor Do?

Tells you what a doctor does when seeing you. How the diagnosis is confirmed, what the treatment options are, and which one may most likely be chosen.

Safety First – You Must Protect Yourself, Others Have Different Priorities ...

This is a highly important issue because it's about staying alive. Yes, it's that serious! I recall a few sportsmen and women who had a severe accident while they were training—some were killed (e.g. South African Olympic cross-country mountain biker Burry Stander) or rendered paraplegic after the incident (e.g. Swiss Triathlete Dr.med. Christian Wenk). So do everything that is reasonably feasible to protect yourself. You may say, 'I cannot prevent everything. When it is going to happen, it will happen.' I don't agree on that, neither do many studies in the field of injury prevention. Certainly, an element of risk remains, but it's up to you to do everything to reduce it to a minimum. What does this mean? Be prepared, plan your training day, have good and safe material, and be well-equipped. Train hard but be alert. Have a cautious attitude in traffic.

Road cycling

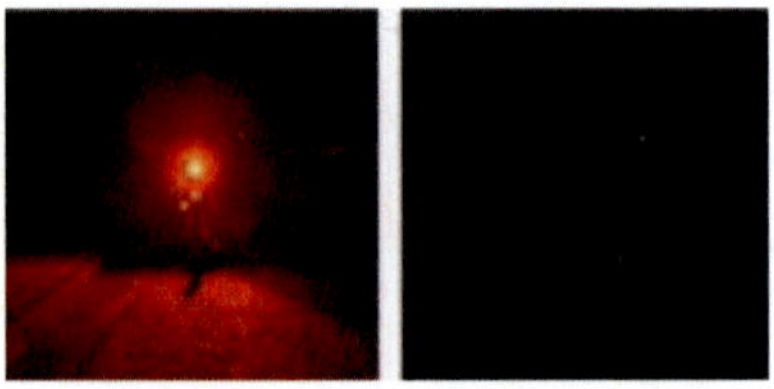

Wear clothes in bright colours and wear a helmet all the time (many studies have shown that wearing a helmet reduces significantly your risk of a severe brain injury). Do your training session in daylight. If it's a long session, take good visible lights with you (there are products that fit on your training bike and you just can leave them on). Wear gloves. Take a raincoat in your jersey (protection against cold and rain, preferably with reflecting colours).

Mountain biking

As above. In remote areas don't bike alone but with a partner, have your mobile phone with you, possibly download specific rescue apps (e.g. Swiss Alps www.rega.ch). Depending on your choice of track for a lot of downhill sessions, you should have more protection. For gravity downhill mountain biking, full protection with a full face helmet, back protector, shoulder pads, knee and shin pads, and gloves are warranted. A Leatt brace (neck protector) is highly recommended.

Running/Jogging

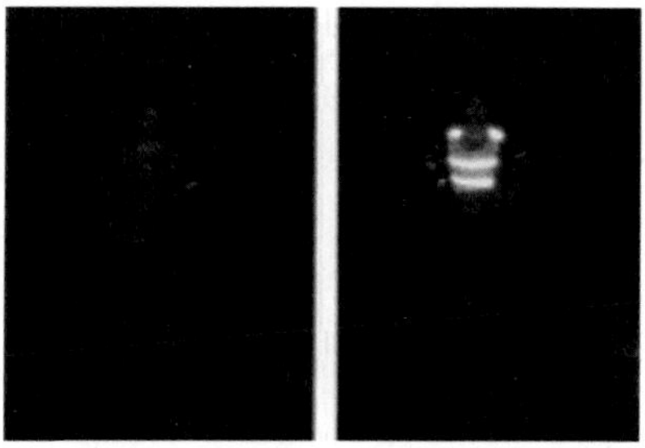

Wear running clothes in bright colours. Do your training sessions in daylight, choose a reasonable route (especially concerning road traffic and mountain hazards) as this reduces the risk of not being seen by car drivers and of unnecessary risk exposure in the mountains. When you consider running at twilight or at night, you must wear a reflective vest and take a torch or head lamp with you.

Alpine snow sports

Wear a helmet, gloves, and, depending on your discipline, a back protector all the time. Be aware of the cold—wear underwear (e.g. Merino wool) that keeps you warm and wicks away the moisture. Follow instructions of the ski station and their safety experts to the letter.

On-water sports

Wear a life vest at all times. You may be the best swimmer but if you're unconscious you will drown! Depending on your discipline you must wear a helmet (whitewater canoe or kayaking).

Equipment

When it comes to your equipment, don't be stingy; don't go for the cheap product. Your sport is your passion, so go for quality. It doesn't have to be the most expensive either, but choose good stuff to a reasonable price.

Heat illness

A very specific topic but to be named in the field of safety, as even today we see athletes die on the field from simple overheating. As it is that important to me, I dedicate two separate chapters to this topic, one focusing on safety aspects (see 'Heat illness') and one focusing on performance (see 'Heat Acclimatisation').

Warming Up – Includes Sport Specific Strength and Proprioception

The warming up is a must! Not only are you preparing for your physical workout by enhancing respiration and blood flow (lungs, heart, vessels including the finest capillaries in your tissues) and are getting all body structures alert and ready for effort (neurons, muscles, tendons, ligaments, cartilage, bone), but you are preventing accidents and severe injuries. Warming-up includes a neuromuscular activation in order to raise your proprioception. The word *proprioception* comes from Latin *proprius* meaning 'one's own', 'individual'; and *capere*, to take or grasp. It is the sense of the relative position of neighbouring parts of the body and sensitises their changes in movement (adapted from Wikipedia).

Many studies, especially those done in Scandinavian countries, show what a good warm-up should look like:

- **General warm-up (5–8min):** Light jogging or cycling to get the circulation and the blood flowing to all the tissues. Also moving shoulders, arms, hands, and trunk to get the whole body involved.
- **Balancing exercises (5–8min):** Related to the demands of your sport. Start in a standing position on uneven ground (wobble-board, etc.) then moving to jumping and landing exercises first with both legs, then making it more difficult on one leg, progressing to including your sports equipment (e.g. playing passes with the ball on uneven ground or while jumping and landing).

- **Sport-specific strengthening exercises (5-8min):** Perform strengthening in two ways:
  1. As close as possible to your sport specific needs, may it be single leg squats or hamstrings lower or another exercise being close to your sports discipline. The Nordic hamstrings lower exercise has the goal to train the hamstrings muscle and seems to be efficient in preventing knee injuries (e.g. rupture of the ACL, anterior cruciate ligament—see this chapter) as well as direct hamstrings injuries (e.g. structural muscle lesion—see this chapter).
  2. By activating your core muscles (see also chapter 'core stability') by integrating a couple of exercises

Examples of balancing exercises:

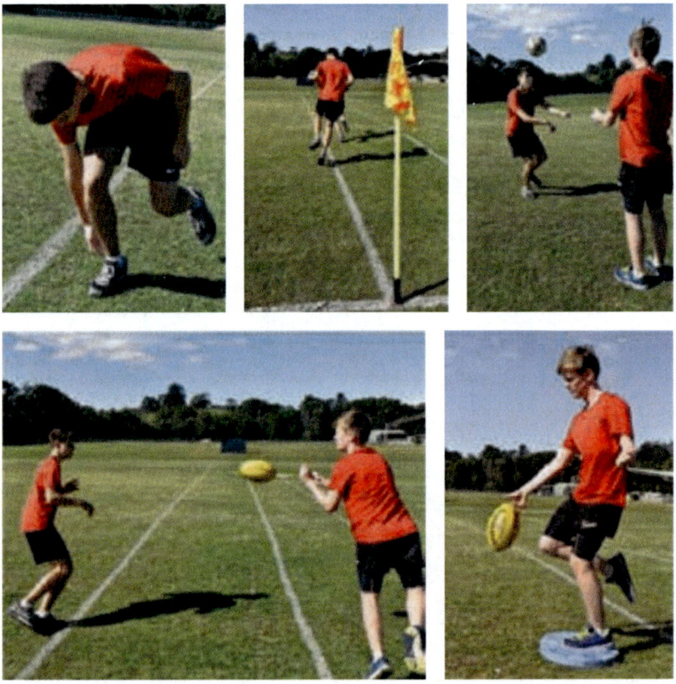

e.g. single leg stance touching heel and touching toes; single leg jumps with line crossing; practicing headers or passes on one leg; partner exercises with one leg jumps; if available practising shots on wobble board

Examples of sport-specific strengthening exercises:

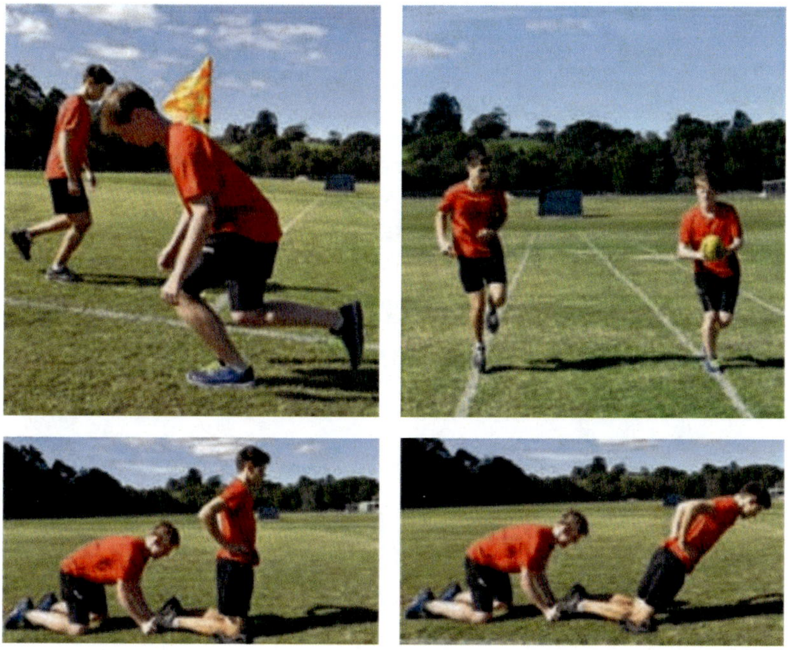

e.g. Single leg squat with good leg axis control "knee over toe"; Nordic hamstrings lower exercise; partner exercise, sport specific single jumps while practising passes, etc.

Literature

Kristianslund E et al. Sidestep cutting technique and knee abduction loading: implications for ACL prevention exercises. Br J Sports Med. 2014 May;48(9):779-83.

Wingfield K. Neuromuscular training to prevent knee injuries in adolescent female soccer players. Clin J Sport Med. 2013 Sep;23(5):407-8.

Myklebust G, Skjølberg A, Bahr R. ACL injury incidence in female handball 10 years after the Norwegian ACL prevention study: important lessons learned. Br J Sports Med. 2013 May;47(8):476-9.

Herman K et al. The effectiveness of neuromuscular warm-up strategies, that require no additional equipment, for preventing lower limb injuries during sports participation: a systematic review. BMC Med. 2012 Jul 19;10:75. doi: 10.1186/1741-7015-10-75.

Engebretsen AH et al. Prevention of injuries among male soccer players: a prospective, randomized intervention study targeting players with previous injuries or reduced function. Am J Sports Med. 2008 Jun;36(6):1052-60.

Myklebust G et al. Prevention of noncontact anterior cruciate ligament injuries in elite and adolescent female team handball athletes. Instr Course Lect. 2007;56:407-18.

Verhagen E et al. The effect of a proprioceptive balance board training program for the prevention of ankle sprains: a prospective controlled trial. Am J Sports Med. 2004 Sep;32(6):1385-93.

Myklebust G et al. Prevention of anterior cruciate ligament injuries in female team handball players: a prospective intervention study over three seasons. Clin J Sport Med. 2003 Mar;13(2):71-8.

Definition of Proprioception: retrieved on the Wikipedia Website 3.6.2016 https://en.wikipedia.org/wiki/Proprioception.

Training and Performance – the Basics of Success

To talk to athletes and coaches about training and performances would seem like carrying coals to Newcastle. But what a training session causes, triggers, and hopefully initiates in our organism is important. Figure 1 shows a typical training session with a training load inducing a certain temporary fatigue and structural load on your body. It's natural that this training stimulus triggers structural, physiological, and neuro-muscular changes, and after the recovery makes the body stronger, faster, more explosive, with more endurance—depending on what has been trained (super-compensation in Table 1).

Table 2 shows how a series of training should enable an athlete's performance to improve. The new training stimulus should allow enough recovery time in order to have a rising training effect.

Having a look at the factors determining performance in sports (Table 3), we come closer to an understanding how comprehensive and complex sport performance needs to be understood. There are a multitude of factors influencing, and sometimes limiting, performance. And that's exactly where the work of the athlete and the coach starts. A detailed training program to improve performance and enhance all contributing factors is established and regularly adjusted in order to reach your top performance.

Table 4 gives already a deeper insight in these processes as it tries to show recovery times and super-compensation from a training stimulus. The intention is to plan the next specific training practice ideally timed in the phase of super-compensation in order to get an optimal rise in level of performance.

Table 1: Effect of Training

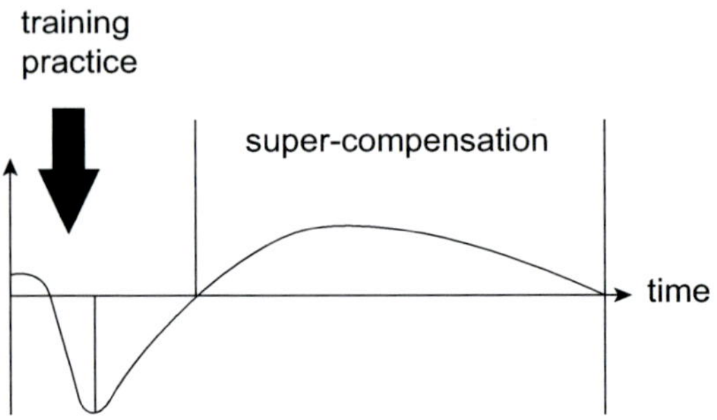

Table 2: Effect of a series of training practices

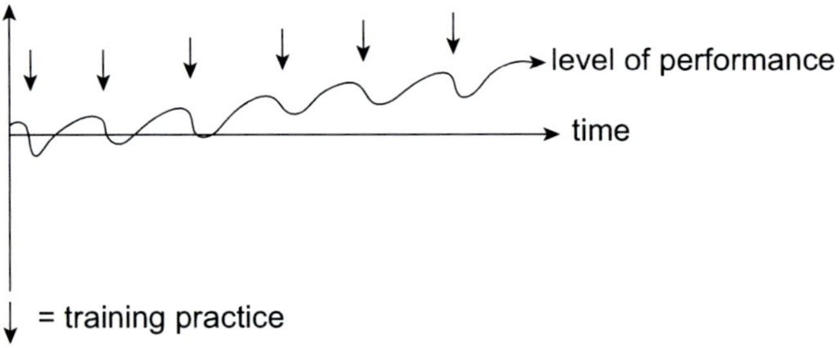

Table 3: Factors Determining Performance in Sports (translated and adapted after Weineck 2009)

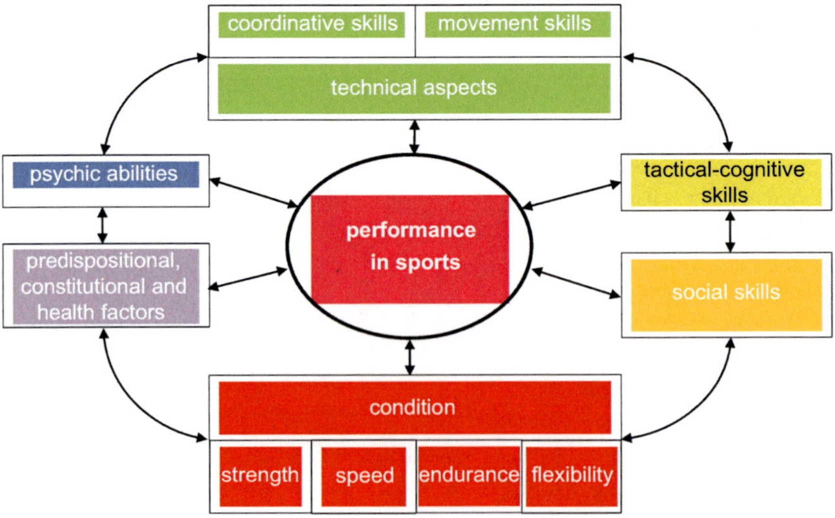

Table 4: Ideal timing of Super-Compensation (courtesy JanOlbrecht).

After a specific training, as indicated with arrows, e.g. extensive aerobic work, the super-compensation will take place in certain range of hours, as indicated in the table below, e.g. extensive endurance from 8 to 12 hours.

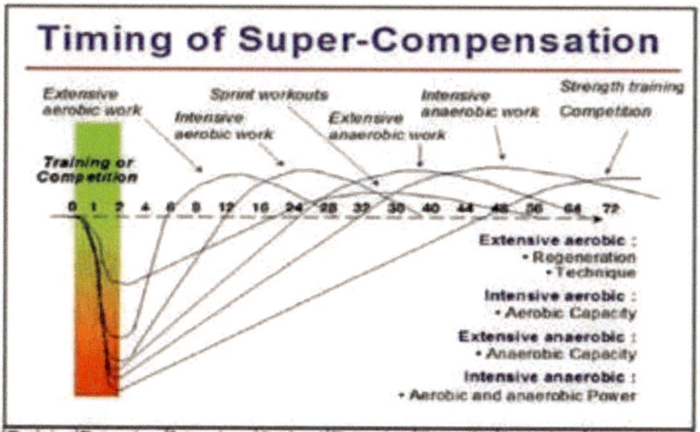

Training types	Extensive Endurance	Intensive Endurance	Sprints/ Short Sets	Extensive Anaerobic Training	Extensive Strength Training	Intensive Anaerobic Training	Intensive/ Strength Training/ Competition
From	8	24	30	36	40	40	48
To	12	30	40	48	60	60	72

Literature

Olbrecht J. The Science of Winning: Planning, Periodizing and Optimizing Swim Training, Dec 17, 2013 Kindle eBook, F&G Partners, 2015 ISBN 9078158069, 9789078158066.

Weineck J. Optimales Training, Spitta; 16th edition (1st December 2009), Balingen Germany, ISBN 978-3-938509-96-8.

Core Stability – Better Performance and Less Backpain

Imagine the vertebral column with all its bony vertebrae, the rib cage in front, just a column of bony bins with a few ligaments to hold things together. To keep our body on the one hand flexible and on the other hand stable if needed, that's the job of our trunk's muscular system, more commonly known as the core muscles.

Let me compare it with a circus tent, which needs to be put up with several poles and secured with tensioning ropes from all sides. The better the tensioning ropes are placed, the stronger they are, and the better they are coordinated in their action, the better the stability. Now with this example it is easier to understand that our body muscles in the rear (back and lumbar muscles), the ones in the front (abdominal muscles), and the ones on each side (lateral muscles) need to work together to hold the core of our body stable (see Figure 1). The advantage of a muscular system, compared to a more stiff construction like a house, is that we are able to move, to change position, to transmit, and even to further develop power. This means, for example, in case of a shot putter, the power of the start-up and the explosivity of the legs can be transferred in the one movement behind the shot to reach top performance.

Naturally core stability is not just about one single performance peak (maximal strength for one movement) as in the shot putter, but also about all adaptations that happen in other sports, like the 110m hurdles sprint (adapted explosive strength for 11–12 seconds) and like the long term stabilisation task in a marathon runner (strength endurance for 2h 10min). It's also about stabilising the body during many hours of training and competition and, last but not least, throughout daily life.

So to understand how this core stability really works, we are talking about global and local systems of muscles. The *global system of core muscles* consists in the rear of the big back and lumbar muscles (erector spinae, longissimus dorsi, latissimus dorsi, quadratus lumborum) and in the front of the big abdominal muscles (rectus abdominis, see Figure 2). Their job is to do the big things, the greatest work; they are involved in all major movements, especially the peak power output (e.g. shotput) and the tasks asking high explosivity (e.g. 110m hurdles). Underlying the global muscle system there is the *local system of core muscles*. This consists of the small back muscles (multifidi) and the transversal abdominal muscles (transversus abominis, partially externus and internus abdominis, see Figure 3). The latter gives the local stabilisation and is ideally able to stabilise the trunk by a co-contraction around the vertebral column on the needed level. This means the contraction of a muscle segment all around the core of our body (i.e. on either side of the vertebral column), helping stability and firmness, but still ready for adaptations if needed. To summarise core stability allows a continuous and focused energy transfer and secures an optimised coordination between the local/global core muscles and the involved muscle chains, and therefore improves power output.

Figure 1: Circus Tent, Core Muscle System of the Body

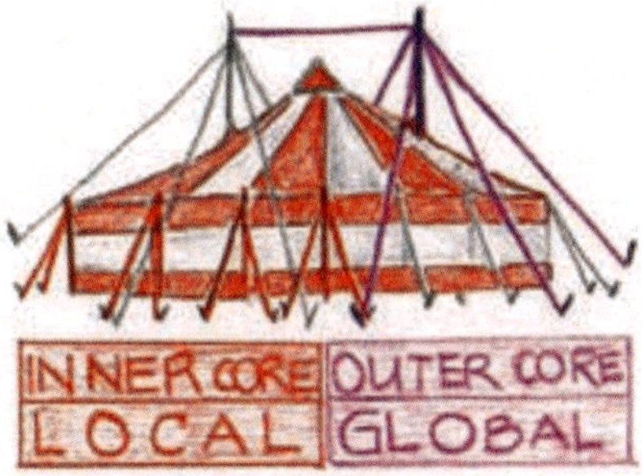

Inner core muscles / LOCAL
1. Multifidus muscle
2. Transversus abdominis muscle
3. Pelvic floor muscles

Outer core muscles / GLOBAL
4. Rectus abdominis muscle (i.e. abdominals; abs)
5. Abdominal external oblique muscle
6. Erector spinae muscle

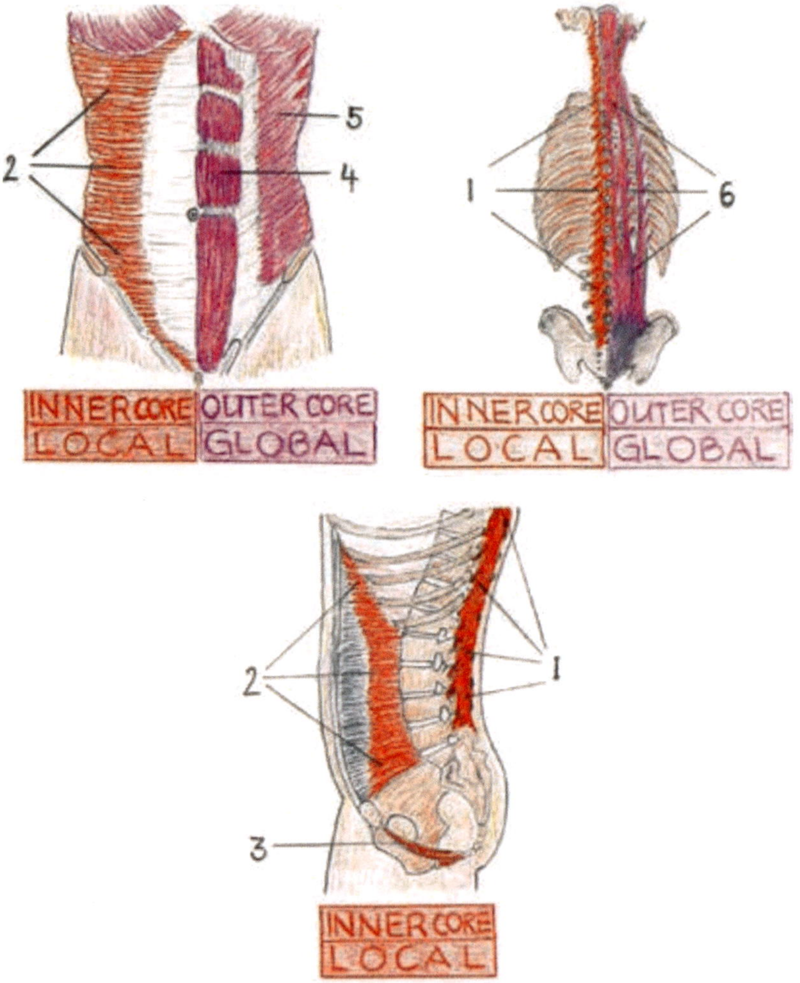

What about back pain? Is it frequent in sports?

Yes, back pain is a quite frequent complaint in both daily life and in sports. Studies clearly show that regular training of core stability and strengthening of endurance of the core and the whole trunk muscle system reduces the number and duration of back pain episodes. So core stability is a must for all athletes (in fact for all human beings). And yes, as athletes have a higher exposure to stop and go movements, to shearing and rotational forces on the trunk, and to impacts of all kind the level of core stability and strength endurance of the trunk muscles needs to be by far superior to that of a normal person. Some sports are even more demanding than others on the core stability system: especially gravity disciplines (e.g. downhill MTB, alpine skiing), martial arts (e.g. judo, taekwando, karate), and team sports with direct opponent contact (e.g. AFL, rugby, handball, ice hockey just to name a few). In these disciplines, core stability is an absolute must, as the core and trunk muscle systems act like a corset in stabilising and protecting the body.

Core stability exercises should be done on a regular basis by every single athlete. So make sure you integrate these exercises in your training program. As an elite athlete starting up, you may go ahead with 3–4 times 30–45min for 2 or 3 months. Once you're on a good level, twice a week 30–45min is sufficient (for master and recreational athletes once a week is fine). And I promise strengthening your core stability will make you feel better.

Practical Exercises – See the following pages

Stage I – BEGINNERS
Stage II – ADVANCED
Stage III – EXPERT

Literature

Prieske O et al. Neuromuscular and athletic performance following core strength training in elite youth soccer: Role of instability. Scand J Med Sci Sports. 2016 Jan; 26(1):48–56.

Stuber KJ et al. Core stability exercises for low back pain in athletes: a systematic review of the literature. Clin J Sport Med. 2014 Nov; 24(6):448–56.

Schmidt CP et al. Prevalence of low back pain in adolescent athletes – an epidemiological investigation. Int J Sports Med. 2014 Jul; 35(8):684–9

Shinkle J et al. Effect of core strength on the measure of power in the extremities. J Strength Cond Res. 2012 Feb; 26(2):373–80

Petering R, C Webb. Treatment Options for Low Back Pain in Athletes. Sports Health. 2011 Nov; 3(6): 550–555.

Core Stability Exercises – Stage I – BEGINNER

Perform three series of these 8 exercises – once you manage them well and your core stability and body awareness have improved, you may move up to the Stage II – ADVANCED exercises.

1. Pelvic tilting

	Instructions	Time
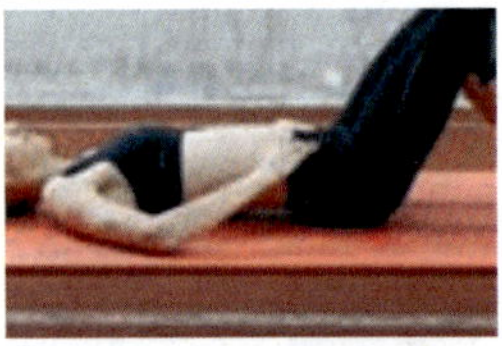 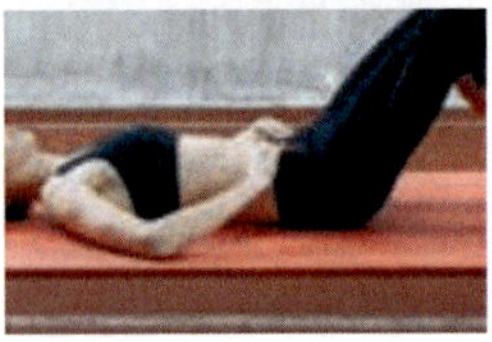	In supine position, tilt your pelvis by releasing and activating your abdominal muscles. Goal: better awareness of the positioning of the pelvis.	12 repetitions

2. Activating the local core muscle system at rest – in different positions

	Instructions	Time
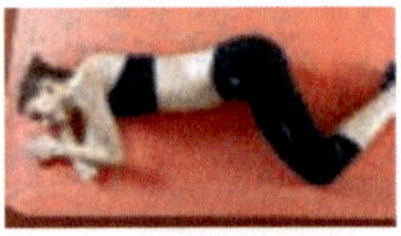 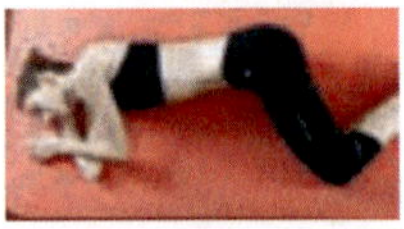	Activate your local core muscles: transverse abdominal (anterior), pelvic floor (below), and multifidus muscles (back). Gents: balls up. Ladies: as you would close the zip of tight jeans.	Activate and hold for 10sec, 5sec rest. Repeat 8 times
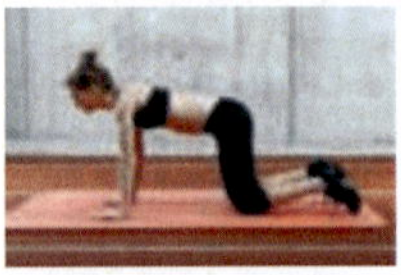 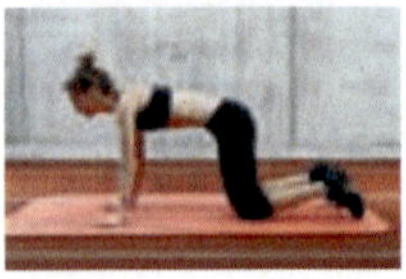	Once you are familiar: a) Do the same exercise in a four point kneeling. b) Do it in upright position.	

3. Train the local core muscle system under slight movement

	Instructions	Time
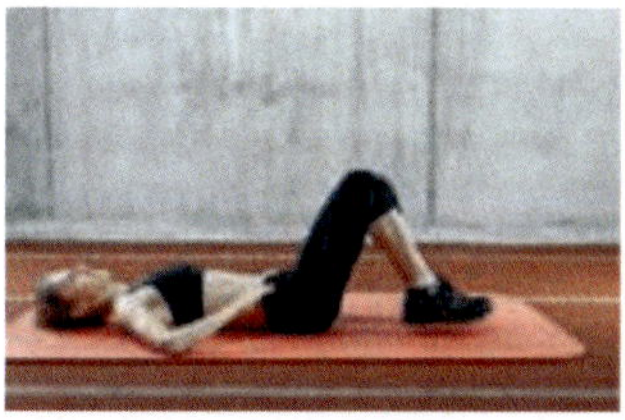 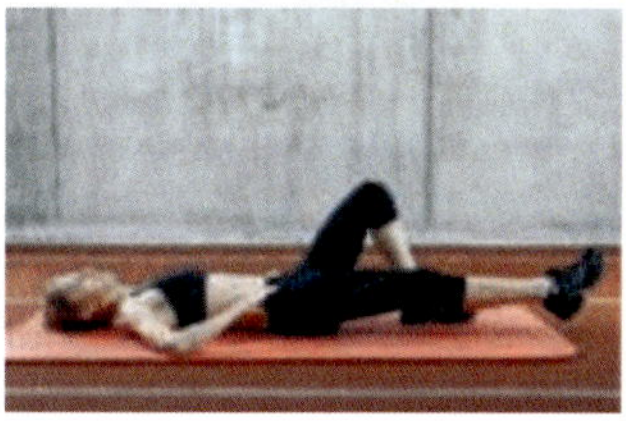	Supine, hip flexed, one foot on the ground the other in the air. After activating the local core muscles move one leg forward, control the firm pressure of the lower, lumbar spine muscles to the ground with one hand, the activation of the local abdominal muscles with the other hand.	Right leg: 30sec Left leg: 30sec

4. Plank exercise (global anterior muscle chain)

	Instructions	Time
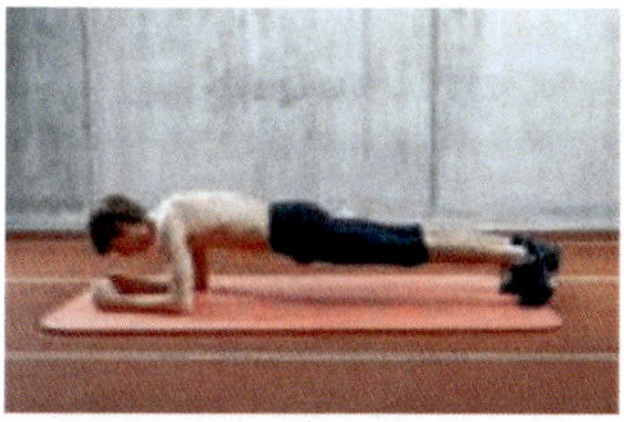 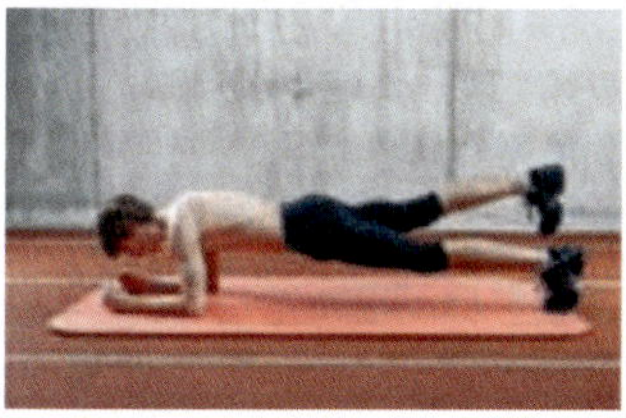 If too hard at the beginning, you may do the same exercise on your knees. A shorter lever will make it easier.	Holding the plank position, raise your right foot about one foot in the air, alternate left-right, keeping your body stable. Important: control your lower back and pelvis by activating the local core muscles. Don't allow your hips to drop.	Start with 45sec, later 60sec

5. Global lateral muscle chain

	Instructions	Time
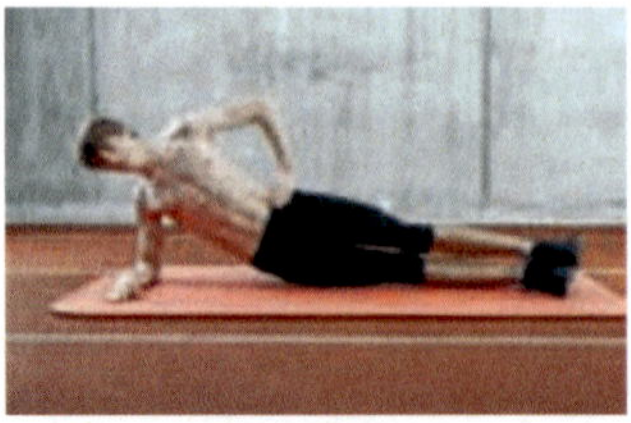 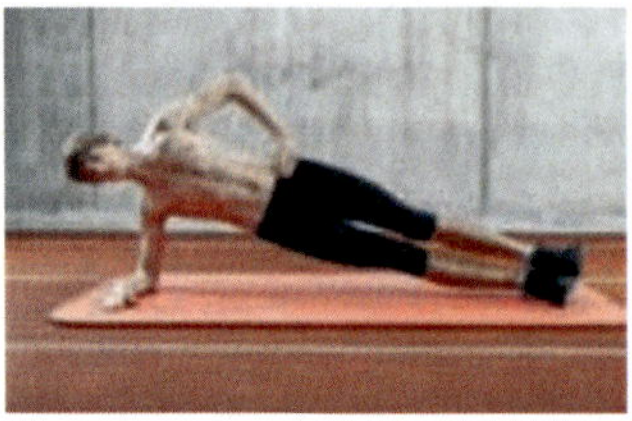 If too hard at the beginning, you may do the same exercise with bent knees, having a shorter lever (only until your knees).	Come up and down in a rhythm of one second per movement.	Start with 20sec, then 30sec, later 45sec

6. Global back muscles (posterior chain)

	Instructions	Time
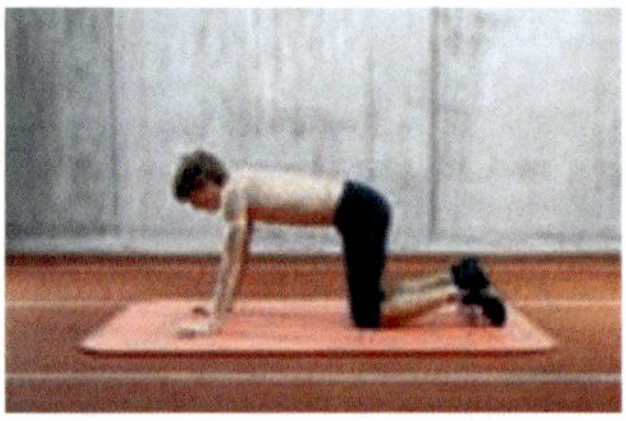 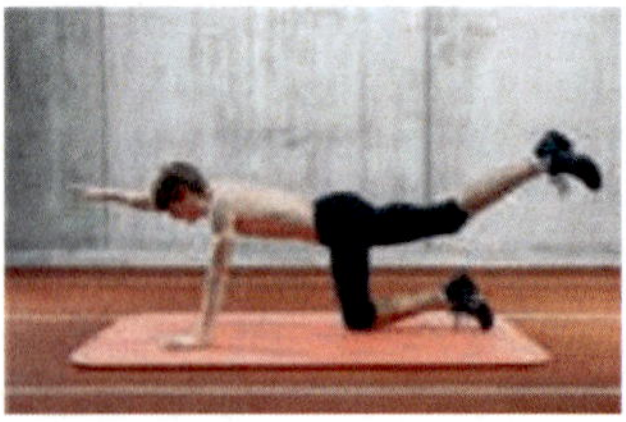	In four point kneeling position. Crosswise lift the right arm – left leg and vice versa, always having a good control of the lower back and pelvis (don't fall into a hollow back).	60sec
	Slightly advanced: stay with the left arm-right leg exercise for 30sec, instead of a rest when coming down, knee and elbow touch under your body, and continue.	30sec R leg – L arm, 30sec for L leg – R arm

7. Global abdominal muscles

	Instructions	Time
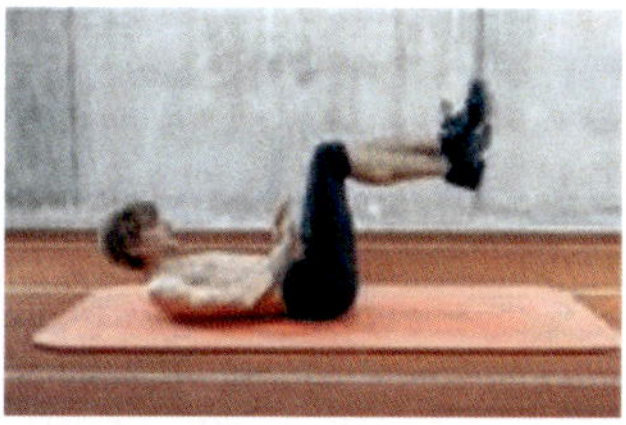 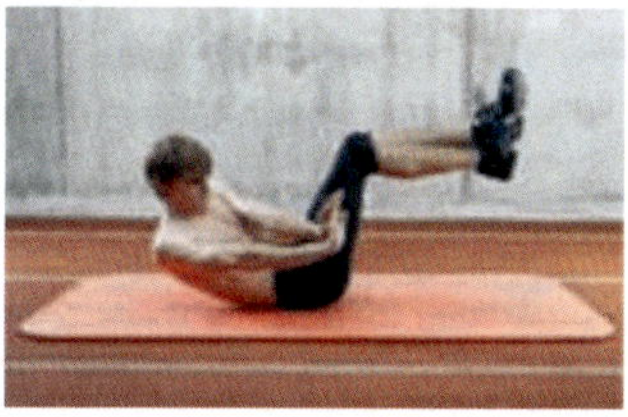	Supine, hip flexed, lower legs in the air, hands together. Come up across your body, changing left and right side, always lifting the shoulder completely off the ground.	60sec

8. Local back muscles

	Instructions	Time
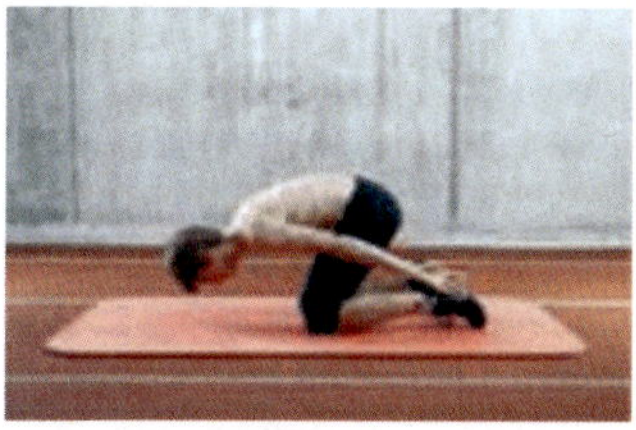 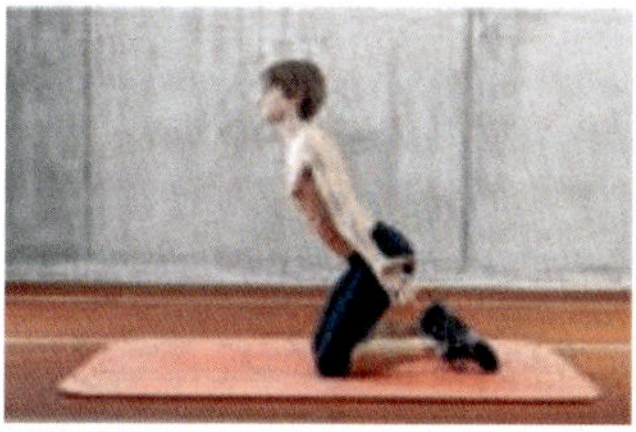	On your knees, bend very slowly forward, 'feeling each vertebra', and come up again. While bending forward, rotate your shoulder inwards. While coming back up again, rotate your shoulder outwards (activation of rhomboid muscles).	60sec Allow a slow execution, counting 1-2-3-4 for 8–10sec for one complete exercise

Core Stability Exercises – Stage II – ADVANCED

Perform three series of these 8 exercises. Once you manage them well, you may progress to the Stage III – EXPERT exercises.

1. Activating the local core muscle system at rest – in different positions

	Instructions	Time
a) 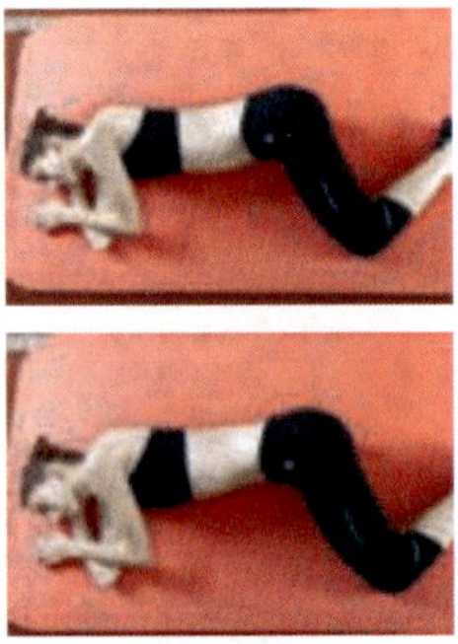 b) 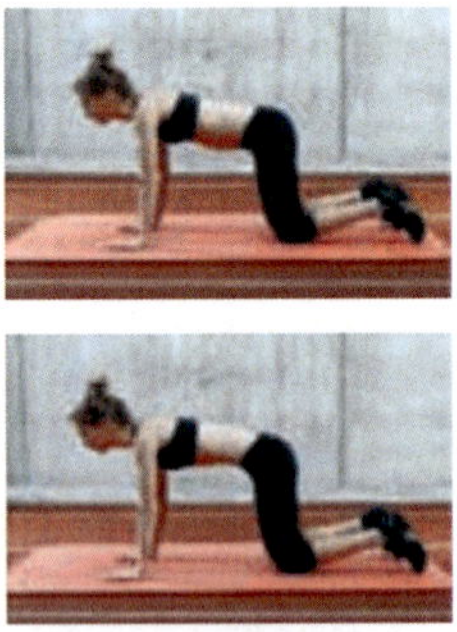 c) 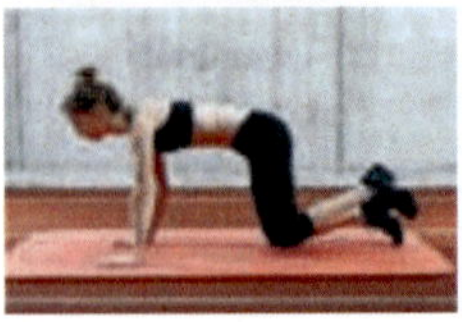	Activate your local core muscles: transverse abdominal (anterior), pelvic floor (below), and multifidus muscles (back). Gents: 'balls up'. Ladies: 'as you would close the zip of tight jeans'. Alternate positions: a) Lying sideways. b) Four point kneeling position c) Four point kneeling position, one knee slightly lifted d) Upright position.	Activate and hold for 10sec, 5sec rest. Repeat 8 times

2. Train the local core muscle system under slight movement

	Instructions	Time
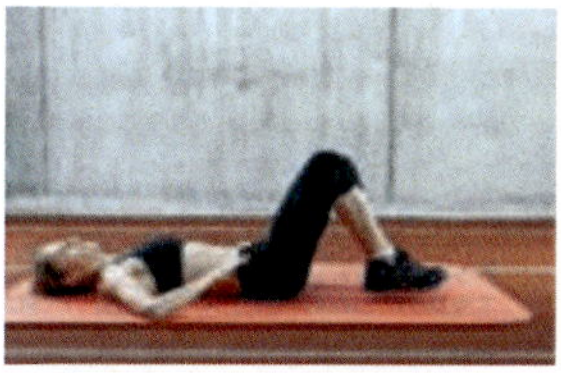 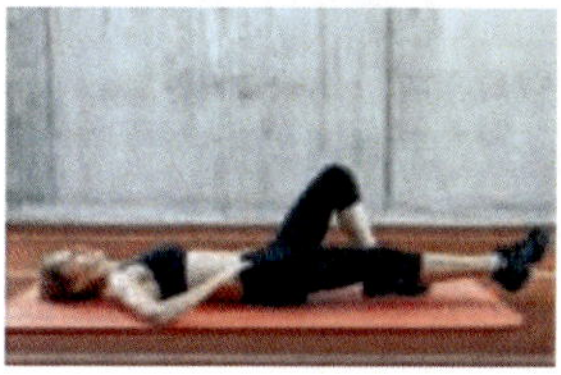	Supine, hip flexed, one foot on the ground the other in the air. Activating the local core muscles, move one leg forward, control the firm pressure of the lower, lumbar spine muscles to the ground with one hand, the activation of the local abdominal muscles with the other hand.	Right leg: 30sec Left leg: 30sec

3. Train the local core muscle system under consistent movement

	Instructions	Time
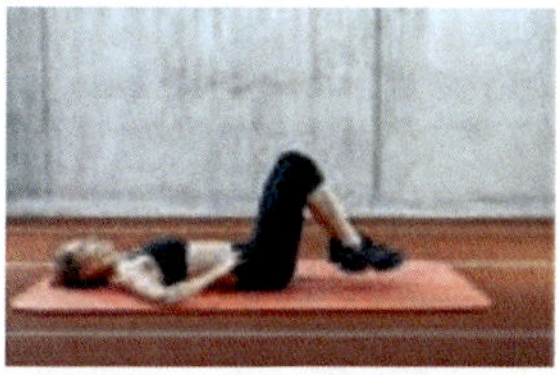 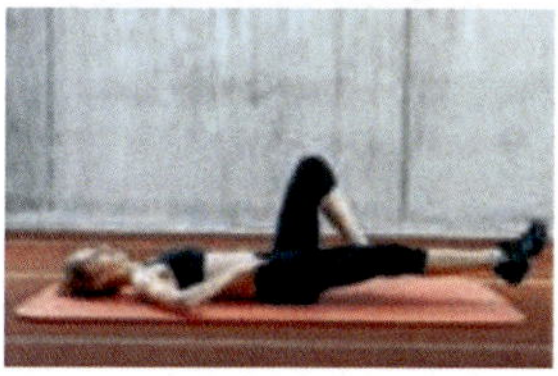 Don't allow your back to come off the ground. Control with one hand in the back a firm pressure towards the ground, and with the other hand on your lateral abdomen the activation of the local abdominal muscles.	With both feet 5cm above the ground, bring one foot forward, in a one-second rhythm, alternating left and right.	Start with 30sec, increase to 45, later 60sec

4. Plank exercise (global anterior muscle chain)

	Instructions	Time
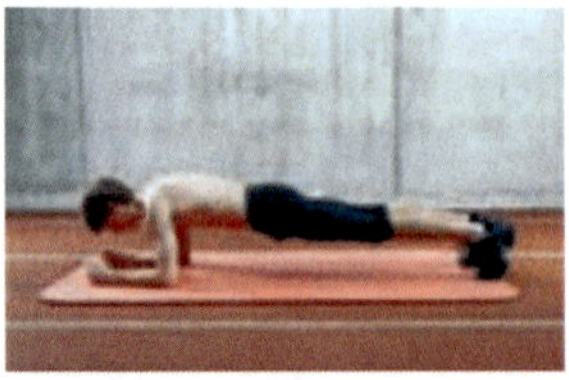 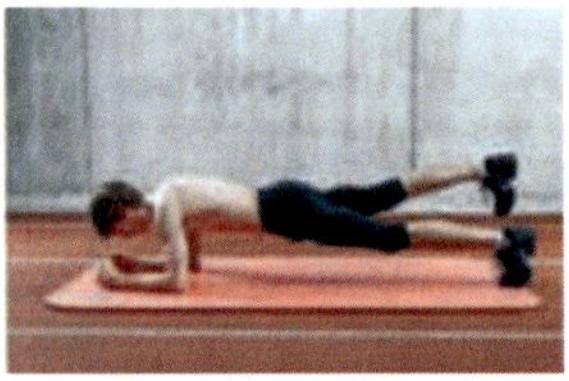	Holding the plank position, raise your right foot about one foot in the air, alternate left-right keeping your body stable in the plank position. Important: Don't allow hips to drop.	60sec

5. Global lateral muscle chain

	Instructions	Time
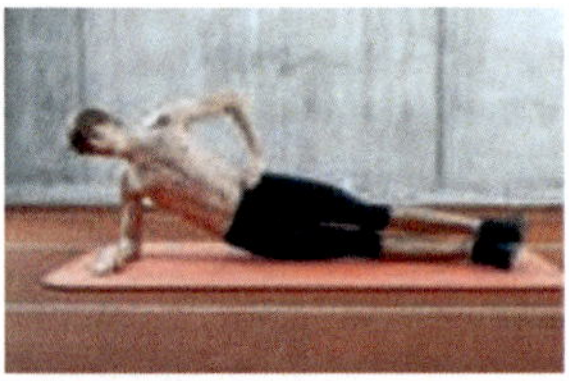 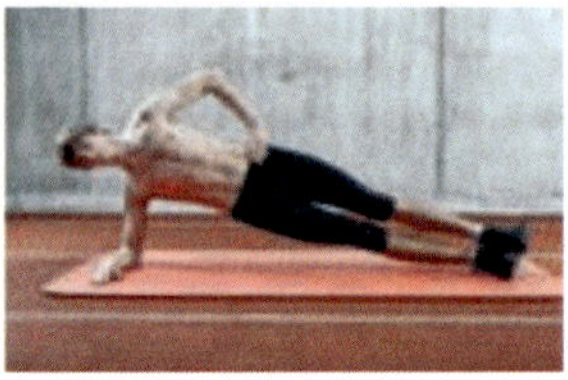	Come up and down in a rhythm of one second per movement	45sec

6. Global back muscles advanced (posterior chain)

	Instructions	Time
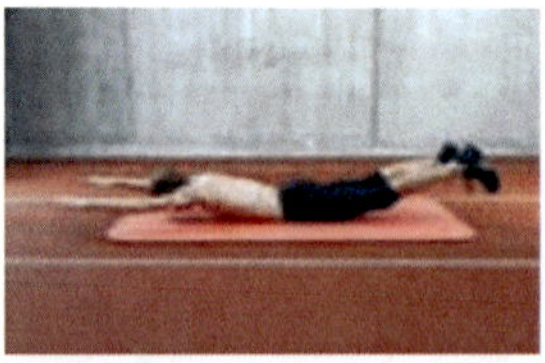 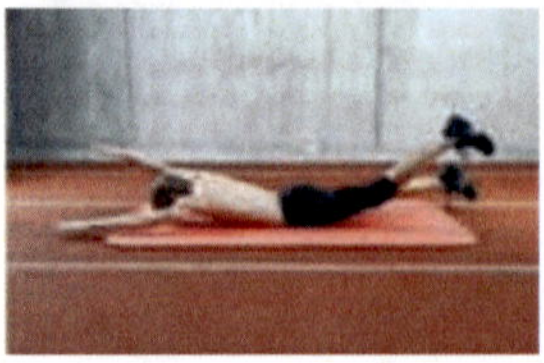	Prone, hold up all four limbs for the whole time of exercise. Lift up left leg – right arm in a one-second rhythm, alternating with right leg – left arm.	60sec

7. Global abdominal muscles

	Instructions	Time
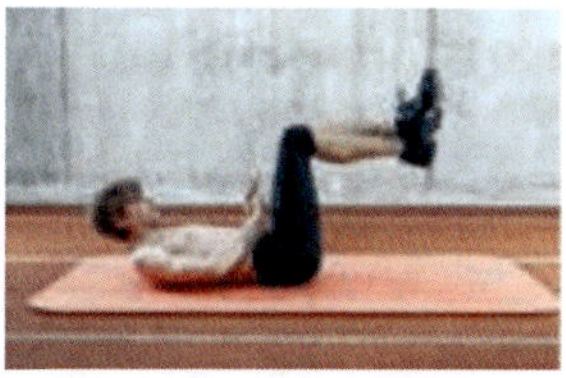 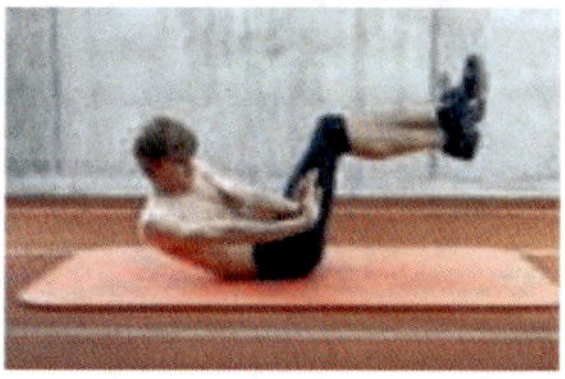	Supine, hip flexed, lower legs in the air, hands together. Come up across your body, changing left and right side, always lifting the shoulder completely off the ground.	60sec

8. Local back muscles

	Instructions	Time
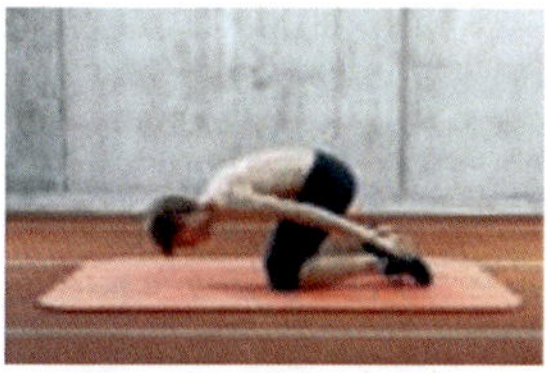 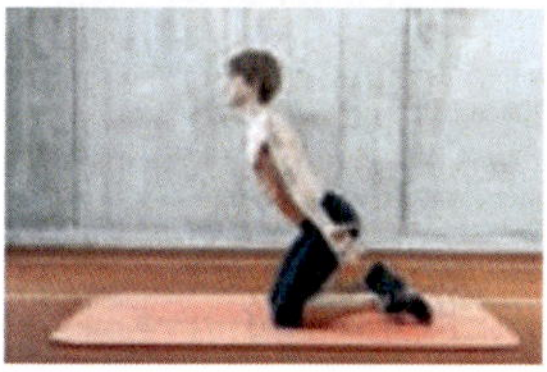	On your knees, bend very slowly forward, 'feeling each vertebra', and come up again. While bending forward, rotate your shoulder inwards. While coming back up again, rotate your shoulder outwards (activation of rhomboid muscles)	60sec Allow a slow execution, counting 1-2-3-4 for 8–10sec for one complete exercise

Core Stability Exercises – Stage III – EXPERT

Perform three series of these 8 exercises, and keep going – core stability is essential.

1. Pelvic tilting

	Instructions	Time
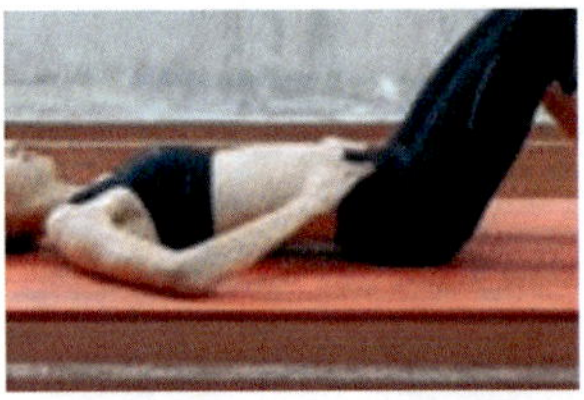 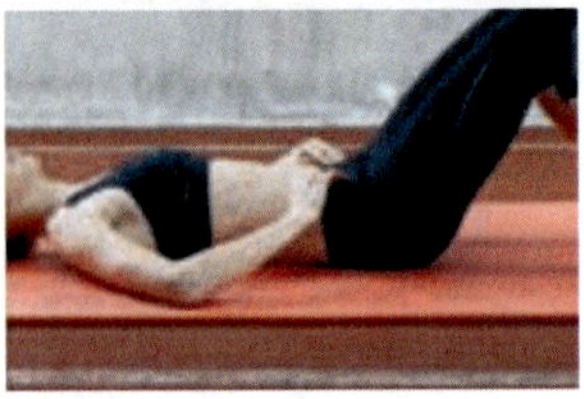	Supine, tilt your pelvis by releasing and activating your abdominal muscles. Goal: better awareness of the positioning of the pelvis. Advanced: Do 12 reps in an upright position.	12 repeti-tions

2. Train the local core muscle system under consistent movement

	Instructions	Time
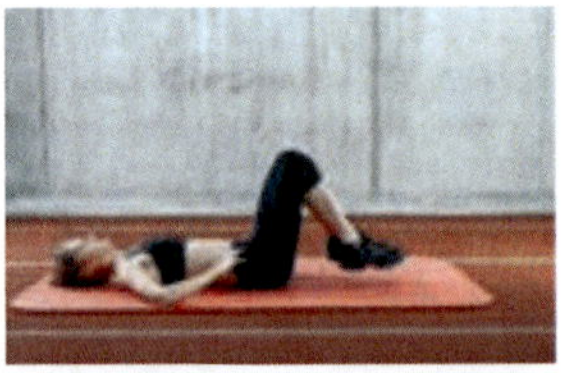 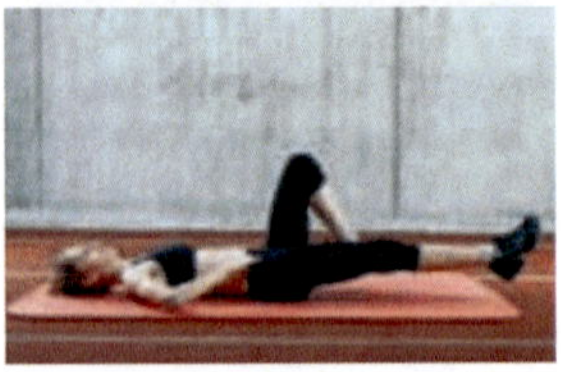 Control with one hand in the back a firm pressure towards the ground, and with the other hand on your lateral abdomen, the good activation of the local abdominal muscles.	Keep both feet 5cm above the ground. Bring one foot forward in a one-second rhythm, alternat-ing left and right.	Start with 30sec, increase to 45, later 60sec

3. Full control of local core muscle system

	Instructions	Time
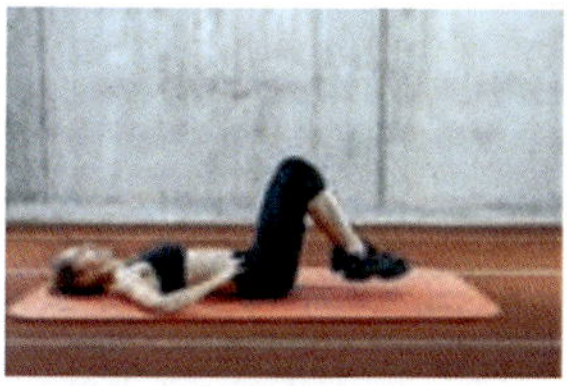 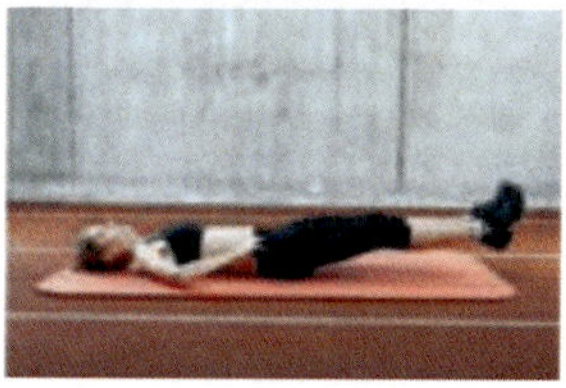 Important: control exact position	Bring both feet forward in one movement but have a perfect control of your pelvis. Go for just a few reps first, when tired, go back to the easier exercise above.	Start with 2–3reps first, then possibly go for 5–6

4. Lizard (global anterior muscle chain, advanced)

	Instructions	Time
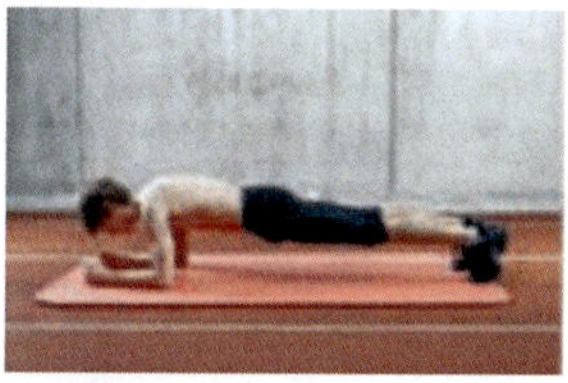 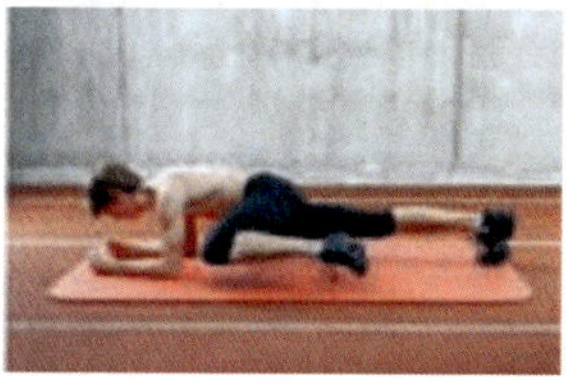	Holding plank position, move one leg laterally forward, alternating left right, rhythm of one second per movement. Keep horizontal position, especially keep a good local pelvic control (don't fall into a hollow back!)	60sec

5. Global lateral muscle chain

	Instructions	Time
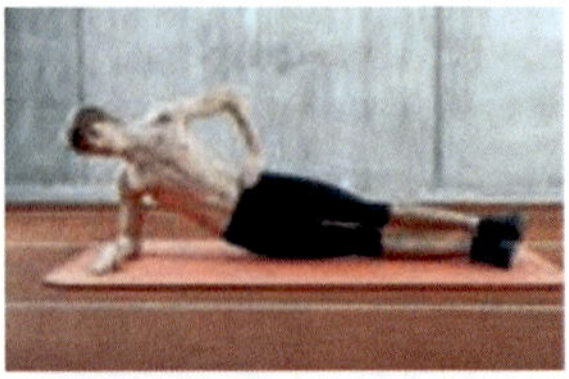 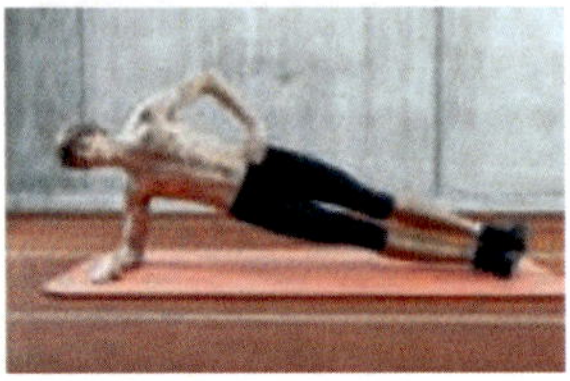 Advanced: a) In the upper position, abduct the upper leg further up to max. b) The upper leg is during the whole exercise controlled free in the air 5–10cm above the other	Come up and down in a rhythm of one second per movement.	45sec

6. Global back muscles advanced (posterior chain)

	Instructions	Time
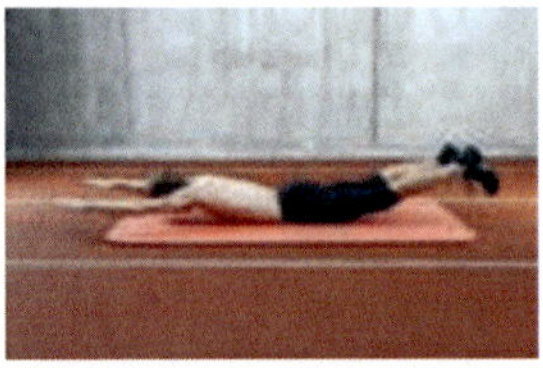 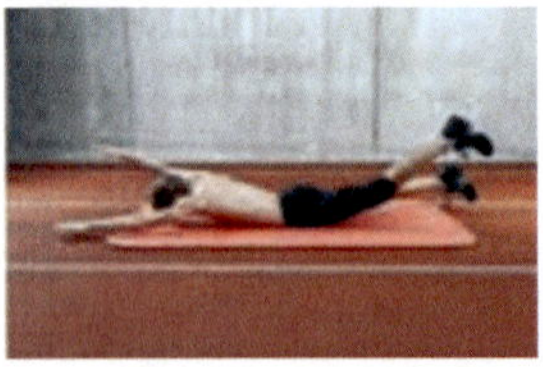	Prone, hold up all four limbs for the whole time of exercise. Lift up left leg-right arm in a one-second rhythm, alternating with right leg-left arm.	60sec

7. Global abdominal muscles

	Instructions	Time
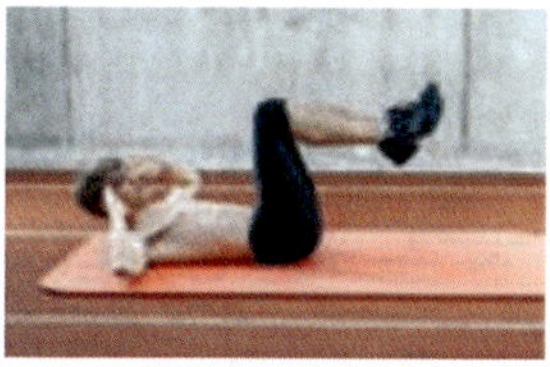 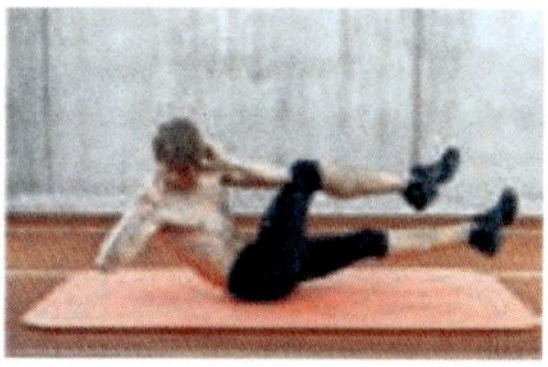	Supine, hip flexed, lower legs in the air, hands close to your head touching the ears, but not holding on to anything. Come up across your body, left elbow touches the right knee and vice versa, always lifting the shoulder completely off the ground and completely stretching out the other leg.	60sec

8. Combined exercises

	Instructions	Time
a) 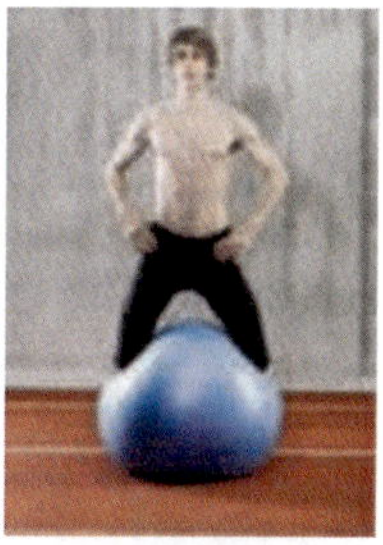 b) 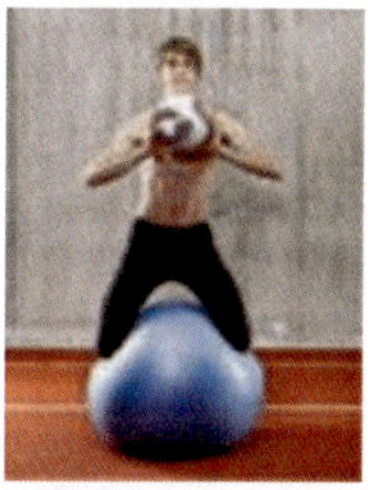 c) 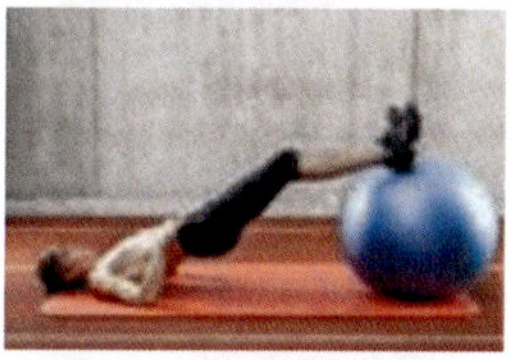 d) 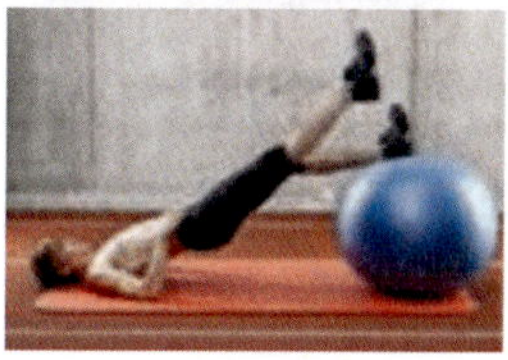	Choose one – and vary a) Balance on a Swiss Ball b) Balance and practice passes, with a partner or against a wall c) On your shoulders, feet on the Swiss Ball, balance d) Same position as c) but lift one leg up high, alternating left and right	60sec

Stretching and Gymnastic Exercises – Flexibility Is Indispensable, Go for 12 in 20

After the broad introduction of stretching exercises in the 1980s, mostly due to Bob Anderson's basic principle of stretching, a never-ending series of studies followed. These studies investigated everything about possible (and impossible) effects of stretching exercises—improvement of performance of any kind, prevention of muscle soreness, changes in muscle strength and length, prevention of injuries, etc. A lot of things stretching exercises were not intended for. Some studies were badly designed and were asking questions that, predictably, would provide negative responses.

Muscle soreness are micro lesions in the muscle ultrastructure

For instance, the muscle soreness. It has been well known for more than 25 years that muscle soreness is a result of micro lesions in the ultrastructure of the muscle due to mainly eccentric muscle action. In eccentric (the opposite of concentric) exercises the muscle is engaged to decelerate the action, e.g. landing after a jump, running downhill. So how could a stretching exercise, especially done after the effort, make any change to these lesions?

Don't stretch immediately before explosive strength is needed!

Static stretching immediately before a competition, which requires explosive strength, is wrong as it reduces your explosivity in sprint and your performance in a jumping discipline. But, most of the studies I referred to above did not reflect what

I see as common sense. It seems quite clear to me, that as a preparation to any explosive activity you need to activate the muscle tone and to get the neuromuscular unit alert in order to perform at your best. If you work on the flexibility in your warming-up before a competition you're better of doing some callisthenics.

Image 1: Muscle Soreness
Ultrastructural picture of the microlesions (courtesy Prof Dr.med. H. Hoppeler, Berne)

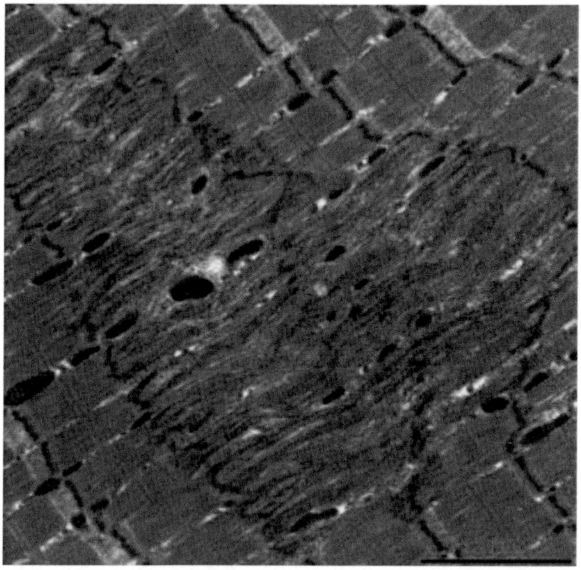

Do your stretching afterwards – optimise muscle length and muscle tone and support recovery

Nowadays, there is a backlash from all this. As a reaction to all these studies published, showing poor or no results, some sportsmen and women, even at top level, rather tend to drop stretching and to abandon any kind of mobility exercise. And that's the wrong behaviour, as poor flexibility is a performance limiting factor.

Figure 1: 12 in 20 – 12 Basic Stretching Exercises in 20min

Superficial calf muscle (gastrocnemius)	Deep calf muscles (soleus, tibialis posterior group)	Quadriceps muscle (anterior thigh)
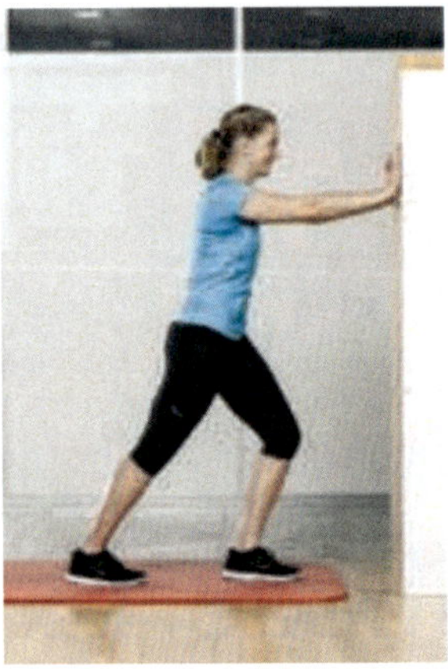	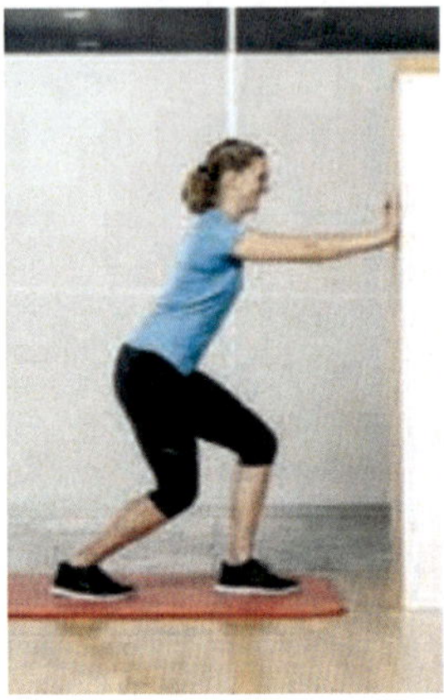	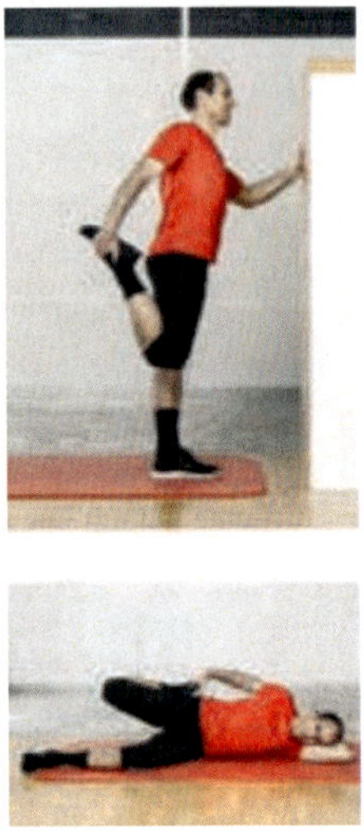
1 R + L – 60sec	**2** R + L – 60 sec	**3** R + L – 60 sec
Hamstrings muscles (posterior thigh)	Hip flexor muscle (iliopsoas)	Piriformis and gluteal muscles (gluteus maximus)
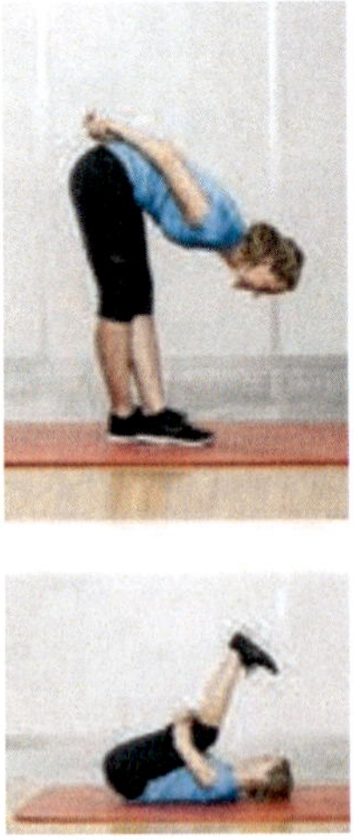	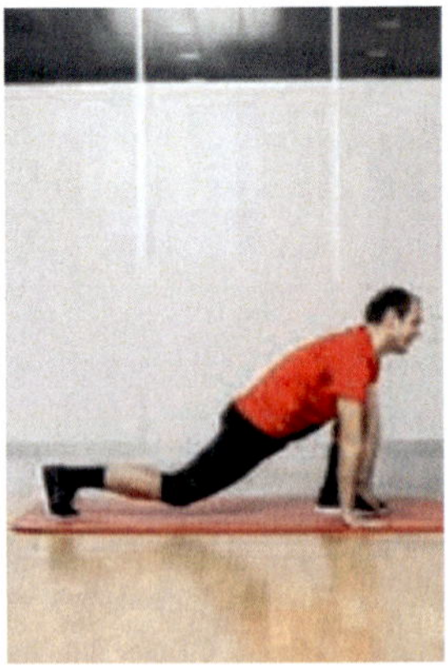	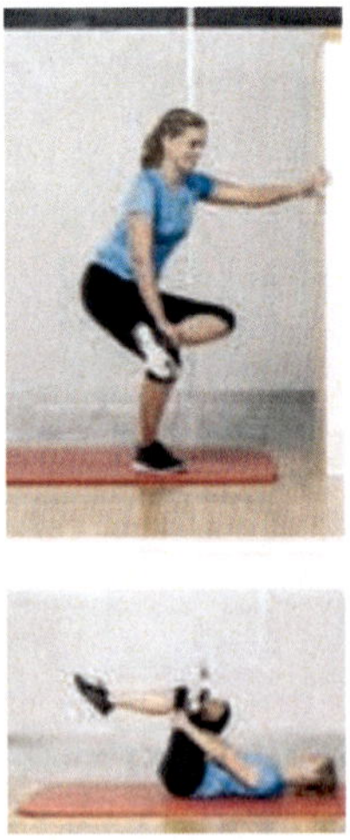
4 R + L – 60 sec	**5** R + L – 60 sec	**6** R + L – 60 sec

Adductor muscles (adductor magnus, longus, brevis, gracilis)	Lower back muscles (erector spinae / quadratus lumborum)	Posterior chest/Upper back muscles (erector spinae and rhomboid)
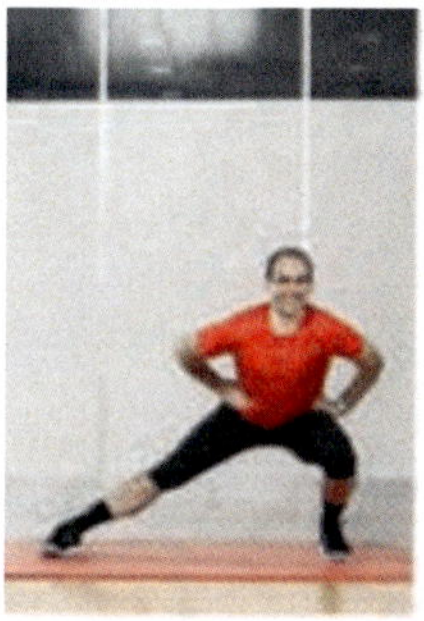 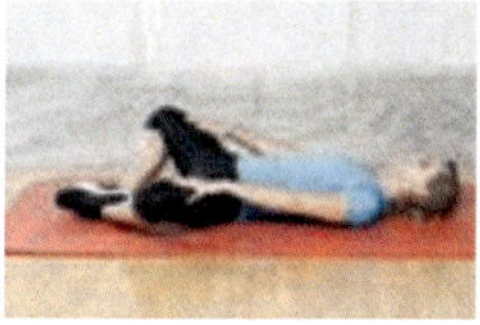	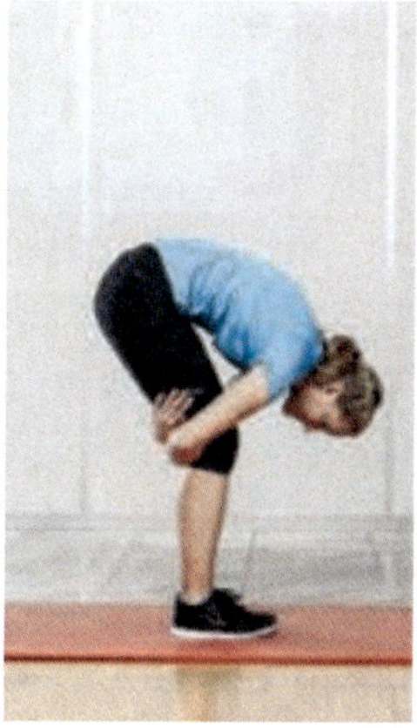	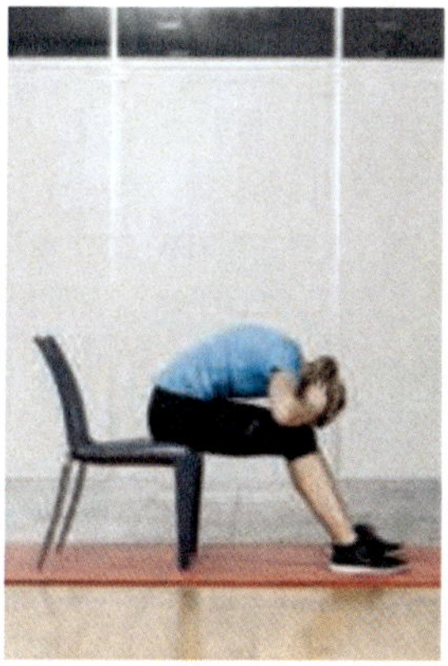
7 R+ L – 60 sec	**8** 30sec	**9** 30sec

Lateral trunk and gluteus muscles (quadratus lumborum, gluteus medius, and minimus)	Anterior chest muscles (pectoralis major and minor)	Neck muscles (trapezius, levator scapulae, scalene)
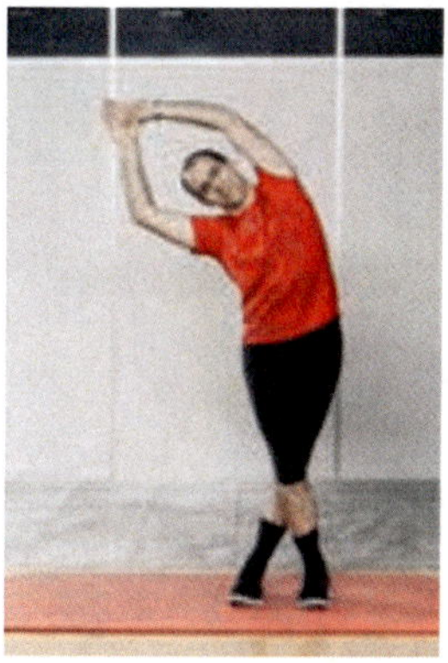	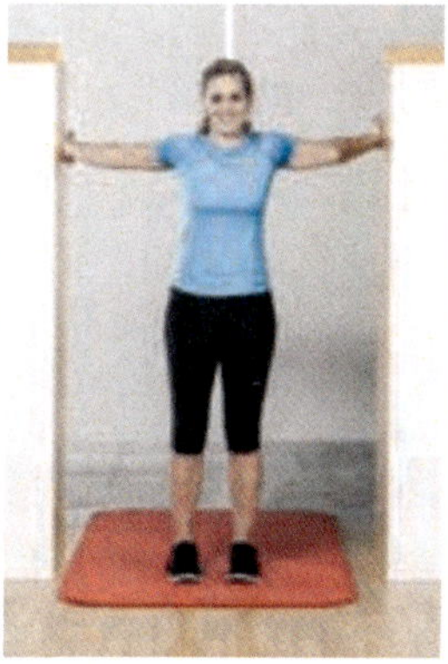	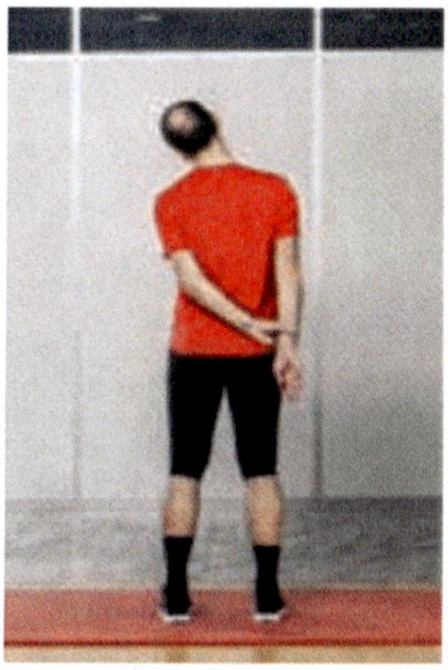
10 R + L – 60sec	**11** 30sec	**12** R + L – 60sec

Stretching has its place, both as an exercise and part of athletes' training (see Figure 1: 12 in 20)—possibly combined with other exercises (see Figure 2: self-myofascial release/deep foam rolling)—as it remains one of the best methods to improve flexibility in order to:

- Optimise muscle length by releasing and slightly lengthening shortened muscles and tendon units
- Contribute to an ideal muscle tone and therefore help in the prevention of trigger point formation and overuse or training error injuries
- Support active recovery after training practice and competition

The ideal way of practicing flexibility exercises like stretching is by integrating them into the training process, e.g. for an endurance athlete, a series of twelve exercises all for 30sec at the end of a session, once daily 20–25min. In others, like gymnastics, athletics, or team ball sports (e.g. soccer, rugby), flexibility exercises should certainly be part of each training session.

Literature

Freitas SR et al. Stretching effects: High-intensity & moderate duration vs. low-intensity & long duration. Int J Sports Med 2016; 37:239-244

Freitas SR et al. Are rest intervals between stretching repetitions effective to acutely increase range of motion? Int J Sports Physiol Perform 2014

Anderson Bob. Stretching. Shelter Publications; 30 Anv edition (April 6, 2010), ISBN-13: 978-0936070469

Hoge K et al. Gender differences in musculotendinous stiffness and range of motion after an acute bout of stretching. J Strength Cond Res 2010; 24:2618-2626

Avela J et al. Altered reflex sensitivity after repeated and prolonged passive muscle stretch. J Appl Physiol 1999; 86:1283-1291

Magnusson SP et al. Biomechanical responses to repeated stretches in human hamstrings muscle in vivo. Am J Sports Med 1996; 24:622-628

Figure 2: Self Myofascial Release/Deep Tissue Foam Rolling

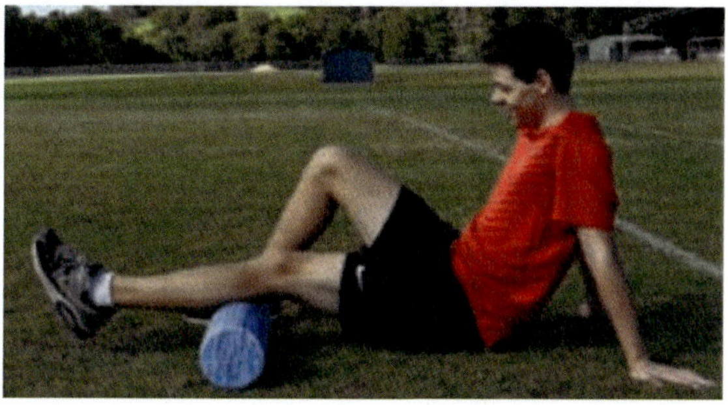

According to a couple of published studies and practical experiences, the self-myofascial release (*myo* means muscle, *fascial* means the fascia, i.e. muscle sheath), mostly performed by a deep tissue foam rolling seems also to improve flexibility. By its slight compression and local massage of muscle and fascia, it may additionally have beneficial effects on recovery. However, there are some important limitations: due to anatomical configurations, some muscle groups are easily accessible for self-treatment (e.g. hamstrings, calf), whereas others (e.g. leg adductors, shoulder muscles) are more challenging and hardly treatable.

To conclude: self-myofascial release is an interesting form of therapy for athletes in elite sports. As it contributes to both flexibility and recovery, it may be used as add-on to other basic flexibility exercises like stretching.

Literature

Schroeder AN, Best TM. Is self myofascial release an effective preexercise and recovery strategy? A literature review. Curr Sports Med Rep. 2015 May-Jun;14(3):200-8.

Behara B, Jacobson BH. The acute effects of deep tissue foam rolling and dynamic stretching on muscular strength, power and flexibility in division I linemen. J Orthop Trauma. 2015 Jun 24. [Epub ahead of print

Regular Medical Checks – an Important Service to Your Health

Here I like the comparison with Formula 1 and cars in general: how often do you bring your car to a garage to have the service done or to repair this or that? Okay, surely once a year, maybe more often if needed? And how often is this done with a Formula 1 race car?

Maybe you like to be compared with a Formula 1 car, maybe not, it just underscores the importance of a regular follow-up. In fact, screening in elite athletes is parallel to the regular screening of others with physically demanding jobs, including firemen, divers, pilots, and military personnel. You're training hard, you're dedicating many years of your life to sports, and you're making many sacrifices to compete and hopefully be on the podium. So you deserve a good and regular service to your health. And there's by far more in it than just injury prevention. It's where we come back to my statement in the introduction about Athletes' Health and the WHO definition. Comparing again the metaphor with the car: You wouldn't expect that your car after the service is now protected for any further accident, would you? But you expect, that everything works well, that the oil has been changed, the engine is fine, the gears work properly, even the turbo is well adjusted, the tyres are in a good condition. Briefly, you invest in the longevity of your car and you don't risk a breakdown in a really unsuitable moment. What does such a service look like? I propose a yearly check done by a sportsmed physician, with an extensive interview, a clinical examination head to toe, including particular focus on your most recent or still active complaints. In the laboratory, blood and urine tests ('Big Sportslab', see Table 2) should be performed (annually), as well as an ECG (every second or third year). For endurance athletes, I would recommend the 'Small Sportslab' twice or three times a year, as hematologic findings and iron are relevant for physical performance. At the end of these investigations you should get a personal report with the main findings (short summary, one page A4, in an understandable language!) and the lab results.

It's part of the empowerment of athletes that the lab results and the written summary with diagnosis and proposed treatment are all discussed so you can take over and initiate the indicated measures. Finally, I strongly recommend that you put this report together with all other medical information (e.g. X-ray or MR report, etc.) in your personal health file or folder. This allows you to show particular findings to your physio or, when travelling, to another doctor, and to compare lab results after treatment or just to observe them over time. Certainly health professionals are keeping your file and they do have all your information in a safe place. In the future an electronic athlete monitoring system (AMS) will possibly take over this role. But as the protection of personal data is a serious issue, there are still hurdles to overcome, until a good and sustainable AMS may be established.

Table 1: Proposed Investigations for Health Check for Athletes

Yearly Sportsmedical Exam

- Extensive interview
- Clinical examination (head to toe)
- ECG (12-lead resting ECG)
- Blood and urine exams (see Table 2 below, 'Big and Small Sportslab')

Table 2: Blood and Urine Results to be Performed—'Big and Small Sportslab'

'Big Sportslab'—once a year, together with the sportsmed exam

- Haemoglobin, hematocrit, MCV (mean cellular volume of erythrocytes), MCH (mean cellular haemoglobin per erythrocyte), leukocytes, thrombocytes
- Ferritin, C-reactive protein
- Creatinin, urea, GPT/ALAT (liver transaminasis), magnesium, cholesterol
- Vitamin B12, vitamin D3
- Urine stix, general overview

'Small Sportslab'—for endurance sports, additionally twice a year

- Haemoglobin, hematocrit, MCV (mean cellular volume of erythrocytes), MCH (mean cellular haemoglobin per erythrocyte), ferritin, C-reactive protein

Literature

Sportaerztliche Untersuchung SGSM nach den Standards von Swiss Olympic, retrieved at the 3.6.2016 http://www.swissolympic.ch/Spitzen-Nachwuchssport/Verbaende/Sportmedizin/Downloads-6

Kriemler S et al. Sportärztlicher Untersuch von Jugendlichen – SPU SGSM Fortbildungstag 2014 Visite médico-sportive annuelle du jeune – Une formation continue de la SSMS 2014. Schweizerische Zeitschrift für Sportmedizin und Sporttraumatologie 63 (3), 6-15, 2015

Bakken A et al. Health conditions detected in a comprehensive periodic health evaluation of 558 professional football players. Br J Sports Med. 2016 Mar 24. pii: bjsports-2015-095829.

Anti-doping – There Are No Shortcuts to Real Success

In elite sports, it's often by a blink of an eye that you're on the podium (or not). So everything needs to be done to maximise your performance. Try harder with all your capacities—**but not beyond!** It's very important to realise, you are the person responsible!

> *'Athletes are responsible for everything that goes into their body!'*
>
> —World Anti-Doping Agency (WADA)

So it's completely your responsibility not to dope. This means you need to be aware of the following:

- Use medications only if necessary.
- If using a medication, tell the doctor or health professional that you are a top athlete and that you're not allowed to take any medication banned by the anti-doping code. Remind your doctor respectively of their duty of care that both of you are fine with the choice of this medication.
- If you're not 100% sure, and if the health professional is unsure, double check that the medication doesn't contain any illegal substance (check with the help of your country's anti-doping agency and their hotline or website. Often there's also an App available
    - o Australia: www.checksubstances.asada.gov.au
    - o Switzerland: www.antidoping.ch/de/medizin-substanzen-und-methoden/medikamente-schweiz-abfrage
- Generally, the National Anti-Doping Agency provides a leaflet with a list of allowed medications for common illnesses, like flu, constipation, etc. This list is renewed on an annual basis. Keep it close by at all times.
- If you need supplementation use only known products that are widely accepted in your country. There are several cases

known where supplements bought on the internet from overseas contained illegal substances. These were mostly accidentally in this supplement, as during the proceedings by the manufacturing process, traces of an illegal medication were still in the production chain and were wrongly integrated. But that's no excuse.

- Be careful with so called 'natural, organic products'. Often it is not clear where they really come from and what they contain.
- Don't accept anything doubtful in training or competition.
- Close to major competitions, be especially aware of what you are eating and drinking. Don't accept anything doubtful. Only let trusted people prepare your meals and don't accept already opened drinks if you don't know their origin.

Do all that, check what your National Anti-doping Agency or the WADA provide as resources for athletes, announce your whereabouts, if requested, and follow the instructions of the anti-doping commissioners. That's always the best course of action.

Let's look quickly at doping. A positive doping test brings terrible consequences—uncovered as a cheat to the sports community, your fans, your country, your family, and finally to yourself. And it will be extremely costly, too—unimaginable, not having talked yet about negative health consequences related to any of these illegal substances. Stay cool, stay clean. Honesty is the best policy.

Literature

WADA Website: Athletes questions and answers: download 26.3.2016 https://www.wada-ama.org/en/questions-answers/athletes-and-medications

Hygiene in Sports – Don't Give Funghis, Bacteria, and Other Germs a Foothold

Another part of the jigsaw to success. You don't need to be perfect, you may even be a bit messy concerning your way of arranging things in your household, but as soon as it touches on personal hygiene, you need to be strict. As an athlete, during training, you're perspiring naturally and you're getting sweaty, so take regularly a shower after training practice. Furthermore brush your teeth, change clothes, and do the laundry, etc. I like to share just a couple of thoughts, as you shouldn't give funghis, bacteria, and other germs a foothold:

- There are still athletes with stinking, moist socks and humid climate in their shoes—no wonder that this leads to a *foot mycosis.* Things like that can easily end up in a serious skin infection. Much easier to dry your feet and your toes after having a shower, change socks, and let shoes dry.
- *Oral hygiene.* Caring for your teeth is another topic to be addressed. Often, athletes' teeth are not as they should be, according to different studies. Possible explanations for this phenomenon are:
    - High sugar and other carbohydrate levels in an athlete's diet provoking growth of dental caries
    - Often high acidity in sports drinks (low pH attacking the dental enamel)
    - Insufficient oral hygiene (not enough teeth brushing)
- As dental infections are source of systemic infectious diseases they may be a performance limiting factor.
- Be organised with your wet clothes in winter. *Don't risk a flu!* Have dry clothes, a towel, and a dry cap ready.
- A simple plastic bag or a tidy plastic box will help *transport your sandwiches and other food.* No need to have them in between shoes and moist training clothes.

- What about the *drinking bottle*? It is important to drink regularly (see also 'Drinking In Sports'). So an athlete's drinking bottle is his or her permanent companion. Wash it regularly out, clean the mouthpiece, and, last but not least, *have your own!* Don't share and don't use somebody else's. In teams, have the drinking bottles clearly labelled with the name (or number) and respect this. Don't share as this can be a major factor in the transfer of infections. And replace the bottle after a couple of weeks.

As elite athletes are more prone to infectious diseases because of the reduced immune response, *it matters!* You will find more information about this topic in the chapter 'Prevention of Infectious Diseases'.

Literature

Needleman I et al. Poor oral health including active caries in 187 UK professional male football players: clinical dental examination performed by dentists. Br J Sports Med. 2016 Jan;50(1):41-4.

Needleman I et al. Oral health and impact on performance of athletes participating in the London 2012 Olympic Games: a cross-sectional study. Br J Sports Med. 2013 Nov;47(16):1054-8..

Solleveld H. Associations between poor oral health and reinjuries in male elite soccer players: a cross-sectional self-report study. BMC Sports Sci Med Rehabil. 2015 Apr 20;7:11. doi: 10.1186/s13102-015-0004-y. eCollection 2015.

Schwellnus M. Illness during the 2010 Super 14 Rugby Union tournament - a prospective study involving 22 676 player days. Br J Sports Med. 2012 Jun;46(7):499-504.

The Athlete's and the Coach's First Aid Kit – a Start Without Delay

You don't need much, but *every athlete* should have a tiny first aid kit in his training bag—to disinfect a small wound or abrasion, to put a plaster on, or to put a cooling elastic bandage on a sprain.

Table 1: Athlete's First Aid Kit

- Tiny bottle of disinfectant (iodine solution like Betadine, or alcohol based like Octenisept) and some clean swabs; or alternatively you may find disinfectant swabs.
- Some plasterdressings of different sizes
- 1 x cooling, elastic bandage
- Small tweezers
- Small scissors

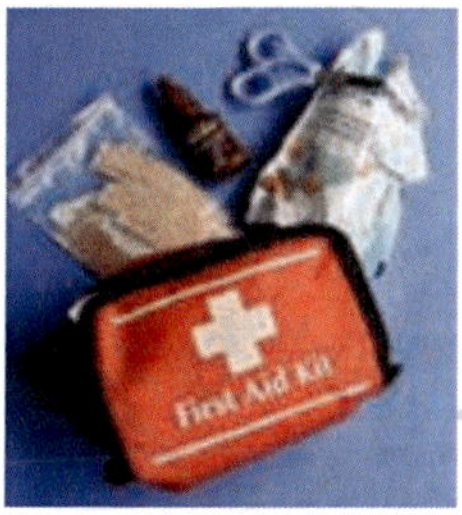

As a coach, you need to be ready at all times—in the daily training, at training camps, and in competition—to do necessary first aid without delay. It's about knowing if your athletes suffer a particular illness (e.g. severe allergy against bees or wasps, asthma, diabetes, etc.) and being prepared, organised, and independent. It actually will save you a lot of time and hassle, you just need to have it with you.

Table 2: Coach's First Aid Kit

- Bottle of disinfectant (iodine solution like Betadine, or alcohol based like Octenisept) and some clean swabs; or alternatively you may find disinfectant swabs.
- 5 x 30ml saline
- 1 x pack plaster dressings (band-aids)
- 2 x packs gauze dressings of different sizes, (e.g. 6x8cm and 10x10cm)

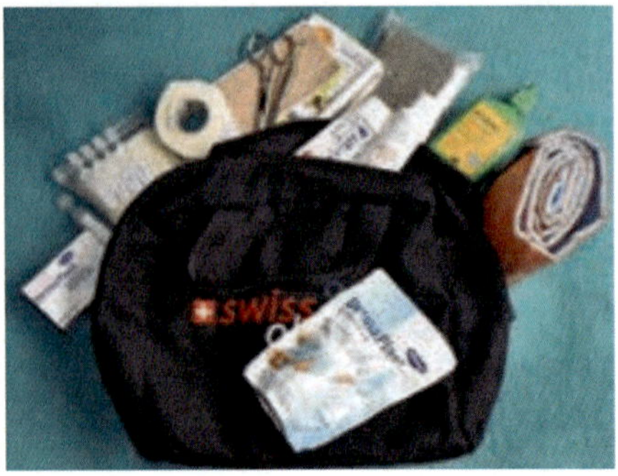

- 2–3 x cooling, elastic bandages (e.g. Physicool, Ice&Go, Coolfix Dermaplast)
- 1 x tube anti-inflammatory cream (e.g. Voltaren)
- 1 x tube antiseptic cream, especially for deep abrasions (e.g. Savlon or Flammazine)
- 1 x flask eye drops (e.g. Visine)
- 2 x normal elastic bandages
- 1 x triangular bandage – evtl 1 SAM Splint
- 2 x rolls rigid tape (Strapit Rigid Tape, Leuko Sportstape)
- 1 x roll kinesiotape (e.g. Kinesio Tex Gold, Leuko K Tape, Rock Tape)
- Medifix/Omnifix 5cmx10m
- Tweezers
- Scissors

Recovery and Regeneration – 'After the Game is Before the Game'

Let's have a closer look at the scheme of the training process in Figure 1. We recognise that if the training practice with its stimulus to adaptations and accompanying fatigue is one half of it, then recovery is the other half of the training process and it lasts much longer than the training session itself.

Figure 1: Training Process

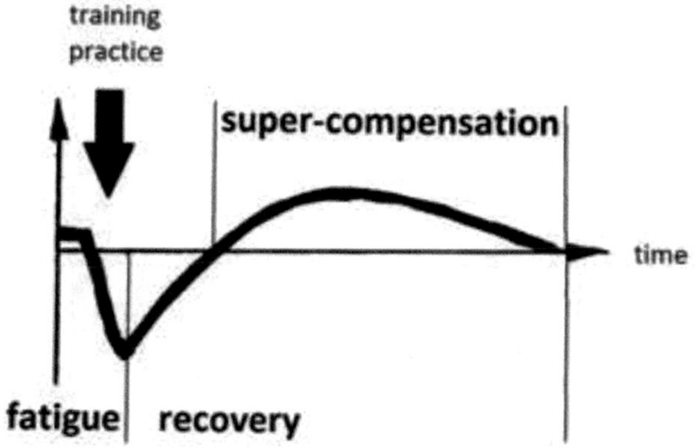

This observation underlines the importance of recovery as an essential part of any sports training. Looking at the definitions of the terms 'recovery' and 'regeneration', which are often synonymously used, we gain further insight into exactly what they are about—'becoming completely well', 'becoming successful', and 'improvement of a system'.

recovery

Definition: the process of becoming successful or normal again after being damaged or having problems; the process of becoming completely well again after an illness or injury.[1]

regeneration

Definition: improvement of a place or system, especially by making it more active or successful.[2]

What makes recovery and regeneration in sports successful?

There is quite a broad knowledge and a couple of recent studies that point us to important strategies allowing an ideal embedding of the training stimulus. The following list gives an overview in the form of a concentrate.

As athlete and coach, it is important to accompany training practices in the best possible way in order to allow optimised training adaptations according to the motto: 'After the game is before the game'. These include the following:

- Cool down immediately after the competition
- Consider cold water immersion, especially in a series of competition shortly one after the other
- Nutritional aspects
    - o Eat and drink regularly
    - o Plan especially your competition day – eat and drink
        - before the competition ("carboloading")
        - if appropriate, during the competition, or at least in the pause (in order not to empty all the glycogen stores)
        - immediately after the competition ("recharging" and boosting the immune system)
- Sleep
    - o The most important contributor to recovery
    - o Have enough sleep and of good quality
- Active regeneration/recovery
    - o Stretching or other flexibility exercises are part of active recovery
    - o Consider self myofascial release
- Passive regeneration/recovery
    - o Massage is a valuable aid and a good passive regenerative strategy
    - o Take a hot bath, consider sauna from time to time

Literature

Recovery definition: online source 26.3.2016 http://dictionary.cambridge.org/de/worterbuch/englisch/recovery

Regeneration definition: online source 2.11.2015, http://dictionary.cambridge.org/dictionary/english/regenerate

Nédélec M et al. Stress, Sleep and Recovery in Elite Soccer: A Critical Review of the Literature. Sports Med. 2015 Oct;45(10):1387-400.

Nédélec M et al. Recovery in soccer : part ii-recovery strategies. Sports Med. 2013 Jan;43(1):9-22.

Versey NG et al. Water immersion recovery for athletes: effect on exercise performance and practical recommendations. Sports Med. 2013 Nov; 43(11):1101-30.

Gunzer W et al. Exercise-Induced Immunodepression in Endurance Athletes and Nutritional Intervention with Carbohydrate, Protein and Fat—What Is Possible, What Is Not? Nutrients. 2012 September; 4(9): 1187–1212

Often-encountered Sportsmedical problems

Unclear Fatigue – A Common Complaint, When to See a Doctor

Symptoms

Feeling tired more than usual, heavy arms and legs, needing more sleep, and still not really fresh and recovered in the morning. In training, you never get the the 'good feeling', never the feel in the 'flow'. Possibly you observe a higher resting pulse rate in the morning (more than 10 beats/min) or distinctly higher pulse rate in training for the same effort (more than 15–20 beats/min).

Figure 1: Fatigue

How tired do you feel today? On a scale from 1–10. 0 = not tired at all, completely fresh; 10 = very, very tired

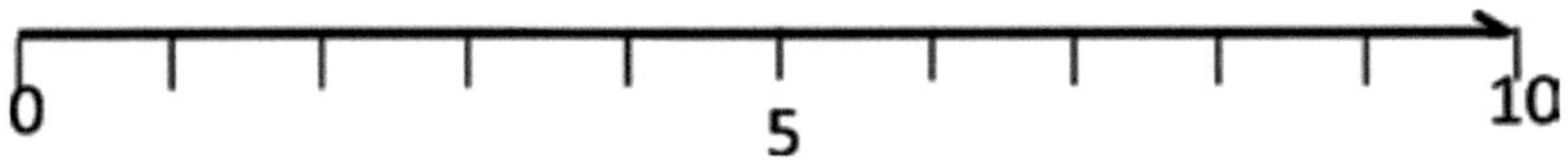

You need to know, that almost everybody feels 'a bit tired'. The average response will be somewhere around 2, ranging from 0 up to 4. However, if you consistently felt a 4 or even >4, then it is recommended to see a doctor.

Background

Unclear fatigue is a frequent complaint among athletes. Studies show in a normal population that even a majority feels 'a bit tired'. It would appear the same of athletes.

For the majority of athletes the diagnosis may be clear and the specific therapy may be started immediately. However, in many cases, unclear fatigue is multifactorial, which means that there is not just one diagnosis contributing to the symptoms, but many different things.

Prevention and Treatment Table for Unclear Fatigue

Prevention	• Allow enough recovery time, as it is part of the training process. Without recovery the training effect (called super-compensation) cannot take place • Plan your days well, but don't overbook them Be particularly careful with other possible stressors beside sports, e.g. study, other work, social issues, etc. • Eat your meals on a regular basis, start the day with a good breakfast suitable for athletic performance e.g. go for muesli, fruits, yoghurt, and not for bacon and eggs (see chapter 'Breakfast, a good start for the day') • If you're an elite level athlete, get your sports-medical exam with blood tests, done once a year • Sleep enough. Ideal sleep duration is individual and may vary, but as an athlete at least 7, but better still 8 hours sleep a night are recommended • Go to bed before midnight (10–11pm is perfect). This allows enough sleeping time and a good start at a reasonable time the next day
Treatment by Yourself	As above.
When is a Doctor Needed?	As soon as you feel that the level of fatigue is just not right anymore (e.g. consistently >4 longer than a week). It's definitely different to what it usually was. Or as soon as you see a real drop in performance, but don't wait too long.
Return to Play/Sports	Depending on the diagnosis, the plan for the return to sports will be made together with your sports medicine physician. Just knowing the diagnosis can help you feel better. If it is about, for example, iron deficiency or Vitamin B12 deficiency, supplementation needs to be planned carefully and high intensity trainings foregone for two or three weeks. However, usual training may be continued on a lower level in order to get back to normal within a few weeks.

What Does the Doctor Do?

The doctor takes the history and performs a clinical examination. The anamnesis will cover the onset of symptoms, the 'how does it feel', sore legs, out of breath, empty batteries? It will include quite a few systematic questions covering different organ systems, recent travel activities, recent infectious diseases, your former medical history, and your family history (e.g. allergies, asthma) and possible additional stress factors—all with the goal of tracking down the source of this fatigue. A blood test is mostly performed the same day (big sports lab and TSH, fT4, serologic testing for Epstein-Barr-Virus and evtl other tests). Depending on these early findings further investigations may be planned (e.g. ECG, lung function testing, prick allergy testing or others).

After this first appointment and analysis, quite often the issues are obvious and can be diagnosed, like iron deficiency, vitamin B12 deficiency, indication for a viral infection, newly discovered exercise induced asthma, hypo- or hyperthyreosis, etc. In some cases, we just find a possible track, where to look in more detail, and the diagnosis will follow some days later. In other cases, the diagnosis is not perfectly clear, contributing factors are found but nothing that explains it completely. Often it is then combined with some stress factors outside the sport (e.g. double stress with ongoing education and high level sport, an approximating exam, an emotional pressure).

Further workup will show how different issues need to be addressed and very often a multimodal treatment plan established (treating and relieving the different issues at the same time). The return to play plan will be designed according to these findings and appointments for a follow up will be fixed.

Literature

Reid VL et al. Clinical investigation of athletes with persistent fatigue and/or recurrent infections. Br J Sports Med. 2004 Feb;38(1):42-5

Viral Infection of the Upper Respiratory Tract (URTI) – How an Athlete Should Cope

Symptoms

Sore throat, running nose, slight coughing, and usually some fever.

Background

Upper respiratory tract infections are the most common illnesses. Because of the volume and intensity of their training regimes, high level athletes are more prone to catch an URTI. It is therefore important to address this topic separately. See also chapter 'Prevention of Infectious Diseases'.

Prevention and Treatment Table for URTI

Prevention	See chapter 'Prevention of Infectious Diseases in Sports'—the recommended measures are discussed and outlined there.
Treatment by Yourself	Good treatment options are: • Drink enough. 2–3 litres of tea (lime blossom is highly recommended) per day. Add some honey (real honey!) directly in the tea • Eat regularly, but according to your appetite. You don't need to overeat • Take echinacea purpurea, e.g. Echinamed tablet (380mg) three times daily to savour on your tongue (important as it is then distributed over the mucosal surfaces and maximises its antiviral action)

	• Take vitamin C and zinc, e.g. combined effervescent tablet as Ascorbic acid 1000mg, Zinc 10mg twice daily (e.g. Redoxon Double Action)
When Is A Doctor Needed?	Usually not needed.
Return to Play/ Sports	*Strictly no sports with fever!* Elevated temperature is a sign of illness and a defense reaction of your body. If you exercise whilst having elevated temperature: • You activate the illness and spread the germs all over your body (due to the risen heart rate, risen blood pressure) • You run a particular risk that the germs contact delicate structures like the heart valves, the heart muscle (myocard), the epi- and pericard (sheats covering the heart), and the risk of an inflammation of one of these structures is significantly elevated, leading to myocarditis, pericarditis • These inflammations (myocarditis, pericarditis) are prone to heart rhythm disorders, which may be fatal! • There is no beneficial training effect • The only thing you achieve is: you lose and you are taking unnecessary risks! If you just have a running nose or a sore throat (*but* normal temperature) you may exercise on a low level, according to how you feel. Usually a URTI resolves within 4–5 days, where a flu would take 7–8 days. Take precautions at the outset and you get rid of it more quickly. Motto: **Less is more!** Be smart! Train harder and smarter, but train harder only when you're completely fit!

What Does the Doctor Do?

Nothing, as there's usually no need for a doctor.

Literature

Dick NA, Diehl JJ. Febrile illness in the athlete. Sports Health. 2014 May;6(3):225-31

Page CL, Diehl JJ. Upper respiratory tract infections in athletes. Clin Sports Med. 2007 Jul;26(3):345-59.

Mononucleosis (Epstein-Barr-Virus-Infection) – Inevitable, but Seek Professional Advice

Symptoms

Usually: fever, really sore throat, enlarged lymph nodes. You are really ill!

Sometimes the symptoms are milder and difficult to differentiate from another upper respiratory tract infection, it presents then with slight fever, slightly sore throat, some enlargement of the lymph nodes.

Figure 1: Typical Features of Mononucleosis (Epstein-Barr-Virus-Infection)

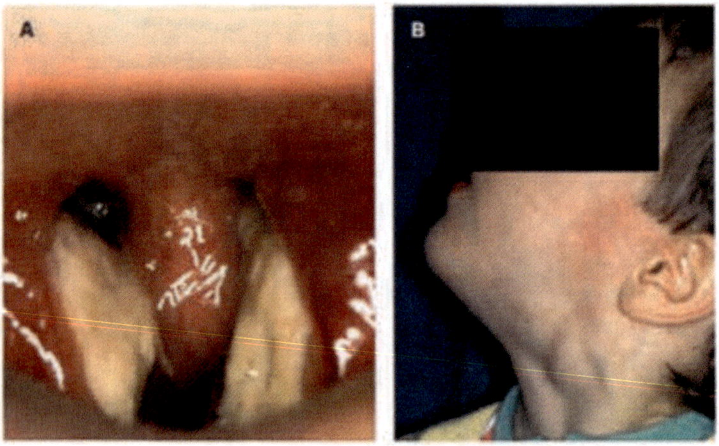

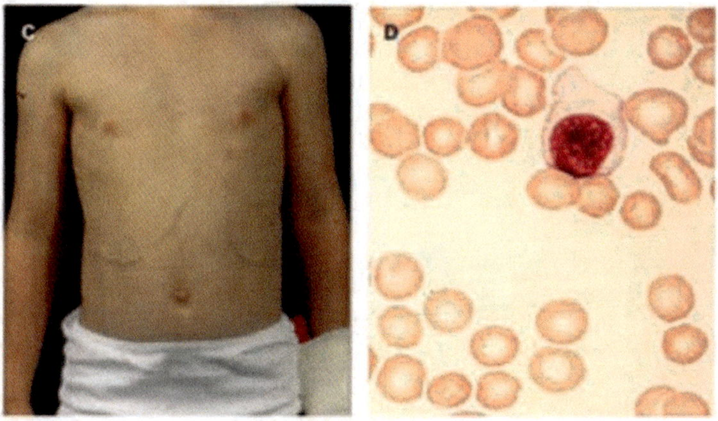

Abildung 1
Typische Befunde bei infektiöser Mononukleose durch EBV.
A Tonsillitis
B Zervikale Lymphadenopathie
C Hepatosplenomegalie
D Atypische Lymphozyten im Blutausstrich

A. Tonsillitis: sore throat with whitish, often smelly, covering
B. Enlarged lymph nodes
C. Enlarged liver and spleen
D. Activated enlarged lymphocytes in the blood

(courtesy Prof D.Nadal, Children's Hospital Zurich, Dr.med. U.Karrer, State Hospital, Winterthur; Schweiz Med Forum 2014;14(11):226–232)

Background

Mononucleosis is caused by an infection with the Epstein-Barr-Virus. This viral illness provokes fever, a really sore throat with painful swallowing, and a massive proliferation of activated lymphocytes (i.e. a particular type of our own body's white blood cells) in the blood stream and within lymph nodes and other lymphatic tissue, leading to enlargement of the lymph nodes and an enlargement of spleen and liver. The name mononucleosis is given due to the distinct microscopic picture of these activated defence cells.

Until the age of thirty-five, almost everybody in the industrialised countries gets Epstein-Barr-Virus infection. So it's kind of unavoidable, an illness you get sooner or later. In most cases the patient interprets it as a flu, which is in fact similar. It's the distinct clinical picture, the duration of the illness, and the blood test that leads to the correct diagnosis. For athletes, it is important to recognise Epstein-Barr virus mononucleosis properly, because this particular viral infection demands a longer lay-off from training.

Although Epstein-Barr virus mononucleosis is a benign, self-limiting disease, it is associated with a small risk of *splenic rupture, which is an emergency and can be life-threatening!* It is recommended vigorous physical activity be avoided for at least 8–12 weeks—rupture of the spleen may occur throughout the whole period of illness, most frequently in week 4, but cases in week 8 have been reported. Spleen rupture presents with abdominal pain, sometimes radiating in the left shoulder, usually after effort or even minor trauma but not necessarily (only 14% of cases reported a former trauma).

Prevention and Treatment Table for Epstein-Barr-Virus-Infection/Mononucleosis

Prevention	No particular prevention recommended as it is kind of unavoidable, *but* certainly go for usual preventive measures before important competitions, as described in chapter 'Prevention Of Infectious Diseases'. Avoid contact to athletes or other persons having this illness.
Treatment by Yourself	Seek professional advice and follow these recommendations.
When is a Doctor Needed?	If Epstein-Barr virus mononucleosis is suspected. With any fever lasting more than four days.

Return to Play/Sports	Competitive sport is not possible for 8–12 weeks after the outbreak and diagnosis of the illness. On the one hand, it is the viral illness itself with its very individual pattern affecting the whole body and organ tissues such as lymph nodes, liver, and spleen that needs to be restored and show signs of improvement (NB: lymph nodes stay enlarged for 2–3 months or even longer), before an uptake of training may be considered. On the other hand it is the enlarged spleen that is at a greater risk of a rupture (for about 8 weeks). So the treatment plan and return to play is individually designed. Getting back into movement and sports is gradual, e.g. once fever is gone, the athlete is feeling well (e.g. after 2–3 weeks) you may go for a 30min walk (just a stroll, not a brisk walk) on a daily basis. If this is okay, extend the walking distance and slightly increase intensity. If this is fine, you may start slight jogging and some core stability strengthening, etc. Motto: Rest first (2–3 weeks). Start slow. Go slow.

What Does the Doctor Do?

The doctor takes the history and performs a general clinical exam. The inflamed throat, the enlarged lymph nodes in the cervical region, in the neck, behind the ears but quite often even in the armpit and groin are typical. A blood test with raised signs of inflammation, the atypical enlarged mononucleotic lymphocytes, often slight inflammation of the liver and the antibody testing for the Epstein-Barr virus (in the first few days of infection not yet positive) will confirm the diagnosis. There is *no* need of antibiotic treatment, as it is a viral and not a bacterial illness. If there is misdiagnosis (sometimes difficult, as sometimes, clinically, a bacterial tonsillitis looks a bit similar) and penicillin-like antibiotics are administered, a typical rash may occur. This is usually harmless but not necessary.

Treatment is symptomatic, meaning the focus is on relieving the symptoms only, as there is no causative therapy. The mainstay of care includes:

- Adequate hydration (e.g. honey sweetened tea). Don't enforce eating in the beginning, try instead milk-shakes, yoghurt, mashed banana, etc.
- Analgesics (paracetamol) if heavy pain is an issue
- In case of heavy swelling, impairment of swallowing, and high fever use anti-inflammatory medication (e.g. ibuprofen)
- Adequate rest
- Treatment with echinacea and vitamin C and zinc, as with other viral infections of the upper respiratory tract, may bring some benefit

Literature

Bartlett A et al. Splenic rupture in infectious mononucleosis: A systematic review of published case reports. Injury. 2015 Oct 31. pii: S0020-1383(15)00688-9.

Becker JA, Smith JA. Return to play after infectious mononucleosis. Sports Health. 2014 May;6(3):232-8.

Karrer U, D Nadal. Epstein-Barr-Virus und infektiöse Mononukleose. Schweiz Med Forum 2014;14(11):226–232.

Putukian M et al. Mononucleosis and athletic participation: an evidence-based subject review. Clin J Sport Med. 2008 Jul;18(4):309-15.

Ebell MH. Epstein-Barr virus infectious mononucleosis. Am Fam Physician. 2004 Oct 1;70(7):1279-87.

Overreaching/Overtraining – When the Batteries are Completely Empty

Symptoms

Persistent fatigue in general and decline in performance in particular. This is often combined with changes in mood (feeling down, depressive), lack of motivation, and sleep disturbances.

Figure 1:

1) Normal training process

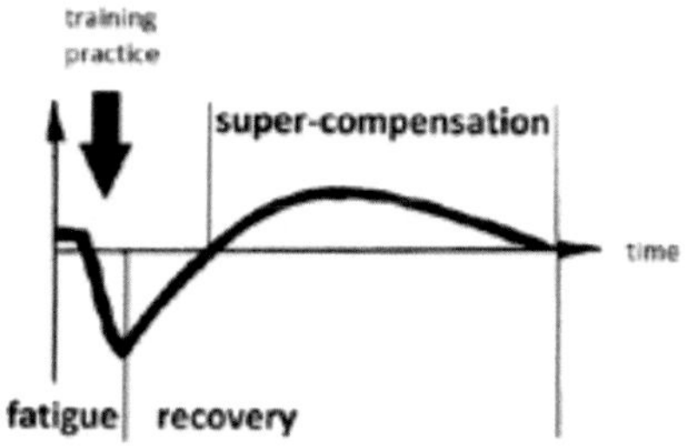

2) Overreaching

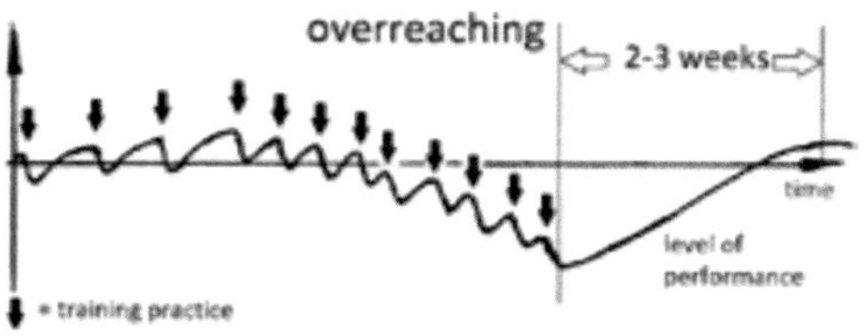

3) Overtraining

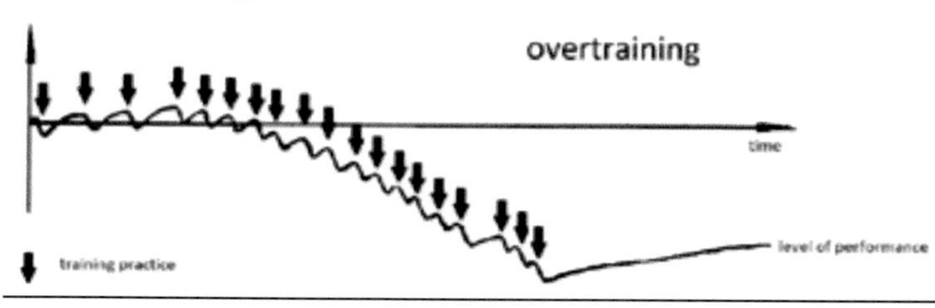

Background

'From an operational standpoint, overtraining can be defined as stress > recovery (regeneration) imbalance, that is, too much stress combined with too little time for regeneration. In this context, stress summarises all individual training, non-training, and competition-dependent stress factors. Particularly, additional exogenous non-training stress factors, such as social, educational, occupational, economic, nutritional factors, travel, and endogenous factors (genetic predisposition) exacerbate the risk of a resulting overtraining syndrome in a completely individual manner. The term overtraining syndrome describes an impaired state of health that is caused by overtraining and characterised by particular findings' (citation Lehmann et al, 1999).

Definitions

Overreaching: A state of experienced general fatigue and impaired performance in competitive athletes typically resolving with a rest period of two weeks.

Overtraining: A state of experienced general fatigue and impaired performance in competitive athletes lasting several months.

Overreaching/Overtraining symptomatology is diagnosed by exclusion. This means the problem is very thoroughly, even meticulously, investigated as outlined in 'Unclear Fatigue' (see corresponding chapter). While always keeping in mind that it could be overreaching/overtraining, all other medical explanations for the symptoms are examined. The rationale for this is twofold. First, there are quite a few frequent sports-related medical diagnoses to be ruled out before you think it is overreaching/overtraining, e.g. iron deficiency, anaemia, vitamin B12 deficiency, mononucleosis to name a few. Second, despite reasonable research efforts, there is still no precise diagnostic tool for overreaching/overtraining. However, some baseline measurements and their comparison in performance decline may assist in supporting the diagnosis of overreaching/overtraining, e.g. an incremental lactate threshold test, testing of explosive strength, and sportpsychological questionnaires.

Prevention and Treatment Table for Overreaching/ Overtraining

Prevention	• In training increase volume and intensity gradually, do not escalate in rapid strides • Plan and observe training and competitions thoroughly in transition phases, as there is particular risk for overreaching and overtraining • Allow enough time for regeneration after training camps. Plan a really easy week, allow super-compensation • As competitive athlete look for a yearly sportsmed exam. Unfortunately there's no warranty on the exam but an experienced sports medicine physician will recognise possible risk factors and you have the great advantage of having baseline clinical findings, lab results, and exercise tests you can rely on in case of an overreaching/overtraining
Treatment by Yourself	Seek professional advice.
When is a Doctor Needed?	As soon as an overreaching or overtraining is suspected.
Return to Play/ Sports	In case of **'overreaching':** A return to play within weeks is usually possible. Please don't be fixed on the 2 weeks recovery, that's theory, and the practice (and athlete's life) is often different. Luckily, I would say, an athlete is first of all a human being and not a freely programmable machine. Again teamwork athlete-coach-sports medicine physician and a good communication is essential.

	In case of **'overtraining':** The return to play takes several months sometimes a year. Also this time needs to be anticipated and I strongly recommend a written document. Even if the plan is, for example, two months no vigorous effort, but just a daily walk of 30min and twice a week a block core stability for 30min. Discussion is more about what needs to be respected. What else should/could I do instead (as there are many training hours free)? What's the exact plan? Where do we have milestones? How do we address the secondary symptoms like feeling depressed, sleep disturbances? When is the next appointment? etc.

What Does the Doctor Do?

The doctor takes the history and performs a thorough clinical exam. The whole regime as outlined in the chapter 'Unclear Fatigue' is undertaken. At this particular moment, a training pause for the duration of two weeks is initiated, as by definition the overreaching resolves after a two week period and shows this late effect of super-compensation.

As these investigations are the basis for any possible further diagnosis, in particular the overreaching and overtraining, it is important that they are done by a sports medicine physician with high interest and competence in this field and a person you trust.

Literature

Carfagno DG1, Hendrix JC 3rd. Overtraining syndrome in the athlete: current clinical practice. Curr Sports Med Rep. 2014 Jan-Feb;13(1):45-51.

Le Meur Y et al. A multidisciplinary approach to overreaching detection in endurance trained athletes. J Appl Physiol. 2013 Feb;114(3):411-20

Meeusen R, et al. Prevention, diagnosis, and treatment of the overtraining syndrome: joint consensus statement of the European College of Sport Science and the American College of Sports Medicine. Med Sci Sports Exerc. 2013 Jan;45(1):186-205..

Halson SL, AE Jeukendrup. Does Overtraining Exist? - An Analysis of Overreaching and Overtraining Research.Sports Med 2004; 34 (14): 967-981

Vogel R. «Übertraining»: Begriffsklärungen, ätiologische Hypothesen, aktuelle Trends und methodische Limiten. Schweiz Z für Sportmed 49 (4), 154–162, 2001

Lehmann M et al. Definition, Types, Symptoms, Findings, Underlying Mechanisms, and Frequency of Overtraining and Overtraining Syndrome in Overload, Performance Incompetence, and Regeneration in Sport, pp 1-6, Springer, Germany, 1999

Muscle Cramps – Some New Theories and Insights

Symptoms

Sudden, involuntary, often painful contraction of a muscle during or after exercise.

Figure 1: Factors Provoking Muscle Cramps

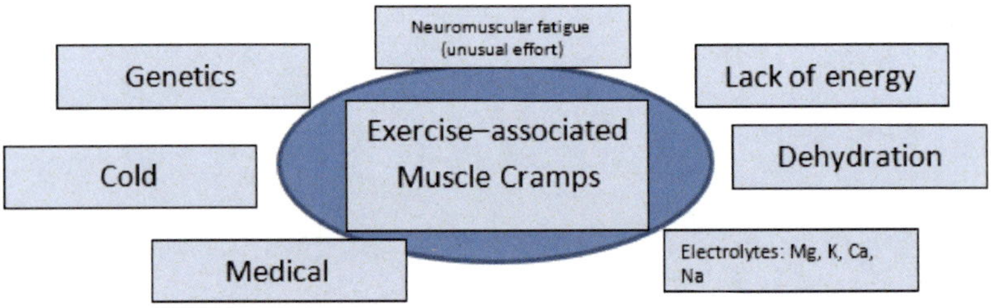

Background

Exercise Associated Muscle Cramps (EAMC) are frequent in sports. Despite many studies, clear evidence on the etiology of muscle cramps is lacking. It is highly probable that it is not a single cause, but many different factors contributing to the genesis of muscle cramps. Figure 1 gives an overview about possible reasons for exercise-associated muscle cramps.

Neuromuscular fatigue (unusual effort): This hypothesis is, according to the literature, the strongest in the field. It means that unusual effort, be in duration, pace, or explosivity, makes the muscles respectively the motor units (the muscle fibre with its individual innervation) more prone to a hyper-excitation. It seems that activating muscle in a shortened state is a stronger trigger than activating it at its normal length. This approach of neuromuscular fatigue is very promising as it is an issue that may be clearly addressed with specific training (and good tactics in competition).

Genetics: A collagen gene as potential marker for EIMA could be identified (COL5A1CC). The finding of a positive family history of athletes with recurrent muscle cramps as well as the fact that a personal history of muscle cramps being a strong predictor for a recurrence are pointing in the same direction.

Cold: Cold, together with exercise, may be a driver of muscle cramps. Especially in water sports or in wet and windy conditions, the cooling out may be a major factor in the genesis of muscle cramping.

Medical: There are medical conditions that should be ruled out, in case of recurrent muscle cramps, e.g. anaemia, iron deficiency, thyroid disorder, diabetes mellitus. Some medications are known to provoke muscle cramps, among them lipid lowering drugs, diuretics, and others.

Electrolytes: Magnesium (Mg^{2+}), potassium (K^+), calcium (Ca^{2+}), and sodium (Na^+) are the usual suspects, but in the literature the evidence is sparse. An important general limitation, which makes a good quality study difficult, is that serum analysis measures what happens in the blood (so called extracellular space) but we are also interested in what happens in the muscle (intracellular space). Additionally, the extracellular and the intracellular levels of these electrolytes differ significantly (e.g. K^+ in muscle 150mmol/l compared to 3.5–5mmol/l in serum; Mg^{2+} in muscle 7–9mmol/kg compared to 0.65–1.05mmol/l in serum). And finally, the blood serum contains only a little fraction of the total body amount (e.g. K^+ only 2% in serum, 98% in cells; Mg^{2+} only 0.3% in blood serum, 99% in cells). These are real handicaps for rational, well-founded evidence about the importance of electrolytes. However there is good theoretical reasoning and anecdotal evidence favouring supplementation of electrolytes in preparation of competitions. But you need to start it early enough (2–3 weeks before the event) and to take appropriate doses (e.g. Mg^{2+} 300–400mg daily, best in combination with K^+). There is also benefit in undertaking laboratory testing for measuring the so called intracellular Mg^{2+}.

Dehydration: Even though research evidence in this field is sparse, and some studies even controversial, it is recommended you start any competition in a eu-hydrated (not over, but sufficiently hydrated) state and drink during and after the competition, usually a sports drink containing carbohydrates and electrolytes.

Lack of energy: A simple lack of energy seems to be an important co-factor in the genesis of muscle cramps.

Prevention and Treatment Table for Muscle Cramps

Prevention	• Prepare your competition thoroughly, be well and specifically trained • Allow a few days (possibly a week) of tapering before longer events • Adapt your pace to your capacities • Be sufficiently hydrated (control it by the colour of urine) • Look for a sport specific nutrition: prepare your competition days with anticipation of your energy needs by planning your eating and drinking for this day, even consider professional advice by a sports nutritionist • Think about your clothing—protect against the cold • In case you want to optimise electrolytes, discuss this issue with your sports medicine physician or your sport nutritionist—throwing in some magnesium tablets is not a bad idea, but neither very constructive nor sufficient
Treatment by Yourself	If you look at the table above, you may hopefully recognise where you have room for improvement
When is a Doctor Needed?	If you have muscle cramps and your self-treatment options are fully utilised

Return to Play/Sports	In acute cramping in a competition: • Static stretching exercises often lead to an immediate release • Re-hydrate with hypotonic electrolyte fluids containing carbohydrates • Take a carbohydrate gel with electrolytes *and* sodium • Eat a little, e.g. banana, bread • If appropriate (e.g. swimming, or cold ambient temperature), protect against the cold • Get your muscles back to work slowly. Adapt your pace: start slow, go slow, try to come back into an adapted rhythm. • Otherwise no general training pause needed. In case of recurrent muscle cramp consider: • Exercising the concerned muscle group with plyometric strengthening (e.g. eccentric jump exercises, as drop jumps) and specific endurance training, both as required by your sport discipline • A diagnostic session with your sports medicine physician and/or a sports nutritionist

What Does the Doctor Do?

The doctor takes a careful history and performs a clinical exam, including stance and gait and muscle length and tone. Usually a blood test is performed to have baseline blood results and in order to rule out possible underlying conditions provoking muscle cramping (e.g. anaemia, iron and vitamin B12 deficiency, thyroid disorder, diabetes mellitus, etc.). The serum electrolytes are usually measured, *but* one must be aware of certain limitations in these measurements as blood serum levels of electrolytes don't represent levels within the muscle.

Literature

Miller, Kevin C et al. Exercise-Associated Muscle Cramps: Causes, Treatment, and Prevention. *Sports Health* 2.4 (2010): 279–283. *PMC*. Web. 3 Mar. 2016.

O'Connell K et al. Collagen genes and exercise-associated muscle cramping. Clin J Sport Med, 2013 Jan;23(1):64-9

Garrison SR. Magnesium for skeletal muscle cramps. Cochrane Database Syst Rev, 2012 Sep 12;9

Schwellnus MP et al. Increased running speed and previous cramps rather than dehydration or serum sodium changes predict exercise-associated muscle cramping: a prospective cohort study in 210 Ironman triathletes. Br J Sports Med, 2011 Jun;45(8):650-6

Stress Reaction/Stress Fracture – the Sword of Damocles

Symptoms

Pain in the lower limb, deep within (the bone), worsening during or after exercise. Local tenderness on palpation and tapping, sometimes with a slight local swelling. Mostly observed in tibia, fibula, mid- or rear-foot, but other locations as femoral head, sacrum, lumbar spine, or ribs are all also possible, depending on the training load and sport.

Background

Stress fractures are common overuse injuries, mostly occurring in lower extremities. Among runners, stress fractures account for 15–20% of all musculoskeletal injuries. The training load (mostly impact related) is the main driver of a stress reaction/ stress fracture. Additional factors, as outlined below, add quite significant risks for the genesis of an overuse injury of the bone.

Risk factors for stress reactions/stress fractures are:

- Sudden increase in physical activities
- Excessive physical activity with limited rest periods
- Female athlete triad (eating disorder, amenorrhea, osteoporosis) respectively RED-S (relative energy deficiency syndrome). See also the corresponding chapter
- Smoking
- Low levels of 25-hydroxyvitamin D
- Previous history of stress fracture

Table 1: An Overview on the Grading of Stress Reactions/ Stress Fractures (according to Kaeding and Miller, JBJS 2013)

Grade	Diagnosis	Symptoms	Imaging	Treatment	Return to competition
I	Stress reaction	No clear or minor symptoms	Visible stress reaction, no microfrac-tures	Conservative	2–3 weeks
II	Pain without fracture	Localised pain deep within, worsening on exercise	Local bone edema, microfrac-tures, but no fracture line	Conserva-tive*	6 weeks
III	Non-dis-placed fracture	+Night pain, +pain with daily activities	Fracture line visible	Conserva-tive**	8–10 weeks
IV	Displaced fracture	As above	Fracture displaced	To be discussed	10–12 weeks, or longer
V	Non-union	+Persistent pain +without success on any treatment	Fracture line, delayed or even missing healing response	Operation	According to tx, 12 weeks and longer

*relative rest, e.g. crutches for 2 weeks (half body weight) and alternative training program

** relative rest, e.g. crutches for 4 weeks (2 weeks 10kg, 2 weeks half body weight) and alternative training program

Figure 1:

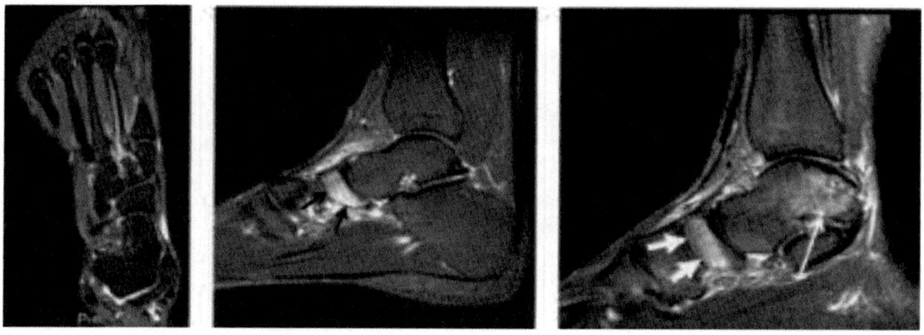

MR images of stress reactions/fractures: II-metatarsal bone (grade II); navicular bone (grade II), navicular and talar bone (grade II-III)

Prevention and Treatment Table for Stress Reaction/ Stress Fracture

Prevention	• In training increase volume and intensity gradually—do not escalate in rapid strides • Plan and monitor training and competitions thoroughly in transition phases, as there is particular risk for overload (e.g. in juniors from regionals to nationals or from U19 to U23, etc.) • After training camps (with justified and planned augmented training volume and intensity) have a really easy week to allow recovery as well as super-compensation • As a team (athlete, coach, junior athlete parents, sports medicine professional) address the above named risk factors • If you're a competitive athlete, discuss this issue in the yearly sports medicine exam with your sports medicine physician
Treatment by Yourself	In case of a suspected stress reaction/stress fracture, seek professional support immediately and follow the given recommendations.

When is a Doctor Needed	If a stress reaction/stress fracture is suspected or if you are at particular risk.
Return to Play/ Sports	Depending on the locality and severity of the stress reaction/fracture. Luckily there are reasonable treatment options—so the allusion with the sword of Damocles is only partially true. In case of an early stress reaction (Grade I), return to sport on a competitive level may take 2–3 weeks, in case of a complete but undisplaced fracture return to competition may take about 8–10 weeks.

What Does the Doctor Do?

The doctor takes the history and performs a clinical exam, including stance, gait, inspection of training and running shoes, and a focused examination of the painful site. Where a stress reaction/stress fracture is suspected, further imaging (MRI) needs to be organised promptly. Where a stress reaction/ stress fracture is confirmed, it will be graded and an individual treatment plan will be established.

Possible etiologic risk factors need to be addressed and treated (e.g. underweight, female athlete triad respectively RED-S, low vitamin D3, insufficient calcium uptake, bad foot alignment, training overload, etc.).

As differential diagnosis (i.e. other explanation for the pain and clinical findings; DD) need to be considered. A periostitis (i.e. inflammation of the bone skin), a tenosynovitis (i.e. inflammation of a tendon and its sheath), and in particular locations: sacrum/lumbar spine DD: SIJ dysfunction/trigger points; shin DD: shin splint/medial tibial stress syndrome; midfoot/rearfoot: plantar fasciitis, metatarsalgia, Morton neuroma.

A written 'return to play' plan is for both athlete and coach extremely helpful, as it allows the whole team following the athlete to have an overview on things to do or not to do. In the first 6 weeks, most of the content is given by the sports medicine physician and the physio. From week 7–12 there is increasing involvement of the coach while health professionals give just recommendations and guide lines on training volume and intensity.

Table 2: Example of a Return to Play Protocol (to be completed and individually designed) e.g. Metarsal Stress fracture Gr III

Activities	1st week	2nd week	3rd week	4th week	5th week	6th week
Weight bearing / crutches	Crutches 10kg	Crutches 10kg	Crutches ½body weight	Crutches ½body weight	Normal daily activities	Normal daily activities
Vitamin D3/ Calcium Fish oil (Omega -3)	Yes Yes	Yes Yes	Yes Yes	Yes Yes	Yes Yes	Yes Yes
Physiotherapy (e.g. proprioception, strengthening, etc.)	Rest	Instruction of alternative training modalities, prevention of muscle atrophy, weekly detail planning, and supervision				
Endurance training	No	e.g. in water, pull buoy swimming	Cycling ergometer, Etc.	Deep water running, etc.		
Strength training	No	Core stability, upper body, other leg	Isometric on index leg	Concentric on index leg		
Running	No	No	No	No	No	No
Team training	No	No	No	No	No	No

Regular follow-up by the physio, intermediate controls after week 2, 4, and 6 with the sports medicine physician.

Literature

Tenforde AS, Kraus E, Fredericson M. Bone Stress Injuries in Runners. Phys Med Rehabil Clin N Am. 2016 Feb;27(1):139-49

Changstrom BG et al. Epidemiology of stress fracture injuries among US high school athletes, 2005-2006 through 2012-2013. Am J Sports Med. 2015 Jan;43(1)26-33.

Kaeding CC, T Miller. The comprehensive description of stress fractures: A new classification system. J Bone Joint Surg Am; 2013 Jul 03;95(13):1214-1220

Fredericson M et al. Stress fractures in athletes. Top Magn Reson Imaging. 2006 Oct;17(5):309-25.

Patel DS et al. Stress fractures: diagnosis, treatment, and prevention. Am Fam Physician. 2011 Jan 1;83(1):39-46.

Special Situations Warrant Special Attention

Prevention of Infectious Diseases – How to Support Athletes' Lowered Immune Response

Symptoms

Infectious illnesses are frequent in competitive athletes. They may present in different ways. The most frequent are:

- Skin infections with bacteria or fungi (mostly red and inflamed part of the skin, often with germ specific skin alteration)
- URTI (upper respiratory tract infections) mostly viral (coughing, running nose, slight fever), or more severe respiratory infections like bronchitis (deep coughing with purulent discharge)
- Gastro-intestinal infections, such as gastro-enteritis (diarrhoea with or without vomiting)
- Others

Figure 1:

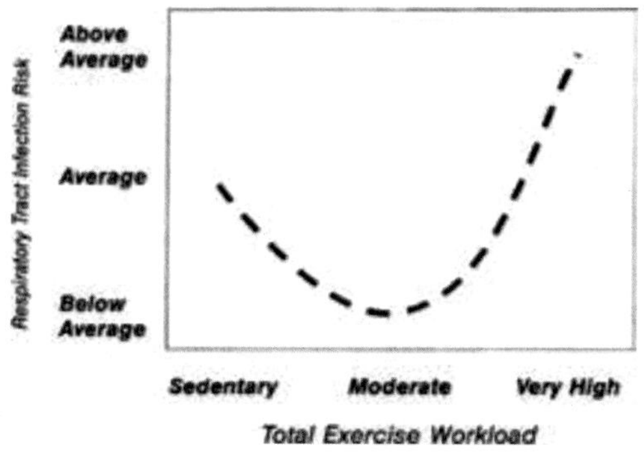

1) J-Shape curve of exercise workload vs upper respiratory tract infection risk (courtesy Prof David Nieman)

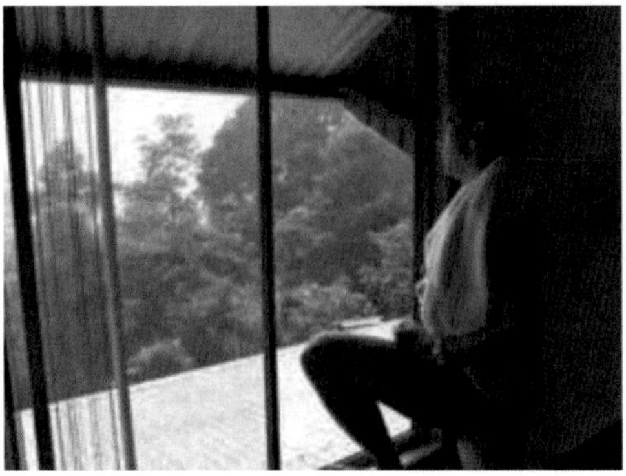

2) OPEN WINDOW in sports

Background

Moderate physical activity boosts our immune system. This is the reason why recreational sportsmen and women are less frequently ill (see J-curve above). On one hand, several studies have shown that regular moderate sporting activity prevents upper respiratory tract infections, on the other hand quite recent immunological research shows that competitive strenuous athletic training leads to a temporary suppression of the immune response called the *open window,* lasting 3–12 hours after marathon-like efforts. These findings were confirmed by studies with elite athletes who indicated air travel and competitions as additional factors to be taken into account.

Respiratory infections, and to some extent, the gastro-intestinal infections, may be caused primarily by an impaired immune response. As a gastro-enteritis often occurs after ingestion of contaminated water or food, a more careful choice of beverages and meals is warranted. As skin infections occur more frequently, they may be due to direct contact, as in wrestling or rugby, with either a fungal (tinea gladiatorum) or viral skin infection (herpes gladiatorum). As they are also observed in quite a few other sports, e.g. gymnastics, orienteering, mountain-biking and road cycling, it is likely they are due to a reduced immune response but possibly also to insufficient wound care.

Prevention and Treatment Table for Infectious Diseases

Prevention (adapted after Nieman)	• Eat a well-balanced diet to keep vitamin and mineral pools at optimal levels. Insist on the 5 servings of vegetables and fruits of different colours per day • Keep other life stresses to a minimum • Avoid overreaching and chronic fatigue • Get adequate sleep on a regular schedule • Keep your body weight stable; avoid rapid weight loss • Before important events, avoid putting hands to the eyes and nose, avoid hand-shaking, sick people, and large crowds. Consider consequent hand disinfection for these time periods • Keep your vaccinations updated. For athletes competing during the winter months, flu shots are highly recommended • Clean and disinfect skin wounds immediately and watch your feet. • Consider special care for your nasal mucosal surface for air travel (use some nose ointment during air travel, keeping the nasal mucosa protected, and rinse the nose with saline after arrival. Wash everything out) • Use carbohydrate beverages before, during, and after competitions or unusually heavy training bouts • Consider vitamin C and zinc (as effervescent) before exhaustive, long lasting sport events. In time-critical moments, shortly before and during major events, consider echinacea (as drops or tablets to suck), vitamin C, and zinc (as effervescent)
Treatment by Yourself	Be strong and disciplined in prevention! As soon as an infection is suspected, seek professional advice.

When is a Doctor Needed?	As soon as an infectious disease is suspected, but be *active* and *creative* in the prevention field (not just *reactive* treating the illness). As an athlete, coach, sports official, sports medicine doctor, sports physiotherapist, sports nutritionist, sports scientist, take up the prevention topic and inform yourself, your mates, and your team athletes about it.
Return to Play/ Sports	According to the illness and the treatment plan. Always take some days of entire rest and then gradual and slow return to practice is the way to go. Discuss the detailed plan with your sports medicine physician.

What Does the Doctor Do?

Where an infectious disease is suspected, the doctor takes the history and performs a clinical exam. Sometimes other examinations as blood tests or germ identifications of the infectious disease will be conducted and only rarely may further investigations be needed. Based on the diagnosis, the treatment and return to play plan will be established. But we definitely don't want to stop here, as we are aware of the vulnerability of sportsmen and women to infectious diseases. *We know about the open window—the risk for mainly respiratory, gastrointestinal, and skin infections—so be prepared!*

Literature

Svendsen et al. Training-related and competition-related risk factors for respiratory tract and gastrointestinal infections in cross-country skiers. Br J Sports Med. 2016 Mar 3.

Hauswirth C et al. Evidence of disturbed sleep and increased illness in overreached endurance athletes. Med Sci Sports Exerc. 2014;46(5):1036-45

Harris MD. Infectious disease in athletes. Curr Sports Med Rep. 2011 Mar-Apr;10(2):84-9.

Kakanis MW et al. The open window of susceptibility to infection after acute exercise in healthy young male elite athletes. Exerc Immunolog Rev, 2010, 16, 119-37;

Shah SA et al. Evaluation of echinacea for the prevention and treatment of

the common cold: a meta-analysis. Lancet Infect Dis. 2007 Jul;7(7):473-80.
Nieman DC et al. Exercise and the common cold. ACSM Current comment. Downloaded 11.3.16. https://www.acsm.org/docs/current-comments/exerciseandcommoncold.pdf
Nieman DC. Risk of upper respiratory tract infection in athletes: an epidemiologic and immunologic perspective. J Athl Train. 1997 Oct;32(4):344-9

Heat Illness: Still Provoking Deaths in Sports! – Goal: Zero Deaths!

'Heat illness is an inherent risk when exercising in hot conditions and can affect even the best-conditioned athlete. Failure to respond to an athlete in distress by removing them from activity, cooling their body and giving them fluids can result in **severe dehydration and, in extreme conditions, death.***'*

(citation M.Nadelen ACSM recommendations 2012)

Symptoms

Exercise (heat) exhaustion: Should be suspected in athletes with a rapid decline in performance or lack of ability to continue exercising. Further symptoms may be extreme thirst, dizziness, headache, weak and rapid pulse, and profuse sweating.

Heat syncope: Occurs at the end of a race or another physical effort after an athlete stands still for a certain period of time. The weakness, the dizziness, and the possible fainting experience is attributed to a so-called blood pooling mechanism in the extremities. This means the available blood in the circulation sinks in the now inactive extremities and overheated skin, the blood pressure drops distinctly, and the athlete faints.

Heatstroke: This corresponds to an elevated core temperature to a level of 40°C (104°F) and above, causing organ failure. This condition is life-threatening unless promptly recognised and treated. Confusion, disorientation, loss of balance, possible loss of consciousness, hot red skin, sometimes profuse sweating (sometimes there is no sweating anymore!), and rapid pulse.

The risk for developing heat illness is greatest when the ambient temperature is greater than 28°C (82°F). And it is not just the temperature but also the humidity, which greatly influences the perceived temperature. In high humidity our sweating is impaired and therefore the perceived temperature rises. For a more accurate appreciation, the heat index has been introduced, combining ambient temperature and humidity, leading to the perceived apparent temperature.

Figure 1: Heat Index in Celsius (courtesy of Environment Canada)

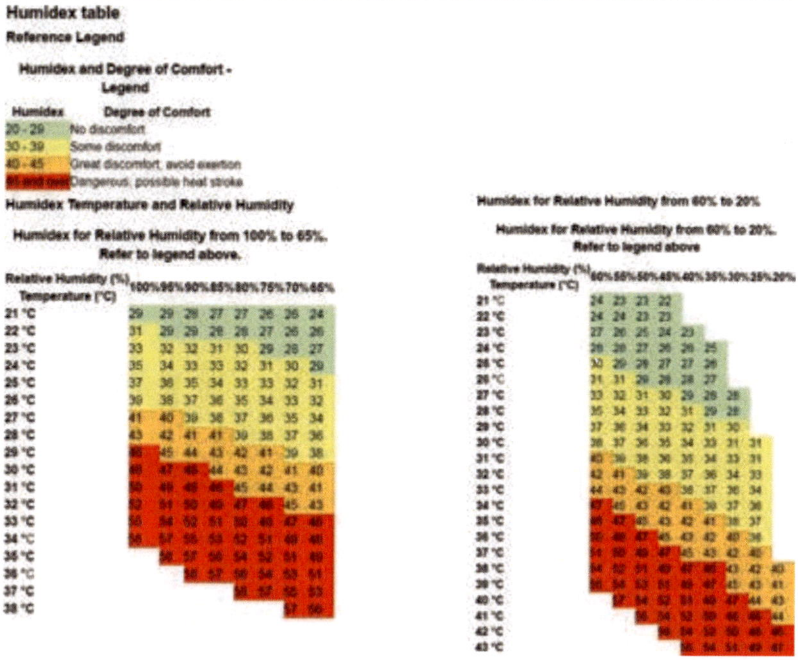

Humidex table

Reference Legend

Humidex and Degree of Comfort - Legend

Humidex	Degree of Comfort
20 - 29	No discomfort
30 - 39	Some discomfort
40 - 45	Great discomfort, avoid exertion
46 and over	Dangerous, possible heat stroke

Humidex Temperature and Relative Humidity

Humidex for Relative Humidity from 100% to 65%. Refer to legend above.

Relative Humidity (%) / Temperature (°C)	100%	95%	90%	85%	80%	75%	70%	65%
21 °C	29	29	28	27	27	26	26	24
22 °C	31	29	29	28	28	27	26	26
23 °C	33	32	32	31	30	29	28	27
24 °C	35	34	33	33	32	31	30	29
25 °C	37	36	35	34	33	33	32	31
26 °C	39	38	37	36	35	34	33	32
27 °C	41	40	39	38	37	36	35	34
28 °C	43	42	41	41	39	38	37	36
29 °C	46	45	44	43	42	41	39	38
30 °C	48	47	46	44	43	42	41	40
31 °C	50	49	48	46	45	44	43	41
32 °C	52	51	50	49	47	46	45	43
33 °C	55	54	52	51	50	49	47	46
34 °C	58	57	55	53	52	51	49	48
35 °C		58	57	56	54	52	51	49
36 °C			58	57	56	54	53	51
37 °C					58	57	55	53
38 °C							57	56

Humidex for Relative Humidity from 60% to 20%

Humidex for Relative Humidity from 60% to 20%. Refer to legend above

Relative Humidity (%) / Temperature (°C)	60%	55%	50%	45%	40%	35%	30%	25%	20%
21 °C	24	23	23	22					
22 °C	24	24	23	23					
23 °C	27	26	25	24	23				
24 °C	28	28	27	26	26	25			
25 °C	30	29	29	27	27	26			
26 °C	31	31	29	28	28	27			
27 °C	33	32	31	30	29	28	28		
28 °C	35	34	33	32	31	29	28		
29 °C	37	36	34	33	32	31	30		
30 °C	38	37	36	35	34	33	31	31	
31 °C	40	39	38	36	35	34	33	31	
32 °C	42	41	39	38	37	36	34	33	
33 °C	44	43	42	40	38	37	36	34	
34 °C	47	45	43	42	41	39	37	36	
35 °C	48	47	45	43	42	41	38	37	
36 °C	50	48	47	45	43	42	40	38	
37 °C	51	50	49	47	45	43	42	40	
38 °C	54	52	51	49	47	46	43	42	40
39 °C	55	54	53	51	49	47	45	43	41
40 °C		57	54	52	51	49	47	44	43
41 °C			56	54	52	50	48	46	44
42 °C				56	54	52	50	48	46
43 °C					56	54	51	49	47

Read more about a heat index in Fahrenheit:

- http://www.momsteam.com/health-safety/hydration-safety/heat-index-measures-risk-heat-illness-for-athletes#ixzz42MQcLvnn
- http://www.momsteam.com/health-safety/hydration-safety/heat-index-measures-risk-heat-illness-for-athletes

Background

Exercising in heat and high humidity, wearing of heavy and closed protective clothing (heating up the body, impairing air circulation, and withdrawing the cooling effect of sweating), and training or competing in direct sunlight bear the risk of overheating and heatstroke. All these factors contribute to one thing, they all rise the body's core temperature. *Athletes at a particular risk* developing heat illness or heat stroke are:

- Very muscular
- Having a heat illness or heat stroke in their history
- Dehydrated
- Overweight
- Under conditioned

Sport officials, coaches, and athletes all need to realise that even our body is quite robust, a rise in body core temperature leading up to 40°C (104°F) must be prevented at all cost. We need to appreciate that exercising physiologically raises our body core temperature by several degrees, often leading to a temperature around 39°C (102°F), so quite close to the critical one, just to illustrate that there's *no* further buffer. So everybody needs to act correctly and responsibly to prevent heat illness and heat stroke. You can save lives!

Prevention and Treatment Table for Heat Illness/Heat Stroke

Prevention	Heatstroke can and must be prevented! The major responsibility in this matter lies in the hand of sport officials and coaches! Watch and protect your athletes, you may save lives!
	• Beat the heat! Be wise, train and compete in cooler hours of the day. Reschedule the day and training session if it's really hotter than expected (compare the heat-index scale) • If it is too hot, skip training and the competition! • Train and compete in the shade, if possible • Drink enough—before, during, and after the training/the game/the competition

	• On hot days, plan additional pauses in the shade, provide cool drinks and enough other cooling possibilities (cold water to pour over head, chest, arms, legs). If available, consider cooling wests. • Consider, if appropriate, not wearing the sport specific protection clothes for selected parts of the training (shoulder pad, helmet, jersey) as they are an additional source leading to heat illness • Think about athletes at a particular risk (compare above)
Treatment by Yourself	*Heat stroke* is an absolute EMERGENCY and professional help must be called. In case of *overheating/heat illness:* • Goal: Cool the patient down • Bring the patient to a sitting position in the shade • Free the patient of heat conserving protective equipment and clothes (remove helmet, jersey, shoulder, breast and back pad) • Continuously cool the patient down with cool water (poured over head, arms, chest, legs) • Provide drinks
When is a Doctor Needed?	In any serious condition. *Immediate* help by emergency professionals needs to be looked for!
Return to Play/ Sports	In case of overheating with any other symptom, even after cooling down, there is *no more* sport activity that day. With heatstroke, *no* further sport and major effort for the following week—a detailed plan for the return to sports needs to be worked out. As people at risk for heatstroke may suffer similar events in the future, particular attention needs to be paid to their prevention.

What Does the Doctor Do?

'Heat stroke is one of the top three causes of death for athletes. Vigilance is required to prevent these illnesses and when faced with an individual who is suffering an exertional heat stroke, the goal is to aggressively cool the patient to 102°F (<39°C) within 30 minutes to optimize survival' (citation Raukar 2013).

The called doctor or paramedic starts emergency appraisal and treatment—primary goal is to cool the patient and secure survival.

Literature

Krohn AR et al. Heat Illness in Football: Current Concepts. Curr Sports Med Rep. 2015 Nov-Dec;14(6):463-71

Tripp BL et al. Exertional heat illness and environmental conditions during high school football practices. Am J Sports Med. 2015 Oct; 43(10):2490-5

Racinais S et al. Consensus recommendations on training and competing in the heat. Br J Sports Med. 2015 Sep;49(18):1164-73

Raukar N et al. Heat Illness - A Practical Primer. R I Med J (2013). 2015 Jul 1;98(7):28-31.

Nadelen M. Preparing for and playing in the heat. Jan 13, 2012. ACSM recommendations download 28.2.2016

Pre-Cooling – a Cooler Engine Works More Efficiently

Background

In every kind of exercise our working muscle is producing additional heat. This leads to a distinct rise in body core temperature of several degrees. If there is additional heat from the environment—due to hot climate, high humidity, the need to wear protective clothing—this effect of heating up the working muscle and the whole body is further boosted, leading to a distinct rise in core temperature.

The comparison with a car engine will give us a better understanding of this topic. The task of a car engine is to lead to a safe drive with a powerful and long running propulsion leading to a good speed. Beside this main task the car engine, as any other engine too, produces quite a lot of heat, which is just an unplanned by-product. Engineers all around the world are doing research to improve engines to be more efficient, more powerful, and more economical fuel-wise, and all without by-producing too much heat. As this heat is to a certain extent unavoidable, the car needs to have a cooling system. Otherwise it would finally blow up or at least show the picture of a stopped car at the side of the road with a steaming radiator in a hot summer day, as we know it from older movies.

Taking this picture of the car engine and the necessity of cooling, we come back to the athlete and we recognise that also in human beings the findings are comparable. To move the body, the muscle is by producing heat, which leads to a rise in the whole body temperature. As in the engine, a warmed up body is perfectly performing but an overheated organism starts to be inefficient. The more intensive the exercise, the hotter the ambient temperature, the more humid the air, the more pronounced is this effect.

Several studies have shown that at an ambient temperature of 25°Celsius (77°Fahrenheit) and above cooling of an athlete's body leads to a measurable improvement of performance. Some facts about pre-cooling and performance:

- Larger effects may be observed in hot (>26°C) compared to moderate temperatures
- Largest enhancements in open-end endurance tests, graded exercise tests, and time-trials
- In intermittent sprints a good effect is observable whereas short-term high intensity sprint showed smaller or no effect
- Cold drinks (e.g. ice slurry), cold room, and cold water immersion may be the most effective, cooling vest moderately effective, simple water application with small effect
- Best effects observed in athletes with the highest aerobic capacity (VO2max) compared to moderate
- The body core temperature gradually increases but compared to athletes without pre-cooling remains lowered for about 45min—having performance enhancing effects for the same time span (and still bringing advantages as it may considerably help saving energy for the further ongoing competition)

Recommendations for Pre-cooling

- If the ambient temperature rises above 25°C, consider pre-cooling methods
- In endurance sports (with time trials or open end competitions), a broader application and a cooling of the whole body seems appropriate
- If you consider using pre-cooling in high intensity sports (sprint, throwing, putting, jumping, etc.), focus on the body core (e.g. cold drinks and cooling jacket)
- Start 45–30min before the competition with the pre-cooling, for the duration of 20–30min
- Conserve the cool core temperature with a cooling jacket, possibly until the starting line
- Be well-hydrated
- Do your other immediate competition preparation as usual

Literature

Schmit C et al. Heat acclimatization and pre-cooling: a further boost for endurance performance? Scan J Med Sci Sports, 2015 Dec 17.

Fukuchi CA et al. Effects of cold water immersion on lower extremity joint biomechanics during running. J Sports Sci. 2015;33(5):449-56.

Brade CJ et al. Effect of pre-cooling on repeat-sprint performance in seasonally acclimatised males during an outdoor simulated team-sport protocol in warm conditions. J Sports Sci Med. 2013 Sep 1;12(3):565-70.

Jones PR et al. Pre-cooling for endurance exercise performance in the heat: a systematic review. BMC Med. 2012 Dec 18;10:166.

Wegmann M et al. Pre-cooling and sports performance: a meta-analytical review. Sports Med. 2012 Jul 1;42(7):545-64.

Cooling Therapy in Sports – How Does This Work?

The use of post-exercise cold water immersion (CWI) with the goal to minimise fatigue and accelerate recovery is popular among athletes. CWI has the ability to decrease tissue temperature and blood flow to the extremities—the exact mechanisms by which CWI supports or even promotes recovery are in discussion.

As main mechanism by which CWI facilitates short term recovery is via ameliorating hyperthermia (i.e. cools the whole body and the working muscles down) and consequently reduces CNS (central nervous system) mediated fatigue and by reducing cardiovascular strain (earlier and 'externally' supported reduction in cardiovascular action). To understand this better, we need to remember that physical activity leads to a distinct rise of the body core temperature (up to 38–39°C) and a massive heating up of the working muscle with distinctly increased blood flow. Then we understand better that the CWI is cooling the whole body and the muscles, and leads to a lesser blood flow and reduction of the workload for the heart.

CWI mediates a parasympathetic reactivation. This means it supports the part of the autonomous nervous system regulating the body's unconscious actions promoting the 'rest and digest' functions. This leads to an improved longer term physiological recovery and better day to day training performances. The cooling supports the body's unconscious actions by the parasympathetic nervous system, this resets the body and brings it quicker in a 'relax' mode.

CWI attenuates the exercise induced muscle damage, dependent on the mode of exercise used. More effective in whole body endurance/intermittent based exercise modalities, less in single-joint eccentrically contractions. The cooling seems to reduce the local muscle leakage, reducing local inflammation and allowing better short time performance (e.g. in a series of competitions).

Figure 1: Mechanisms of CWI

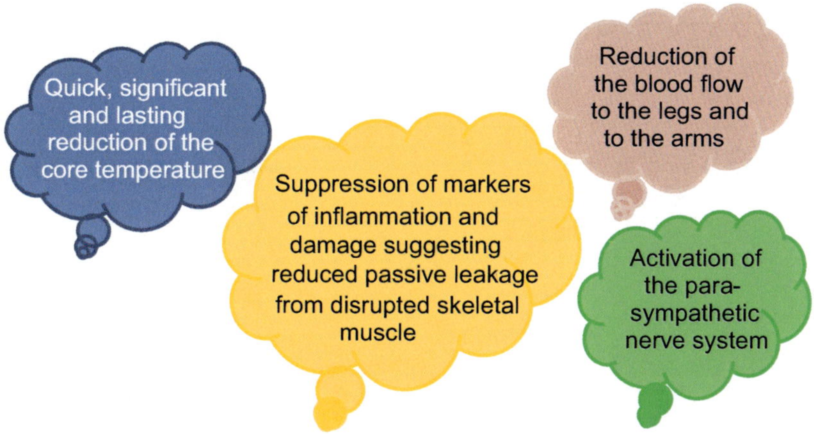

Practical Recommendations for Cold Water Immersion

- After an intensive training session, drink first, then perform an active cool down (10–15min)
- Drink and eat a bite, ideally a recovery shake, containing carbohydrates and proteins
- Apply 15min of cold water immersion at 10–15°C, lower limb until belly button (navel)
- Depending on your sports discipline, include shoulders and arms, eventually adapt in that case water temperature to 15–18°C (because of the involved parts of the chest)
- Perform stretching exercises and roll out (self-myofascial release)
- Shower
- Have lunch or dinner
- Relax

Literature

Ihsan M, Watson G, Abbiss CR. What are the Physiological Mechanisms for Post-Exercise Cold Water Immersion in the Recovery from Prolonged Endurance and Intermittent Exercise? Sports Med. 2016 Feb 18.

Marquet LA et al. Comparison of between-training-session recovery strategies for world-class BMX pilots. Int J Sports Physiol Perform. 2015 Mar;10(2):219-23

Pournot H et al. Short term effects of various water immersions on recovery from exhaustive intermittent exercise. Eur J Appl Physiol. 2011 Jul;111(7):1287-95.

Vaile J et al. Effect of cold water immersion on repeated cycling performance and limb blood flow. Br J Sports Med. 2011 Aug;45(10):825-9.

Acclimatisation to the Heat – How to Optimise Sports Performance?

To be able to perform in the heat good acclimatisation is essential. Certainly we want to prevent heat illness or even heatstroke (see corresponding chapter 'Heat Illness') but as a competitive athlete we also aim to optimise performance. Here good preparation pays, as well adjusted athletes perform at their top (or close to) while non-adapted athletes do not measure up and never reach their potential.

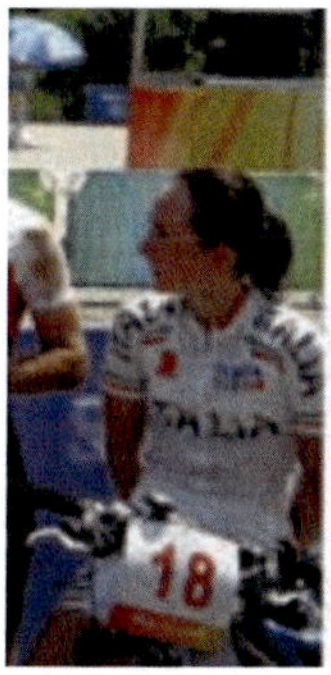

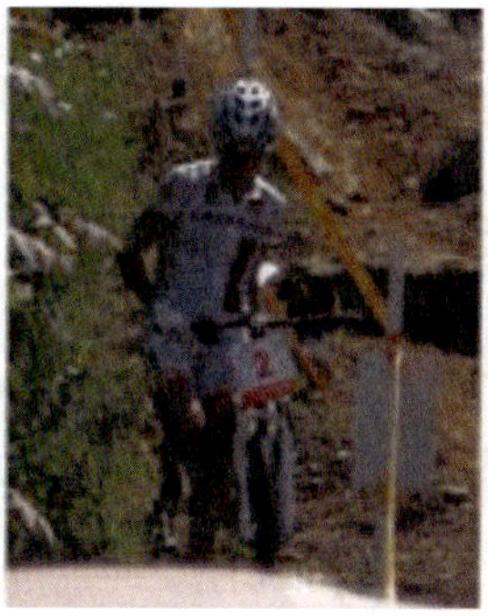
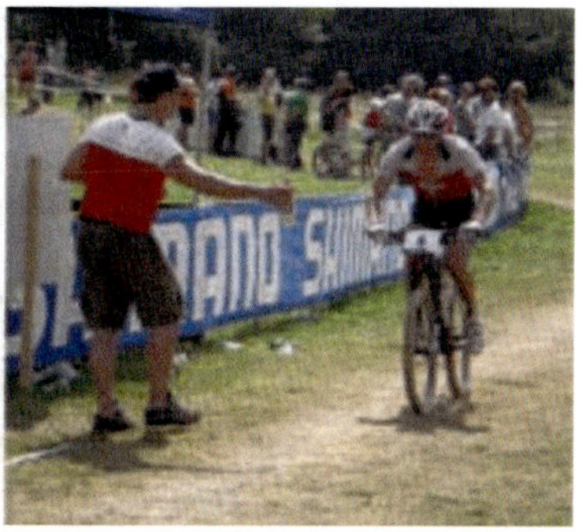

Background

Adapted from the ACSM guidelines, 'Preparing for and playing in the heat' by M. Nadelen 2012:

Coming from a cooler environment, our body is not adapted to the high temperature; the humidity and the heavy sunlight exposure and many body functions need to adapt to the new circumstances. Heat acclimatisation needs quite a lot of time, as many organ systems need to adapt: the cardiovascular system (regulation of the pump function of the heart, blood pressure, blood flow to muscles and different body organs), blood flow to the skin and body extremities, function of the sweat glands, tolerance to heat in general, and in particular the cardiorespiratory system and the energy metabolism of the muscle, etc. To fully adapt coming from a colder country to a hot environment, a period of 10–14 days seems to be ideal.

Practising in the environment the athlete will be playing in, starting already at the first or second day after arrival with just a short and low-intensity session (e.g. 15–40min), two sessions on day 3 and gradually increasing over the following days (for sprint athletes: first intensity then duration; for endurance athletes: first duration then intensity) will allow the body to adapt to the warm environment. This leads to a better heat tolerance and an improvement in performance.

Prevention and Treatment Table for Good Heat Acclimatisation

Prevention	Athletes and coaches should: • Progressively increase the intensity and duration (compare above) of their training sessions over a 10–14 day period to become fully acclimatised • Initially plan training sessions lasting 15–40min for the first couple of days leading, two short session on day 3, progressively up to a two 2–3h hour training sessions by day 14 • Maintain hydration by drinking before practice 2–3dl (7–10oz) 20min before exercise; during practice 2–3dl (7–10oz) every 15min; within two hours after practice 6–7dl (24oz) for every pound lost. • In long lasting efforts (>3h) and extremely hot conditions you must supply your body with a sufficient amount of electrolytes, especially sodium, either by sports drinks or electrolyte containing gels or other food. • Monitor an athlete's level of hydration by the colour of his or her urine (athlete), which should be clear to light yellow, and by monitoring pre- and post-practice body weight (staff).

	• If exposed to direct sunlight, and if possible (at least in training), wear a hat or a cap • Choose clothing and equipment that is light-coloured, loose-fitting, and moisture-wicking (as this will help to keep the athlete cool) • For athletes who must wear protective equipment, allow time to start training in shorts and t-shirts and gradually add equipment each day, as their bodies acclimatise. The body's ability to cool itself through the evaporation of sweat decreases significantly as the amount of equipment increases • Remove equipment during breaks • Take breaks in cool, shaded areas
Treatment by Yourself	Heat acclimatisation is in the hands of the athlete and the coach. By following the recommendations above you will acclimatise, allow an optimisation of performance, and prevent heat illness.
When is a Doctor Needed?	Only if a heat illness is suspected or in preparation for an event.
Return to Play/ Sports	Training starts on the first or second day after arrival, as described above—follow the recommendations. An individual properly acclimatised should be able to train in the warm environment for one or two hours at an intensity equal to competition.

What Does the Doctor Do?

In general there's no need for a doctor in heat acclimatisation.

As contemporary elite and professional athletes are travelling a lot also to hotter countries there's a need for good planning to be ready for the heat. Your sports medicine physician or a sports scientist may assist you in this preparation. As far as teams or a whole delegation are concerned, a thorough preparation pays:

- By sensitising athletes and team officials months in advance, even in the planning session for the new season
- Having a talk about acclimatisation, e.g. by your sports medicine physician, 2–3months before the event
- Distributing a fact sheet with the most important facts and discussing it 3–4 weeks before departure
- Sending an electronical reminder one week before departure

Literature

Racinais S et al. Consensus recommendations on training and competing in the heat. Br J Sports Med. 2015 Sep;49(18):1164-73

Nadelen M. Preparing for and playing in the heat. Jan 13, 2012. ACSM recommendations retrieved 28.2.2016 https://www.acsm.org/public-information/articles/2012/01/13/preparing-for-and-playing-in-the-heat

Schmit C et al. Heat acclimatization and pre-cooling: a further boost for endurance performance? Scan J Med Sci Sports, 2015 Dec 17.

Jet Lag – Good Coping Strategies

Symptoms

Feeling tired in the new local daytime and yet unable to sleep at night. Waking in the new night and unable to get back to sleep. Feeling less able to concentrate or to motivate oneself. Decreased mental and physical performance and increased incidence of headaches and irritability. Loss of appetite and general bowel irregularities (Waterhouse et al, 1997).

Figure 1:

1) Melatonin secretion – the 'darkness-hormone'

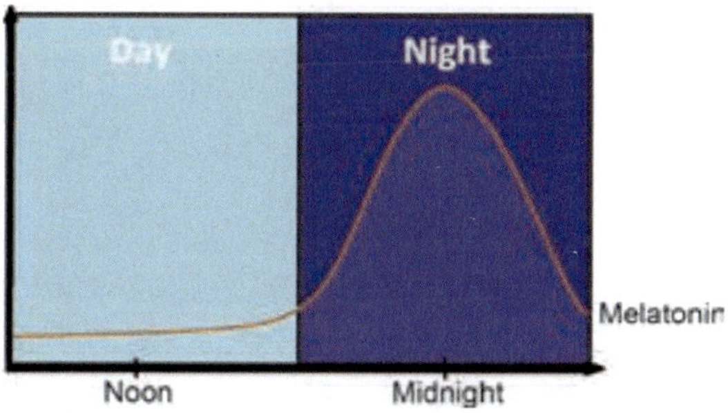

Background

Elite athletes today travel across multiple time zones for training and competition. These journeys place a physiological and psychological burden on those athletes who have to adjust to a different time zone (and different climate), and then have to re-adjust back to their home time zone after their return. The usual travel fatigue may be quickly overcome, but crossing multiple time zones is associated with a desynchronisation of our circadian rhythm.

'Jet lag is a temporary sleep disorder among air travellers who rapidly cross >3 time zones. Jet lag occurs as a result of the slow adjustment of the body clock to the destination time. Consequently, the daily rhythms and the internal drive for sleep and wakefulness are out of synchronization with the new environment. The secretion of melatonin by the pineal gland is responsible for setting our sleep-wake cycle. Its synthesis and release are stimulated by darkness and suppressed by light.'

(citation R.Henry, Jet-Lag, CDC 2016)

Eastward travel is associated with difficulty falling asleep at the destination bedtime and difficulty arising in the morning (i.e. as it is shortening the day of travel). Westward travel is associated with early evening sleepiness and predawn awakening (i.e. as it is lengthening the day of travel). Usually flying eastward requires a longer time for adaptation.

Coping and Prevention Table for Jet-Lag

Coping/ Prevention	To cope best with jet lag athletes and coaches should: • Allow a sufficient number of days in the new time zone to adapt, to regain training levels, and thus facilitate peak performance. As a rule of thumb, allow the number of days to adapt equal to the number of time zones crossed Before travel: • Start travelling in good physical condition: exercise, eat a healthful diet, and get enough rest
	• Begin to reset your body clock by shifting your timing of sleep a few days before your leave by doing the following: o Travelling westward: seek bright light in the evening and shift sleeping 1–2hours later o Travelling eastward: shift sleeping 1–2hours earlier and seek bright light in the morning

	During travel: • Avoid large meals, alcohol, and caffeine • Remain well hydrated—drink enough water • Move around the plane (to keep active and to protect against deep vein thrombosis) • Wear comfortable shoes and clothing • If possible, sleep during long flights On arrival: • Adapt to the local daytime rhythm and schedule as soon as possible (most important advice!) • Eat meals regularly and appropriate to the local time: breakfast, lunch, dinner • Optimise exposure to sunlight after arrival bright light in the morning wakes you up, exposure to light in the evening encourages later sleep. A detailed plan for recommended exposures to light according to flight direction and time zones travelled is available (Reilly et al 2007) • Short naps (20–30min) to increase energy are allowed, but keep them short otherwise you interfere with night-time sleep If the travel period is <2 days, remain on home time
Treatment by Yourself	Follow the recommendations above and be patient. The body clock takes a few days to adapt
When is a Doctor Needed?	Usually not needed. Possibly discuss the use of *melatonin* (in many countries available as a nutritional supplement, but unfortunately *not* controlled) with your sports medicine physician. A few studies support the use of 2.0–5.0mg of melatonin before going to bed the first few days after arrival. As contaminants have been found in commercially available products, possible advantages and risks need to be seriously taken into account. One preparation (Circadin, 2mg of Melatonin) is available as medication in some countries.

	If jet lag symptoms are more severe, consult your sports medicine physician or your GP and discuss the use of a nonaddictive sedative hypnotic. This may support a longer period of high quality sleep. The interaction of such medication with alcohol needs particularly be mentioned and should be avoided.
Return to Play/ Sports	Training is part of the new schedule and new local daytime rhythm. Initially, training sessions are lowered in volume and intensity and gradually increased over 5–7 days back to the normal level.

Literature

Reilly T et al. Coping with jet-lag: A Position Statement for the European College of Sport Science. European Journal of Sport Science, March 2007; 7(1): 1-7

Henry R. Jet Lag. In Traveler's health. Center for Disease Control and Prevention. online download 9.3.2016 http://wwwnc.cdc.gov/travel/yellowbook/2016/the-pre-travel-consultation/jet-lag

Waterhouse J. et al. Jet-lag. Lancet 1997, 350,1611-1615

Altitude Training – Stay Healthy and Get a Return on Investment

Background

Altitude training is the practice—used mainly by endurance (and some team sport) athletes—of training for several weeks at high altitude, preferably 1500–2400m above sea level. At these altitudes, the air still contains the 20.9% oxygen and 79% nitrogen, but with the reduced barometric pressure, the partial pressure of oxygen, and therefore the availability of oxygen in the same amount of air, are reduced.[1] In other words: at sea level air is denser and there are more molecules of gas per litre of air, i.e. in one normal breath you get more oxygen, compared to high altitude where the air is less dense (due to the lower atmospheric pressure) and you get significantly less oxygen in one breath. Thus, the main effects of altitude training are based on the acclimatisation of the body to this relative lack of oxygen, by increasing the mass of red blood cells and haemoglobin and by altering muscle metabolism. The lower oxygen saturation in the blood, the muscle metabolism, and the whole body is called hypoxia.[1] This stimulates, through a regulating protein (HIF 1, hypoxia inducible factor 1), the production of erythropoietin (EPO) in the kidney and adaptations in the working muscle. EPO stimulates the production of red blood cells in the bone marrow and thus increases haemoglobin saturation and oxygen delivery. In the muscle, the adaptions consists in a switch to a more economic model of oxygen utilisation and more efficient metabolism in different ways.[2]

Altitude training can also be simulated through the use of an altitude chamber, an altitude simulation tent, or by a mask-based hypoxicator system by a reduction of the oxygen content still with the same barometric pressure (usual technique extracts some oxygen and replaces it by nitrogen).

The natural secretion of EPO by the human kidneys can be increased by training at a natural or simulated altitude, leading to this beneficial increase of haemoglobin and red blood cells, all within natural limits. EPO can also be synthesised to help treating patients with severe kidney failure and anaemia or suffering from cancer and anaemia.[1] But cheating athletes and their management teams have abused EPO to gain illegal advantages. Abuse of EPO, however, can be dangerous. It leads to increases of the red blood cells beyond normal levels, thus increasing the viscosity of blood. This possibly leads to hypertension and increases the likelihood of blood clotting in any part of the body eventually causing a thrombosis and pulmonary embolism, heart attack, or stroke.[1] Luckily, the blood passport of the WADA, with regular blood and EPO testing among competitive athletes, allows detection of many of these illegal, unfair, and, for athletes, potentially harmful procedures.[4][5]

If athletes are at too high altitude (typically above 2500m), the risk of an acute high altitude illness increases. This may include the acute mountain sickness (AMS), high altitude pulmonary edema (HAPE), and high altitude cerebral edema (HACE).[3] The altitude training period itself is already a substantial stress for the athlete's organism and the risk of an illness increases, so follow the recommendations of experienced scientists in the field and don't risk potential negative effects of altitude.[6]

Different training regimens

Live high, train low: This idea involves living at a higher altitude, e.g. 2400m above sea level (*live high*), which is not too high, in order to avoid bad sleeping, headache, and other medical issues due to high altitude. But it is high enough to induce a good 'hypoxic effect' on the formation of red blood cells and on adaptations in muscle metabolism. Secondly, it includes training at a distinctly lower altitude, e.g. 1200–1500m above sea level (*train low*), in order to be able to maintain the same exercise intensity as usual.[1][7]

Live low, train high: This training regimen involves living at low altitude, e.g. 500–900m and training at high altitude, e.g. 2400m (or even more). It is mostly performed with artificial altitude. The idea is to induce a hypoxic effect in the moment of exercise in order to eventually promote changes in the cell metabolism of the working muscle. It is well-known that live low-train high has basically no or just a very little effect on red blood cells, and it is at present unclear whether the theoretically interesting hypoxic effect onto the working muscle is relevant for sports performance or not.(1).

Live high, train high: In live high, train high, an athlete lives at the chosen altitude. The stimulus on the body is constant because the athlete is permanently in a hypoxic environment and any given workload must be performed at a higher relative intensity. Theoretically, we would expect adaptations of mainly the muscle metabolism, as for instance a shorter recovery time in repeated sprints.(1)(2) This is underlined by the findings that even after longer periods of training at altitude with the live high, train high regimen no change in haemoglobin mass or red blood cells could be observed. Further research seems to be necessary for a better understanding of this regimen, as, at present, results for endurance athletes seem to be less promising.(1)

Practical recommendations

- Plan the altitude training camp well in advance and follow professional advice from an experienced sport scientist or sports medicine physician
- 'Live high, train low' seems to be the most promising training regimen. Plan to sleep around 2400m and to train on 1200–1500m. There are different locations around the world offering good facilities at these altitudes(1)(7)
- Plan roughly 14h in the 'live high' zone and 10h in the 'train low' zone(1)(7)
- A period of at least 3 weeks in a row (21 x 14h = 294h, ideal hypoxic exposure) or a chain of 2 x 2 weeks (with only a few days break) are the most recommended (14 x 14h = 196h, short break, and another 196h)(1)(7)
- Have a medical check and a blood test 5–6 weeks before the altitude training camp. Blood parameters and iron stores

need to be sufficient, according to recent recommendations (see chapter 'Iron Deficiency'). One week before and during the training camp, the intake of an iron supplementation and a sport adapted multivitamin seems to be beneficial.[9] Talk to your sportsmed physician and/or your sport nutritionist

- First three days of training camp 'start slow, go slow' with the training. The body needs to adapt well
- Monitor hours and quality of sleep and perceived training stress and fatigue of your athletes on a daily basis. It is essential to be able to adapt training load individually (and risking neither overreaching nor illness in an athlete)
- Allow enough time for individual recovery and have a good social follow-up throughout the camp (e.g. shared meals, daily briefing sessions, group activities other than sport every other day)[7]
- Have reasonable expectations: in a three week altitude training camp an average 5% improvement in haemoglobin mass is observed in studies, but may vary from 0–10%. In performance (e.g. 3000m run), an improvement in time of 3–4% may be expected[8]
- Take precautions to prevent infectious diseases (see chapter 'Prevention of Infectious Diseases in Sports'). There is a reportedly higher risk for illness in an altitude training camp 25–30% of all athletes![3] One very important tool: monitor training stress and fatigue
- Allow ten days after the training camp until your 'main event' takes place and perform at your best[7]

Literature

(1) Wikipedia 'Altitude training' download 10.3.2016, p.1-7 (last update 23.2.2016)

(2) Gore CL et al. Nonhematological mechanisms of improved sea-level performance after after hypoxic exposure. Med Sci Sports Exercise Sept 2007, 39(9):1600-9

(3) Álvarez-Herms J et al. Popularity of hypoxic training methods for endurance-based professional and amateur athletes. Physiol Behav. 2015 May 1;143:35-8.

(4) Biological Passport WADA Website, download 14.3.2016 https://www.wada-ama.org/en/athlete-biological-passport

(5) Saugy M et al. Monitoring of biological markers indicative of doping: the athlete biological passport. Br J Sports Med. 2014 May;48(10):827-32.
(6) Khodaee M et al. Athletes at High Altitude. Sports Health. 2016 Feb 10. pii: 1941738116630948.
(7) Wehrlin JP et al. Live high-train low for 24 days increases haemoglobin mass and red cell volume in elite endurance athletes. J Appl Physiol (1985). 2006 Jun;100(6):1938-45.
(8) Hauser A et al. Similar Haemoglobin Mass Response in Hypobaric and Normobaric Hypoxia in Athletes. Med Sci Sports Exerc. 2015 Nov 4.
(9) Clénin GE et al. Iron deficiency in sports, definition, influence on performance and therapy. Swiss Med Wkly. 2015 Oct 29;145:w14196.

Musculoskeletal System

Flat Valgus Foot (Pes Plano Valgus) – When is Strengthening Not Enough?

Symptoms

A flattening of the longitudinal arch (pes planus) and an inward tilting of the whole foot (pes valgus). This alteration of the stance is, per se, not painful, but depending on its severity and on the training load, especially in sport disciplines with a lot of impacts on the feet (e.g. many team sports, sports with a lot of running and jumping), overcharge problems at different parts of the locomotor system may be expected, e.g. Achilles tendinopathy, shin splint, tenosynovitis in the ankle region (tibialis posterior tendon), stress fractures of the foot, and bursitis of the pes anserinus (see also these chapters).

Figure 1: Pes Plano Valgus

Figure 1.1 Drawing of the foot with two longitudinal and one transversal arches

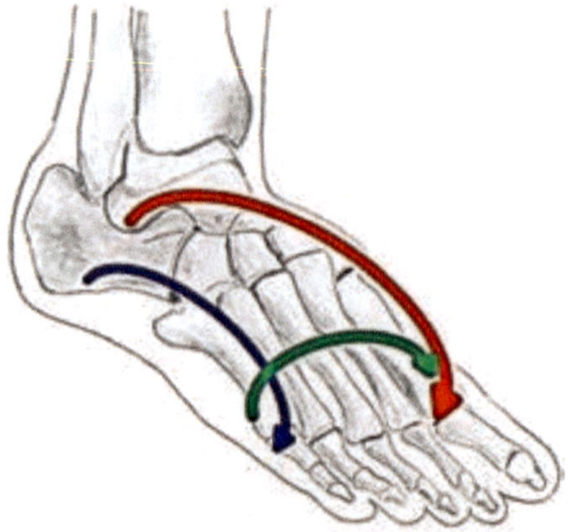

Figure 1.2 picture of a foot with pes plano-valgus (juvenile form; photo courtesy of Chris Kohler, Orthozone, Berne)

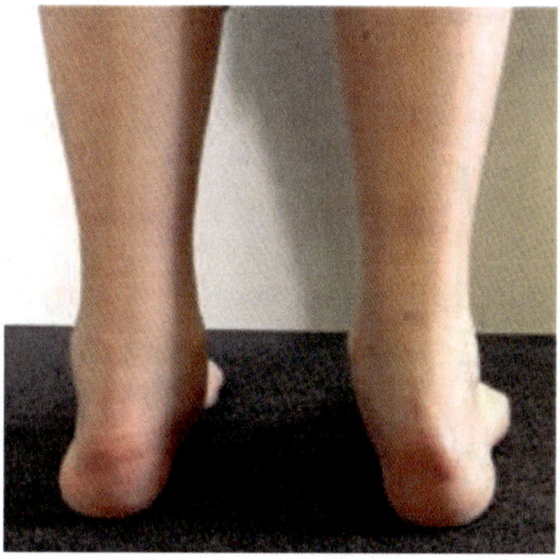

Background

The longitudinal arch of the foot helps to distribute and absorb the impact of every stride we make. When the arch is flattened out and an inward tilt of the foot occurs, the impact of running and jumping still needs to be absorbed by the foot, but due to lost balance and lost alignment overcharge problems will occur.

Two types of flat valgus foot are differentiated:

- Congenital juvenile form, which is inherited
- Acquired adult form, which is due to an insufficiency of the tibialis posterior muscle (i.e. controlling muscle supporting the arch)

Flat valgus foot may already be present while standing straight, in these cases mostly recognised and addressed by strengthening exercises and appropriate footwear. Quite often, however, it shows a dynamic presentation, meaning while standing straight there's a good alignment of the rear foot and an intact arch. But in this dynamic form of flat valgus foot, the inward tilt and the flattening of the arch occur only while pushing off the ground.

Prevention and Treatment Table for Pes Plano Valgus

Prevention	• Regular balancing and strengthening exercises for your foot and your calf (especially in all running sport disciplines), e.g. twice a week, 20–30min. Do some barefoot running from time to time as this also strengthens your foot and calf muscles (e.g. 20min per week). • Always wearing good shoes, not just for sport, and changing them from time to time.
Treatment by Yourself	As above. Look for appropriate footwear, in case you have a slight form of a flat valgus foot a medially supported and reinforced sport shoe may be indicated. Don't get orthotics yourself, ask for professional advice by a sports medicine physician or a podiatrist.
When is a Doctor Needed?	As soon as you feel concerned and bothered. The options of exercises, appropriate footwear (medially supported and reinforced sportshoes) or in severe cases orthotics, can be discussed with the sports medicine physician during your regular sportsmed exam. If orthotics are indicated, get them done by a professional. Either a podiatrist or an orthopaedic technician, they must be of best quality and customised to your foot.

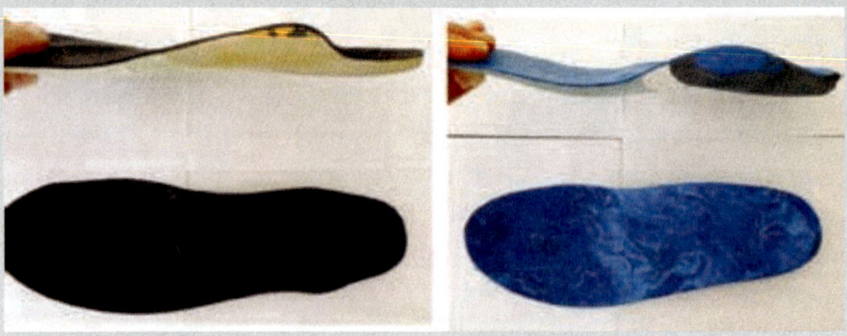

	Get used to them, in the beginning wear them for periods of half an hour a day, then go ahead with 2 or 3 times half an hour, continue with 2–3 times an hour until you get your feet used to the new support. Possibly orthotics need slight adjustment; you will feel that after 2 weeks. Most professionals want to see you again to precisely discuss this issue. Mostly orthotics should be worn for the whole day, not just for sports. Usually orthotics are good for 1–1½ years. Try to have more than one pair at a time to be able to change. Renew orthotics before they are completely worn out.
Return to Play/ Sports	If addressed in time no further pause needed.

What Does the Doctor Do?

The doctor takes the history and performs a clinical exam looking at your gait, your stance, your feet, and your shoes (bring them with you!). In severe cases a further gait analysis by a podiatrist is helpful and occasionally further investigations and a consultation with an orthopaedic surgeon may be indicated.

Figure 2: Strengthening Exercises in Case of a Pes Plano Valgus

Perform three series of these 6 exercises, twice or three times a week.

1. Press and raise	2. Sunrise	3. Balance	4. Penguin
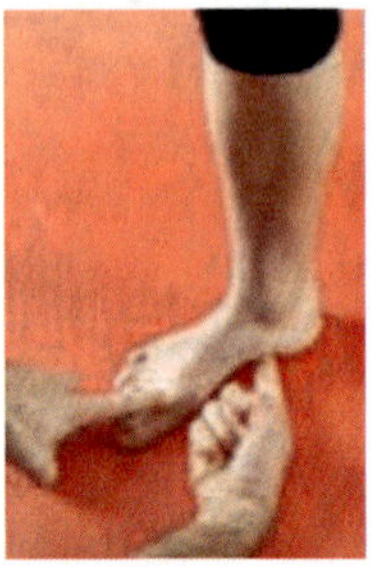	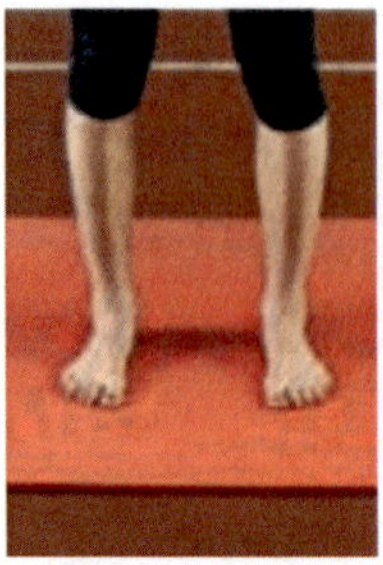	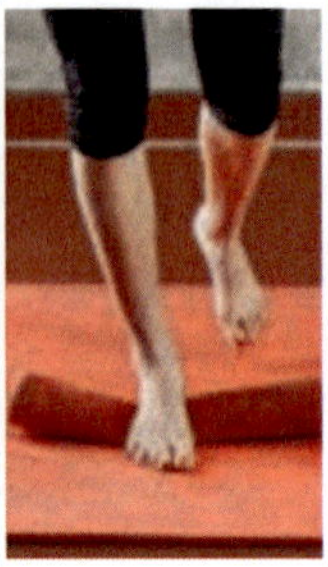	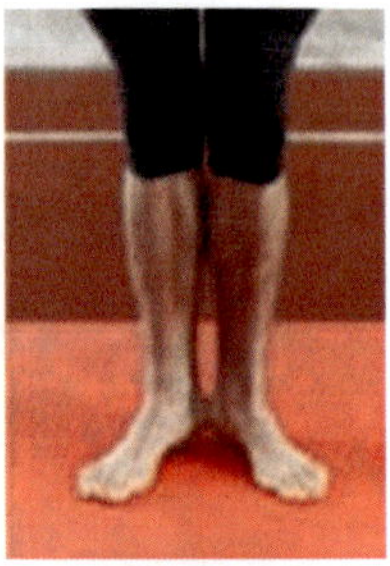
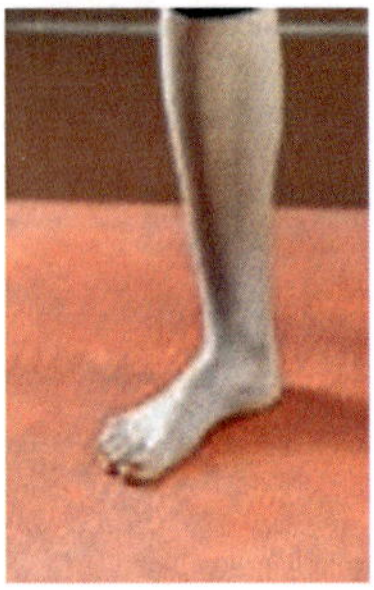	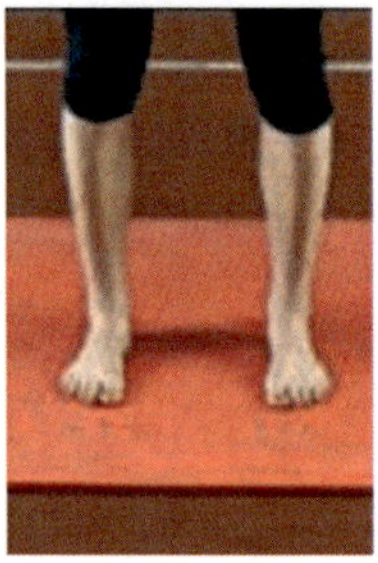		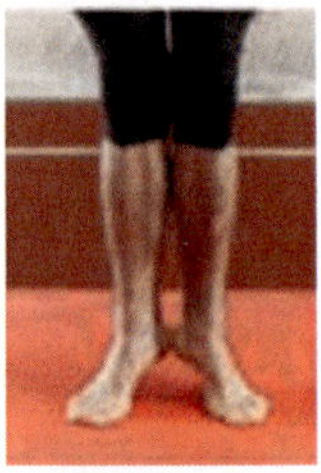 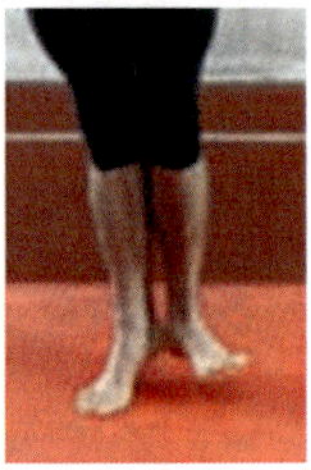
Press your big toe firmly on the ground, lift the medial arch in a kind of twisting movement.	Activate your foot muscles in order to raise your medial arch in both feet. Use the technique from "Press and raise"	Balance on a towel, control your foot position and your leg axis (knee over toe)	Start in the shown position. First raise in tip-toe position, then lift up left foot completely, go back to start. Do the same again eventually lifting the right foot, etc.
Activate 10 sec, 3 reps L + R	Hold for 10sec, 3reps	30sec L + R	60sec

5. Flamingo	6. Happy landing
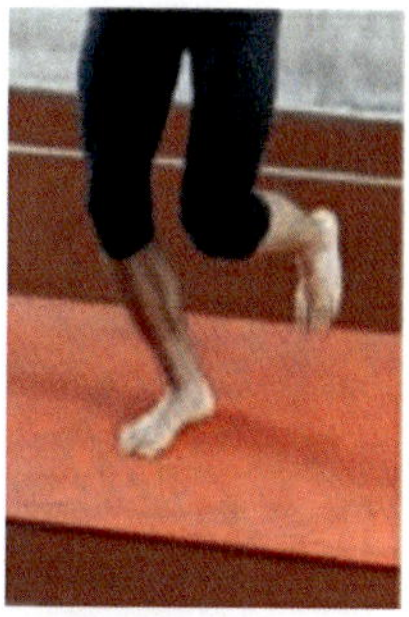	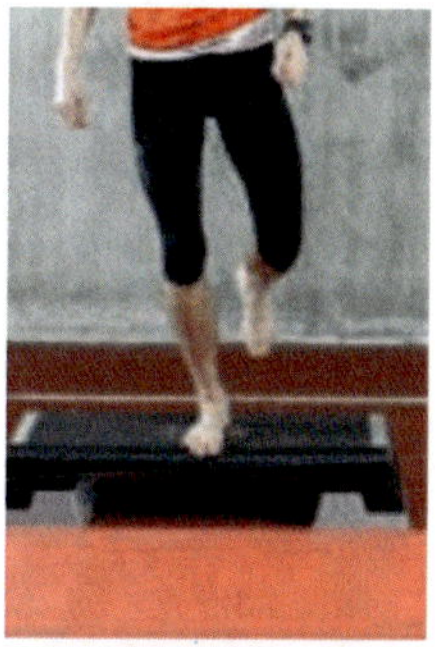
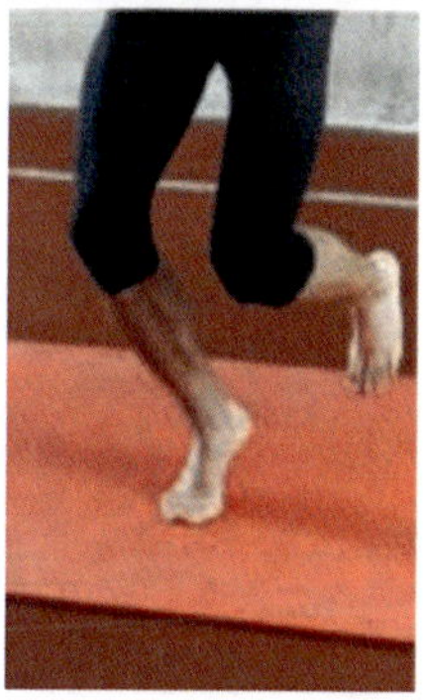	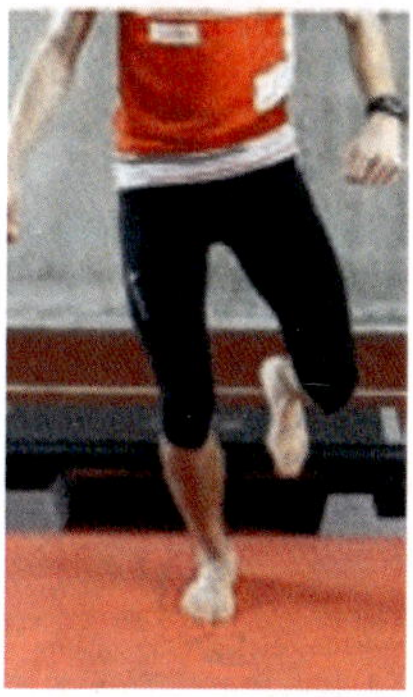
Activate the deep calf flexor muscles (tibialis posterior group). Single leg stance, slightly bend your knee, and perform heel raises.	Jump from a step or a stair and land, keeping your balance. Control your foot position and your leg axis (knee over toe).
60sec L + R	15 jumps L + R

Literature:

Neville CG, Houck JR. Choosing among 3 ankle-foot orthoses for a patient with stage II posterior tibial tendon dysfunction. J Orthop Sports Phys Ther. 2009 Nov;39(11):816-24.

Kulig K et al. Nonsurgical management of posterior tibial tendon dysfunction with orthoses and resistive exercise: a randomized controlled trial. Phys Ther. 2009 Jan;89(1):26-37

Kulig K et al. Effect of foot orthoses on tibialis posterior activation in persons with pes planus. Med Sci Sports Exerc. 2005 Jan;37(1):24-9.

Klingele J, Hoppeler H, Biedert R. Statistical deviations in high-performance athletes. Schweiz Z Sportmed. 1993 Jun;41(2):55-62.

Painful Sesamoid Bones – Pain Underneath the Big Toe in Runners

Symptoms

Plantar forefoot pain, with a most delicate zone underneath the big toe. Getting worse with loading, especially in running when pushing-off. Mostly occurring in running disciplines, e.g. orienteers (powerful long distance running in terrain).

Illustration 1: Sesamoid Bones Underneath the Head of the First Metatarsal

X-ray:

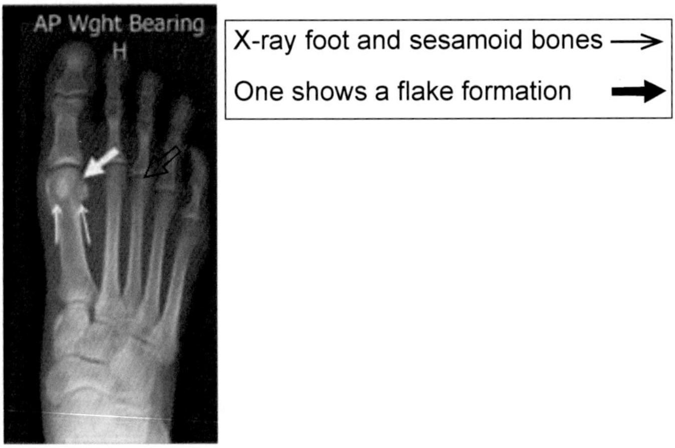

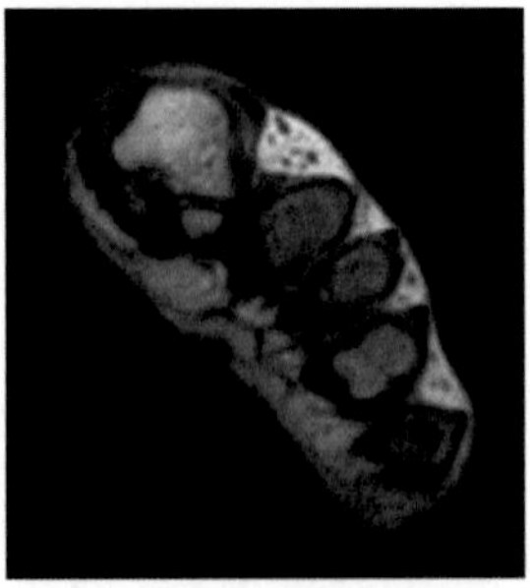

MRI forefoot with stressreaction in the medial sesamoid bone

Background

Two sesamoid bones are underneath the head of the first metatarsal, close to the first metatarso-phalangeal joint, and are an integral part of this articulation. They are integrated in the short toe flexor tendons and are comparable to the knee cap in the quadriceps tendon. Their function is to reduce friction (they have an articular surface to the metatarsal bone), to absorb pressure, and to protect the tendon. Due to an acute injury or chronic overuse, these sesamoid bones may be irritated and painful. It is important to know that in 10–30% of the cases the sesamoids may consist of two or more parts (bipartite or multipartite form).

Prevention and Treatment Table for Acute or Chronic Injury to the Sesamoid Bones

Prevention	Wear good running shoes. Adapt your training load to your capacities. If you enhance your training intensity and increase your training volume do it carefully and slowly.
Treatment by Yourself	Icing, local massage of the foot muscles, anti-inflammatory cream (e.g. Voltaren).
When is a Doctor Needed?	If it doesn't get any better.
Return to Play/ Sports	Depending on the severity.

What Does the Doctor Do?

The doctor takes the history and performs a clinical exam looking at your gait, your stance, your feet, and your shoes (bring them with you!). Additionally x-rays will be taken. Depending on the history (acute vs chronic), clinical picture, and the x-ray, possibly a CT scan or an MRI will be necessary.

Therapy consists primarily in relief of the first metatarso-phalangeal joint and the sesamoid bones. Training adaptation (less or no impact for a certain time; in stress reaction or stress fractures, a complete training pause needs to be discussed, in order not to provoke a chronic stress fracture or even worse avascular necrosis (i.e. die off of the sesamoid because of bad blood supply). Alternative training options include cycling and deep water running.

Local treatments, orthotics with a softer superficial bedding underneath the sesamoids (reduce local pressure), and/or a stiffer insole underneath the whole first metatarsophalangeal articulation (distribute the load) are promising treatment options. With orthotics, underlying foot malalignment may be corrected additionally (e.g. Pes cavus). In recurrent persistent painful situations, an injection with local anaesthetics and cortisone or surgical treatment options may need to be considered.

Literature

Mayer SW et al. Stress fractures of the foot and ankle in athletes. Sports Health. 2014 Nov;6(6):481-91.

Miltner O. Stress reactions in bones of the foot in sport: diagnosis, assessment and therapy. Unfallchirurg. 2013 Jun;116(6):512-6.

Ingrown Toenail (Uncuis Incarnatus) – Nasty Infection of the Nailwall

Symptoms

Painful, reddish toe (mostly the big toe) with a swollen lateral or medial nail fold, often discharging matter (pus).

Background

As soon as the toenail is twisted in and downwards by more external pressure, the skin surface is harmed and an infection with bacteria and fungi occurs.

Prevention and Treatment Table for Ingrown Toenail

Prevention	Always wearing shoes that are large enough, not just in sports. Cutting toe nails regularly (can help to prevent them from being twisted inwards and growing in). Cut them quite straight horizontally and not too short in the corners.
Treatment by Yourself	If getting reddish, slightly irritated, and painful, disinfect locally—best done with a good disinfectant with iodine solution or a local iodine bath (cold tap water + iodine solution = colour of a black tea, bath the toe for 10–15min, dry the foot with a towel, and leave it in fresh air for another 10min). Possibly put a black ointment on (e.g. Ichtholan 20%) and cover or wrap it well with a dressing (black colour).
When is a Doctor Needed?	In a more inflamed state. Or in a perseverative condition, then an excision needs to be considered.

Return to Play/ Sports	If treated sufficiently early, the toe recovers within a few days. If a severe infection occurs, local therapeutic measures and a systemic antibiotic treatment may be necessary.

What Does the Doctor Do?

The doctor takes the history, performs a local clinical exam, and diagnosis is confirmed. Treatment as described above. In perseverative conditions, the surgical wedge resection of the toenail removes the ingrown portion while conserving the majority of the nail.

Morton Neuroma – Pain, Tingling, and Numbness of the Forefoot

Symptoms

Painful mid- and fore-foot, particularly while squeezing the midfoot or on direct local pressure. Pain is sharp, electrifying, and usually radiating towards the toes.

Background

More often in splayfoot, but also occurring in the balanced foot. The etiology is not perfectly clear, but a possible explanation is as follows: one of the nerves serving forefoot and toes may be chronically squeezed and irritated within two metatarsal bones. This recurrent friction and pressure leads to the formation of a thickening of the nerve called neuroma. Once this neuroma is established it may be quite easily provoked by any external squeezing, pressure or particular movement.

Prevention and Treatment Table for Morton Neuroma

Prevention	Always wearing good shoes, not just in sports. Change them often enough. People suffering severe splayfoot are more at risk and may therefore seriously consider orthotics to re-establish the transverse arch of the foot Exercises for the foot—strengthening the foot and calf muscles
Treatment by Yourself	Once it is established, orthotics may be helpful. But discuss the treatment options with your sports medicine physician.

When is a Doctor Needed?	If you do have severe forefoot pain, getting worse with direct pressure or squeezing, it may be a Morton Neuroma. Other possible diagnosis with this picture may be: tenosynovitis, local bruise, stress reaction. If this pain persists for three or more days, see a doctor.
Return to Play/ Sports	If it is a Morton Neuroma, usually a training adaptation but no pause is needed.

What Does the Doctor Do?

The doctor takes the history and clinical exam, if unclear, possibly adds further investigations. Treatment options are: orthotics to support the transverse arch, wearing shoes that are large enough, injection of the region of the neuroma, usually done with local anaesthetics and cortisone (this often calms the situation and reduces the swelling of the nerve). In really large neuromas and recurrent severe pain episodes, despite orthotics and injections, surgery may be indicated.

Literature

Ferkel E et al. Entrapment Neuropathies of the Foot and Ankle. Clin Sports Med. 2015 Oct;34(4):791-801

Splayfoot (Pes Transversoplanus) – Reason for Plantar Forefoot Pain and Bunion Deformity

Symptoms

Localised plantar forefoot pain on loading, especially after or while running or jumping. Due to the flattened transverse arch and the broadened forefoot, the big toe (hallux) is turned inwards with a prominent, often painful, bone formation called bunion (hallux valgus).

Background

The foot has longitudinal and transversal arches. This construction helps to absorb and distribute the impact of a stride or a jump on the different parts of the foot. In case of a flattening out of the transverse arch, the so called splayfoot, the load arrives on one or two metatarsal bones only. Due to the flattened transverse arch, the heads of the metatarsal bones are directly in contact with the ground and don't have any further absorbing system. The repetitive impact in running and jumping leads then to a metatarsalgia (i.e. painful metatarsal bone).

The transverse arch keeps the whole forefoot in balance. When it is flattened out, the metatarsal of the big toe turns outwards, the big toe twists inwards, and a very prominent bone formation starts to be visible: the bunion or hallux valgus. The foot is now, due to the splayfoot and the valgus formation of the big toe, larger and often a local pressure problem on the bunion occurs.

There seems to be a familiar predisposition for splayfoot and bunion deformity.

Prevention and Treatment Table for Splayfoot, Metatarsalgia, Hallux Valgus (Bunion)

Prevention	• Regular balancing and strengthening exercises for your foot and calf muscles, especially in all running sport disciplines, e.g. twice a week 20–30min • Do some barefoot running from time to time as this also strengthens your foot and calf muscles (e.g. 20min per week) • Always wearing good shoes, not just in sport. Change them from time to time. A wide toe box is good. • Avoid pointed shoes and high heels, use them sparsely.
Treatment by Yourself	As above.
When is a Doctor Needed?	As soon as you feel concerned and bothered. The options of exercises, good quality footwear, and/or orthotics can be discussed with the sports medicine physician during your regular sportsmed exam. Strengthening exercises and good footwear alone have a limited range of action, so to prevent further deterioration of an already established splayfoot, customised orthotics are indicated. See chapter 'Flat Valgus Foot' about how to get used and how to proceed with orthotics. In some severe bunion deformities an operation may be needed.
Return to Play/Sports	If addressed in time, no pause needed.

What Does the Doctor Do?

The doctor takes the history and performs the clinical exam looking at your gait, your stance, your feet, and your shoes (bring them with you!). In severe cases, a further gait analysis by a podiatrist is helpful. Treatment options as discussed above.

Figure 1: Strengthening Exercises in Case of a Splayfoot (Pes Transversoplanus)
Perform three series of these 6 exercises, twice or three times a week.

1. One caterpillar	2. Two caterpillars – both feet	3. Lift up a towel
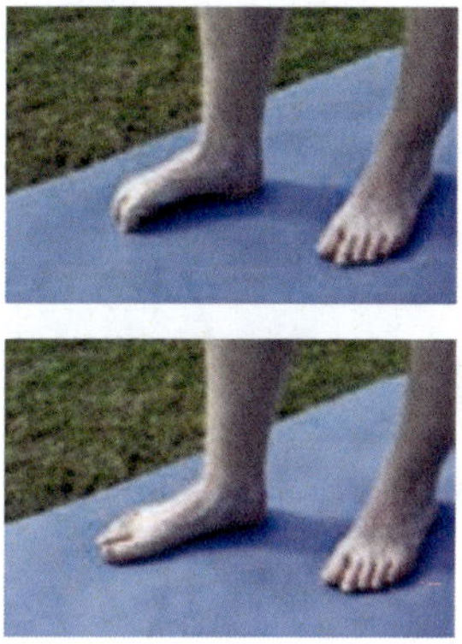	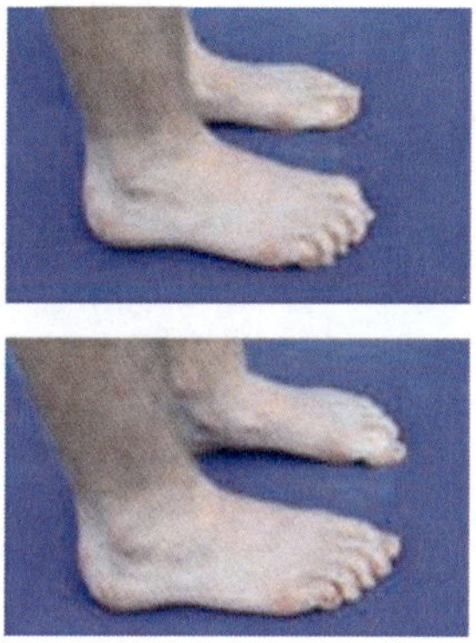	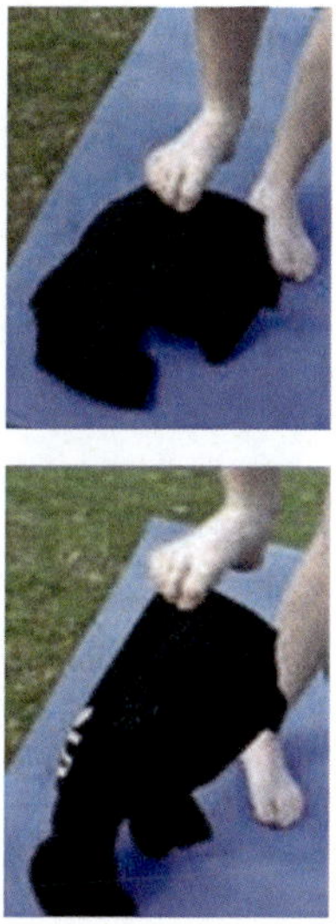
Move one foot forward by making caterpillar-like movements using your foot muscles, flexing and extending your toes.	Move first one foot forward by activating your foot muscles and trying to pull forward with your toes (not to push with your leg), then the other, etc.	Grab a towel (or a shirt) with your toes and lift it up.
30sec L + R	60sec	30sec L + R

4. Roll a ball in a circle	5. Sunrise	6. Stimulate the sole of your foot
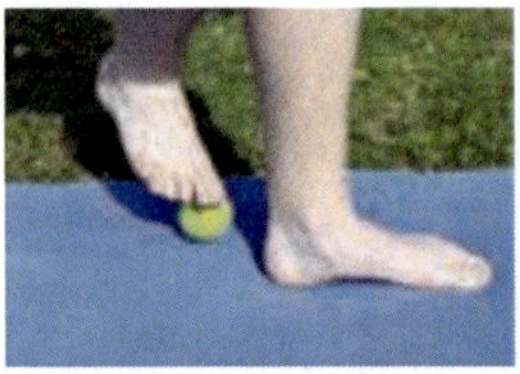 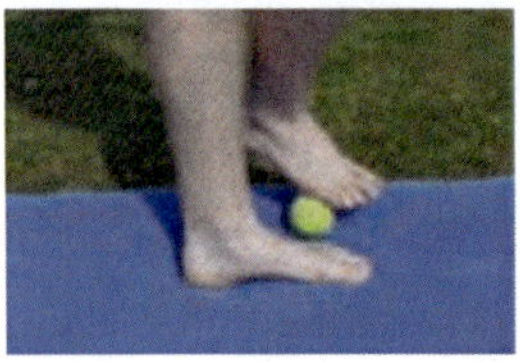	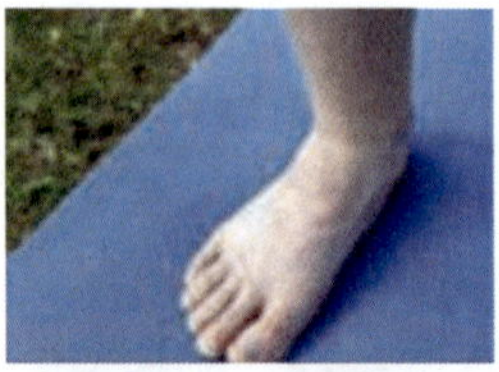 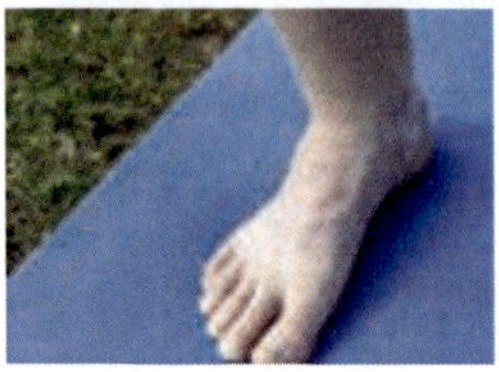	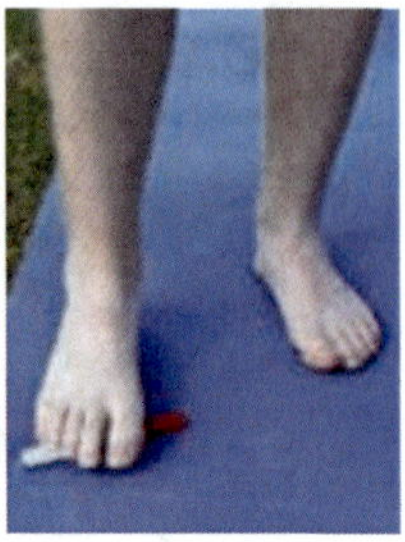
Single leg stance, roll a tennis ball around the other foot, but guide it closely.	Activate your foot muscles in order to raise your medial arch. Press your big toe firmly on the ground, lift the medial arch in a kind of twisting movement.	Roll the sole of your foot on a pen or a wooden stick in order to stimulate the foot.
60sec L + R	Hold for 10sec, 3reps L + R	30sec L + R

Plantar Faszitis ('Heel Spur') – When the Heel Hurts While Getting Out of Bed

Symptoms

The very classical symptom is the acute plantar pain close to the heel when taking the first step while getting out of bed. Improves after a few steps, but still aching. The plantar region a bit further than the heel is also tender on local pressure. Usually symptoms get worse after jogging the day before.

Background

The sole of our foot has a flat-ligament like structure stretched out longitudinally under the skin called the plantar fascia. It gives stability to the foot and protects the deeper structures. Its origin is at the inner lower part of the heel bone (calcaneus) and it is stretched out towards the metatarsals and the toes. The origin of the plantar fascia gets irritated and inflamed due to repetitive, extraordinary loading, such as running and jumping. And it is this local inflammation causing the pain. This ailment also occurs quite frequently in professions with a lot of walking, (e.g. nurses, waiters).

'Heel spurs'—wrong name, wrong concept. In earlier days, doctors took a lateral x-ray to see if a calcification from the calcaneus pointing towards the foot sole was visible. *But* many people have plantar faszitis without calcification and many people have calcification but no planter faszitis, so wrong concept.

Prevention and Treatment Table for Plantar Faszitis

Prevention	• Don't change your training loads too rapidly • Do regular stretching exercises • Do specific balancing and strengthening exercises for your foot and your calf muscles, especially in disciplines with a lot of running
Treatment by Yourself	Do stretching exercises, for all leg muscles, but in particular calf and hamstrings, more frequently and follow the prevention measures. Reduce the impact on your feet (by limiting jumping and running activities) and replace these trainings by with cycling or deep water running, etc.
When is a Doctor Needed?	If this doesn't work out and doesn't get any better in 2–3 weeks.
Return to Play/ Sports	Be prepared: it usually takes weeks and months to get rid of it! Training and competition are usually possible, but in severe cases training load and the type of training needs to be adapted as the pain may be difficult to stand.

What Does the Doctor Do?

The doctor takes the history, performs the clinical exam looking at your gait, your stance, and your feet, and usually diagnoses the illness without any further imaging. Therapeutic measures may include: physiotherapy, shockwave treatment, taping, adaptation of the training load, and a night splint sock. During the night, our feet are mostly slightly pointed, meaning the calf muscles and the foot soles are unloaded and possibly even a bit 'shortening'. So wearing a splint sock ('Strassburg-Sock') during the night gives you a slight permanent stretch on your calf and the foot sole. But don't apply more flexion than 90°, slightly less is optimal. Going higher probably means that you will be so discomforted by it during the night that you just take it off.

Injection with local anaesthetic and cortisone is usually not a first line treatment, but may be an option later on.

Figure 1: Splint Sock (type 'Strassburg-Sock') and Ideal Positioning

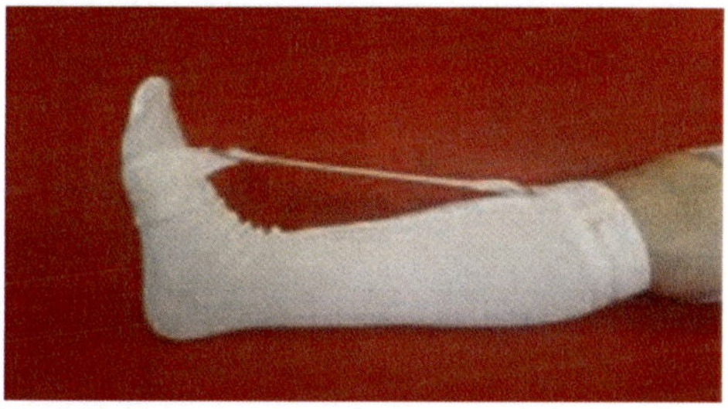

Literature

Ryan M et al. Comparison of a physiotherapy program versus dexamethasone injections for plantar fasciopathy in prolonged standing workers: a randomized clinical trial. Clin J Sport Med. 2014 May;24(3):211-7.

Rompe JD. Plantar fasciopathy. Sports Med Arthrosc. 2009 Jun;17(2):100-4.

Achilles Tendinopathy – Already Achilles Was Vulnerable on This Tendon

Symptoms

Tenderness, swelling, and pain in the Achilles tendon. Sometimes heavily swollen and enlarged (in comparison to the other side). Sometimes 'sandpaper'-like feeling in the tendon while activating the calf muscles.

Background

Achilles tendinopathy (AT) describes the entity of activity related tendon pain, focal tendon tenderness, and intratendinous imaging changes. In athletes and non-athletes alike, it is a considerable issue and a common condition. Basically the name says what it is about: it's a pathology (i.e. an illness) of the main calf tendon. This may include:

- An injury to the tendon, e.g. a partial rupture
- A more acute strain of the calf muscles leading in this tendon (soleus muscle and gastrocnemius muscles) or the tendon itself
- A more chronic onset of an inflammation of the peritendinous tissue; a peritendinitis or of the tendon itself; a tendinitis or a combination of both
- An inflammation of the bursa subachillea
- An inflammation and chronic irritation of the insertion of the Achilles tendon to the calcaneus, due to the Haglund exostosis (a prominent bone formation, putting the Achilles tendon locally under permanent stress)

Symptoms can occur at the mid-portion or insertion of the tendon, with basically a failed healing response, whether it may be of inflammatory or degenerative origin. Macroscopically (i.e.

as we may observe and feel), we find a tendon thickening, loss of mechanical properties, and pain. Microscopically (i.e. under the microscope/ultrastructural changes), there is degeneration and disorganisation of collagen fibres (i.e. important for tendon structure and stability), increased cellularity with formation of matrix metalloproteinases (i.e. enzyme observed in alternating tissues), and often just minimal inflammation. The more chronic degenerative overuse AT is called 'tendinosis'; the more acute inflammatory AT is called 'tendinitis'. However, a clear differentiation is often difficult. To make the right choices in therapy, it is important from the beginning to have a clear diagnosis in order to be able to get an adequate treatment plan ready. With this background and the understanding of the often multifactorial etiology of the AT and the complex healing response of a tendon, a successful treatment clearly consists of several pillars, including the return to sports protocol.

As risk factors for Achilles tendinopathy may be named: foot malalignment, low quality (unstable, wobbly) sport shoes, use of new and badly fitted high shafted shoes (pressure onto the tendon), prominent calcaneal bone formation (i.e. Haglund exostosis), former injections close to or into the tendon, former administration of fluoroquinolone antibiotics (e.g. ciprofloxacin).

Prevention and Treatment Table for Achilles Tendinopathy

Prevention	• Always wearing good shoes, not just in sports • Being careful with new shoes, especially shoes with high shafts. Don't allow painful pressure on your Achilles tendon, this may provoke inflammation • Getting your gait and your stance assessed in the regular sportsmed exam. If the alignment is seriously impaired and out of balance, orthotics or sport shoes with a medial support may be indicated • Doing regular strengthening, balancing, and stretching exercises

Treatment by Yourself	• Avoid all shoes and footwear provoking pain • Local anti-inflammatory treatment (Voltaren cream and during the night a poultice with Antiphlogistine or Pasta Boli is extremely efficient) • Follow the recommendations of your treating doctor and physio
When is a Doctor Needed?	As soon as you feel it is an established Achilles tendinopathy. I tell my patients, 'Don't wait too long!' and this goes along with my experience. The treatment lasts as long as the problem took to develop! So see your doctor early.
Return to Play/ Sports	Depending on the severity. If it is bad enough, Achilles tendinopathy may take very long to heal properly.

What Does the Doctor Do?

The doctor takes the history and performs a clinical exam looking at your gait, your stance, muscle lengths, your feet, and your shoes (bring them with you!). If the history is short, the onset slow and without any injury, and the finding clear, treatment may be started immediately. If the problem has been present for a while and the history is not that clear, then further imaging is probably helpful, usually with an ultrasound of the tendon, the peritendinous tissue, and the bursa. Sometimes an additional MRI may be indicated.

Treatment includes:

- Avoiding all shoes and footwear causing pain
- Local anti-inflammatory treatment as above
- Stretching exercises of soleus and gastrocnemius muscle
- Eccentric strengthening exercises (calf raises first on flat ground 3 x 15 rep per day, raising to 3 x 20, 3 x 25, then change the exercise to calf raises on the stairs again 3 x 15 rep per day, raising to 3 x 20, 3 x 25)
- Possibly fish-oil capsules (EPA 500, 2 x 2cps daily) to have a slight systemic anti-inflammatory effect

- Physiotherapy with instruction of eccentric exercises, stretching, trigger point therapy of the concerned calf muscles (soleus, gastrocnemius), possibly shock wave therapy
- Training adaptation (usually no running, no jogging, but probably cycling (put the cleats as far back as possible to reduce traction on the Achilles tendon), swimming, later on deep water running)
- Eventually shock wave therapy
- *Don't* let any cortisone injection be done! This is harmful, as the cortisone will weaken your tendon.
- Even if it is a severe Achilles tendinopathy, a conservative treatment is the mostly the right therapy management. Remember that the inventor of the eccentric exercises had even a partial rupture of the tendon. His initial plan was to provoke the tendon by doing eccentric exercises and as a consequence, sooner or later, rupture his tendon, but he was completely healed without any surgery as the eccentric strengthening makes the tendon stronger and more robust!
- But there are cases, especially with a prominent and irritated Haglund exostosis (i.e. bony prominence in the heel bone), where surgery is the treatment of choice, as without it the tendon remains mechanically irritated and cannot heal

Eccentric strengthening on flat ground

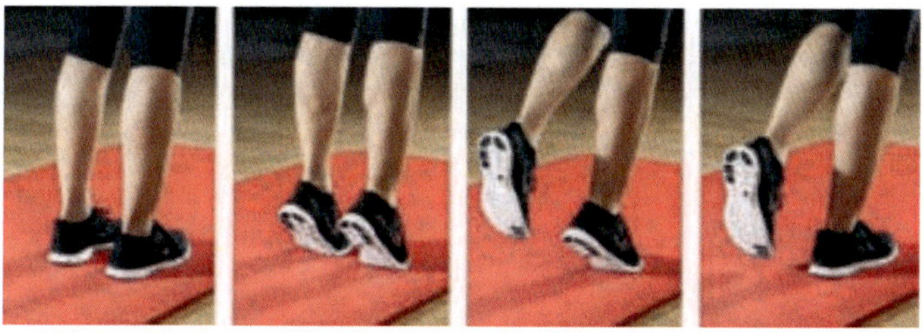

Eccentric strengthening on the stairs

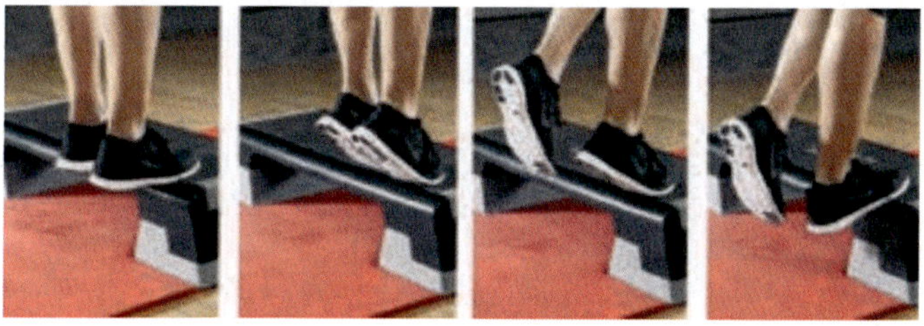

As you see, there are plenty of things to do and to think about. The best way to manage is to write this plan down. You are certainly working with a smart sport physiotherapist and sports medicine physician, so do it together, as it is not too difficult, but part of being successful

Activities	1st week	2nd week	3rd week	4th week	5th week	6th week
Anti-inflammatory therapy, local and systemic						
Individual stretching and eccentric exercises						
Physiotherapy (triggerpoint, shock wave, exercise instructionl, etc.)						
Endurance training						
Strength training						
Specific training						

Literature

Sussmilch-Leitch SP et al. Physical therapies for Achilles tendinopathy: systematic review and meta-analysis. J Foot Ankle Res. 2012 Jul 2;5(1):15

Brett M et al. Treatment of Tendinopathy: What Works, What Does Not, and What is on the Horizon? Clin Orthop Relat Res. 2008 Jul; 466(7): 1539–1554.

Shin Splint – Painful Tibia in Runners

Symptoms

Shin pain, usually in the middle or lower third of the shin bone (tibia), getting worse on loading. Local tenderness, sometimes slight local swelling.

Background

Especially in running and jumping disciplines, shin splint is a frequent problem and is mostly a result of a local overcharge. In case of a pes plano valgus, shin splint occur more frequently and may be more prominent. Two interesting theories may, in general, explain the symptomatology:

Medial compression stress theory: Due to the load by repetitive impacts in sports, the medial part of the shine bone (tibia) is compressed (more than the lateral part). This compression leads to a local ischemia with a secondary inflammation. In case of a pes planovalgus, the stress is even more medially located and the symptoms even more pronounced.

Periost (skin of the bone, very sensitive) overload theory: The load and the repetitive impacts in sport are mainly absorbed by the deep calf muscles (e.g. tibialis posterior, flexor digitorum longus muscle, flexor hallucis longus) which support the medial malleolus and the longitudinal arch. The impact is transmitted from the muscle to its periostal origin at the backside of the shin bone. This leads to a local periostal irritation.

It's even plausible that both mechanism and theories contribute to the findings.

Prevention and Treatment Table for Shin Splint

Prevention	• Wearing good running shoes, changing them from time to time • If you're having a severe pes planovalgus, discuss with your sports medicine physician whether regular strengthening and balancing exercises are sufficient or whether running shoes with medial support or even orthotics are indicated (e.g. during the yearly sportsmed exam)
Treatment by Yourself	• Adapt your training load by reducing the impact (avoid jumps if possible, reduce running, do more cycling or deep water running instead) • If tender on the shin, start a local anti-inflammatory treatment with a cream (e.g. Voltaren) • If available, have a professional massage, especially of the deep calf muscles. If not, take a regenerative bath and self-massage the tight and hardened muscles, possibly roll the calf muscles out (self-myofascial release).
When is a Doctor Needed?	When the shin pain is severe and doesn't get any better by your own treatment options.
Return to Play/ Sports	Shin splint usually requires a training adaptation that is about good planning of the volume and intensity of impact on the shin bone and its periost. So avoid jumping, if possible, or in athletics, count and try to reduce the number of jumps.

What Does the Doctor Do?

The doctor takes the history, performs the clinical exam looking at your gait, your stance, your feet, and your shoes (bring them with you!). Depending on the history and clinical exam, no further imaging is usually necessary and treatment may be started. If the findings are particular, possibly an MRI is indicated.

Literature

Fullem BW. Overuse lower extremity injuries in sports. Clin Podiatr Med Surg. 2015 Apr;32(2):239-51.

Franklyn M et al. Aetiology and mechanisms of injury in medial tibial stress syndrome: Current and future developments. World J Orthop. 2015 Sep 18;6(8):577-89.

Kahanov L et al. Diagnosis, treatment, and rehabilitation of stress fractures in the lower extremity in runners. Open Access J Sports Med. 2015 Mar 27;6:87-95..

Craig DI. Current developments concerning medial tibial stress syndrome. Phys Sportsmed. 2009 Dec;37(4):39-44.

Runner's Knee/ITB-Syndrome – When the Ilio-Tibial Band Rubs and Causes Lateral Knee Pain

Symptoms

Lateral knee pain with local tenderness on the outer femur condyle, slight, often palpable (but mostly not visible), swelling. Often accompanied by a muscle shortening and trigger point in the tensor (tensor fasciae latae muscle) and the quadriceps muscle (vastus lateralis muscle).

Background

The ilio-tibial band, a large ligamentous structure on the outer side of the thigh, is, during exercise with knee flexion and extension, rubbing on the bony surface of the outer femoral condyle. This results in friction and inflammation on the periostal surface of the outer condyle, often combined with a small bursitis (inflammation of the bursa) in between band and bone.

Abrupt changes in training amount, running on uneven surfaces, poor quality running shoes, and a shortened tensor and quadriceps muscle seem to worsen the symptoms and may even lead to this clinical picture in experienced runners.

Prevention and Treatment Table for Runner's Knee/ ITB Syndrome

Prevention	• No abrupt changes in training volume. Always wear good sport and running shoes • Be aware of your muscle length and regularly practice stretching and flexibility exercises

	• Regularly practice strengthening exercises to control leg axis: double leg squats and single leg squats with knee over toe position, balancing exercises on one leg, single leg jumps with leg axis, etc.
Treatment by Yourself	• Perform stretching and flexibility exercises for the tensor and the quadriceps muscle • Use a local anti-inflammatory treatment on the outer femur condyle where the pain occurs. Local massage of the named muscles, possibly roll out (e.g. black roll)
When is a Doctor Needed?	If pain is so strong that a training needs to be interrupted or when symptoms persist for 2–3 weeks
Return to Play/ Sports	Depending on the severity. At an early stage, training may be continued in an adapted form, possibly with a certain reduction in duration and intensity, pain free movements are all allowed. In an advanced stage, a more detailed plan for the return to sports needs to be made, sometimes with no, or just very limited, running for a few weeks.

What Does the Doctor Do?

The doctor takes the history and performs a clinical exam. An examination of stance, gait, and the measurement of muscle length, as well as the localisation of possible trigger points, complete the clinical investigation. Diagnosis is made clinically and in clear findings no further imaging is needed. The treatment plan is usually made with combination of local anti-inflammatory treatment, stretching and flexibility exercises, physiotherapy for trigger point and local treatment, and adaptation of training. At this stage, physiotherapy takes the lead response as there are different therapy modalities possibly engaged (e.g. trigger point therapy and fascial release, eventually ultrasound or electrotherapy, possibly shockwave treatment), depending on the healing response. If it's getting better after 3–4 sessions, this therapy may be continued until complete return to sports.

If even after 8–9 sessions, it has just slightly improved, or has remained the same, other therapeutic strategies need to be considered (e.g. Cortisone injection/PRP injection) following prior imaging.

Literature

Baker RL, Fredericson M. Iliotibial Band Syndrome in Runners: Biomechanical Implications and Exercise Interventions. Phys Med Rehabil Clin N Am. 2016 Feb;27(1):53-77

Phinyomark A et al. Gender differences in gait kinematics in runners with iliotibial band syndrome. Scand J Med Sci Sports. 2015 Dec;25(6):744-53.

Aderem J, Louw QA. Biomechanical risk factors associated with iliotibial band syndrome in runners: a systematic review. BMC Musculoskelet Disord. 2015 Nov 16;16:356.

Osgood-Schlatter Disease – Frequent Reason for Knee Pain in Teenagers

Symptoms

In sporty children and adolescents, an anterior knee pain at the proximal part of the tibia (tibial tuberosity) may occur. Often quite tender on palpation and more painful after intensive training sessions with either a lot of stop and go or a lot of jumps. Occurs mainly in sports with a lot of running and jumping.

Background

Often in growth periods (e.g. growth spurt in adolescence) but already in later childhood the insertion of a tendon to the bone needs to absorb a lot of impact and shearing forces. This leads to inflammation of this ossicle and the whole growth zone. The inflammation causes tenderness, swelling, and quite often a sometimes transient, sometimes persisting prominence at the site of the tibial tuberosity (apophysitis, i.e. inflammation of the apophysis).

It seems that impacts (i.e. jumps, landings) and stop and go activities provoke this condition much more than any other exercise. A shortening of the muscle-tendon length, as observed in growth periods, or in case of insufficient stretching and flexibility exercises, often worsens the condition.

This overuse injury may also occur in other body parts:

Anterior Hip Pain: Origin of rectus femoris muscle (one of the quadriceps tendons) in soccer players, AFL, gymnasts.

Heel Pain (Sever's Disease): Insertion of the Achilles tendon (on the calcaneum) in gymnasts.

Prevention and Treatment Table for Osgood-Schlatter Disease

Prevention	Is all mainly about the training load. As explained above repetitive impacts, shearing forces, and muscle shortening contribute to the overuse. Therefore: • Practice regular stretching and flexibility exercises • With Osgood-Schlatter disease, it's mainly about the quadriceps muscle. But integrate the whole lower limb and muscle chain including the iliopsoas muscle, greater and medium glutaeus, adductors, hamstrings, and calf muscles in your stretching and flexibility program • Adapt the training load. Count jumps and limit them in numbers • Count and limit 'stop and go' exercises, as short sprints with movements back and forth
Treatment by Yourself	• Regular flexibility and stretching exercises • Local treatment with anti-inflammatory ointment, like Voltaren cream or a poultice with Pasta boli (extremely effective overnight for 8–10h)
When is a Doctor Needed?	If symptoms persist and/or even walking up and downstairs becomes uncomfortable.
Return to Play/ Sports	Often a reduction in the training program is necessary. This means continue some of the regular training sessions, cancel a few, *but* remove all jumps (or at least reduce them in numbers) and/or remove the stop and go sections

What Does the Doctor Do?

The doctor takes a history and performs a clinical exam. Mostly no other examination is needed, as diagnosis may be made on history and clinical exam only. A more detailed treatment plan will then be worked out integrating certainly physiotherapy (possible with further local treatment, muscle release treatment, stretching, and other exercises improving flexibility).

Literature

Launay F . Sports-related overuse injuries in children. Orthop Traumatol Surg Res. 2015 Feb;101(1 Suppl):S139-47.

Yanagisawa S et al. Assessment of Osgood-Schlatter Disease and the Skeletal Maturation of the Distal Attachment of the Patellar Tendon in Preadolescent Males. Orthop J Sports Med. 2014 Jul 18;2(7):2325967114542084

Yen YM. Assessment and treatment of knee pain in the child and adolescent athlete. Pediatr Clin North Am. 2014 Dec;61(6):1155-73.

Jumper's Knee – Found in All Sorts of Athletes

Symptoms

Anterior knee pain, mostly located in the patella tendon at the lower pole of the patella (kneecap), with a local tenderness and worsening on intensive exercise.

Background

The jumper's knee is an overuse injury at the origin of the patella tendon. It seems that impacts (i.e. jumps, landings) and stop and go activities provoke this condition much more than any other exercise. A shortening of the muscle length, as observed in growth periods or with insufficient stretching and flexibility exercises, often worsens the condition. In children or younger adolescent athlete, the tibial tuberosity with its growth zone is the weakest link and leads to the Osgood-Schlatter disease (apophysitis of the tibial tuberosity). In adults, it's the origin of the patella tendon at the patella (kneecap) which is the most delicate zone. First of all, the origin of the tendon on the bone and the adjacent proximal tendon react to the greater stress and exposure with an inflammatory response with pain, local tenderness, and slight swelling. If this excessive loading with repetitive high impacts persists, then micro-lesions of the tendon typically at its origin and a further inflammatory response may occur.

Prevention and Treatment Table for Jumper's Knee

Prevention	Is mainly about the training load. As explained above, repetitive impacts, shearing forces, and muscle shortening contribute to the overuse. Therefore: • Regularly practice stretching and flexibility exercises. As far as jumper's knee is concerned, it's mainly about the quadriceps muscle. But integrate the whole lower limb and muscle chain including the iliopsoas, greater and medium glutaeus, adductors, hamstrings, and calf muscles in your stretching and flexibility program • Adapt the training load. Count jumps and limit them in numbers • Same for stop and go exercises, and short sprints with back and forth movement
Treatment by Yourself	• Regularly practice flexibility and stretching exercises • Do a local treatment with anti-inflammatory ointment, like Voltaren cream or a poultice with Pasta boli (extremely effective overnight for 8–10h).
When is a Doctor Needed?	If symptoms persist and/or when walking up and downstairs becomes uncomfortable.
Return to Play/ Sports	A reduction in the training program is necessary, which means continue some of the regular trainings, but remove all the jumps (or at least reduce them in numbers) and/or remove the stop and go sections.

What Does the Doctor Do?

The doctor takes a history and performs a clinical exam. If the history is short and there's no acute injury, no further imaging is usually needed. If the history is either longer or with an acute injury or if symptoms do not improve with the given treatment, it is wise to undergo some imaging with a closer look at the tendon and its insertion, probably with an ultrasound first, and if inconclusive, possibly an MRI. A detailed treatment and return to play plan will be worked out: local and possibly systemic anti-inflammatory treatment prescribed, and stretching and other flexibility exercises, integrating certainly physiotherapy (e.g. possible local treatment, muscle release treatment, shockwave therapy, focused eccentric muscle exercise) introduced; and recommendations about the return to play protocol. In case the treatment is not effective, the treatment plan needs to be adapted with a further load reduction in training but possibly more focused eccentric strengthening and consideration of further treatment options (e.g. PlateletRichPlasma injection).

Literature

Ackermann PW, Renström P . Tendinopathy in sport. Sports Health. 2012 May;4(3):193-201.

Gisslén K et al. Normal clinical and ultrasound findings indicate a low risk to sustain jumper's knee patellar tendinopathy: a longitudinal study on Swedish elite junior volleyball players. Br J Sports Med. 2007 Apr;41(4):253-8.

Gisslèn K et al. High prevalence of jumper's knee and sonographic changes in Swedish elite junior volleyball players compared to matched controls. Br J Sports Med. 2005 May;39(5):298-301.

Patellofemoral Pain Syndrome – When It Hurts Under the Kneecap

Symptoms

Anterior knee pain under or around the kneecap. Worsening on knee loading and deep squat movements. Mostly provoked in a very particular flexed knee position, with no or much less pain before and after going through this really painful flexion position.

Figure 1: Normal X-Ray of a Knee, Showing Knee Anatomy and the Patella (Kneecap) and the Patellofemoral Joint

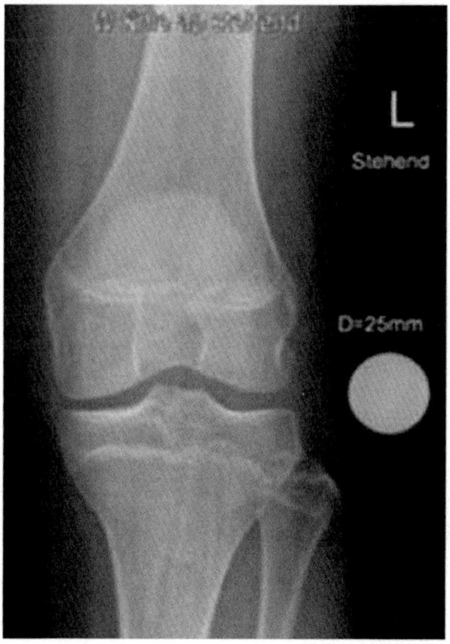

X-ray of the knee, normal (L)

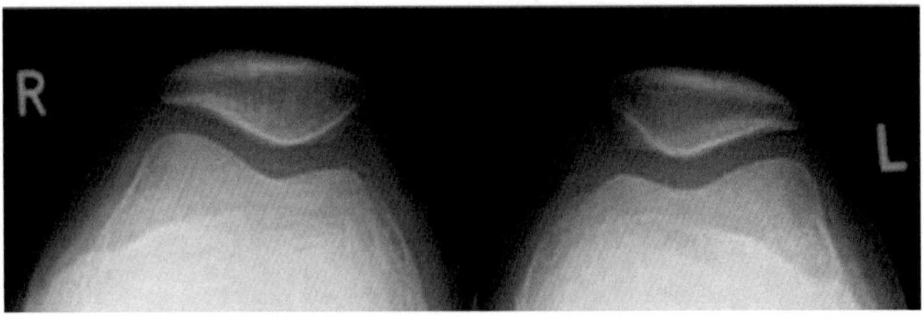

X-ray of the knee, normal

Figure 2: Patellofemoral Pain Syndrome in the Following Case after an Injury in a Soccer Player – Usually More an Overuse or Training Error Injury

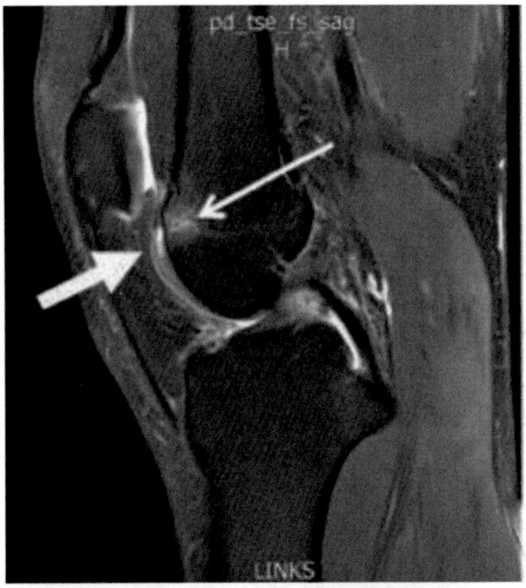

MRI of the knee lateral view

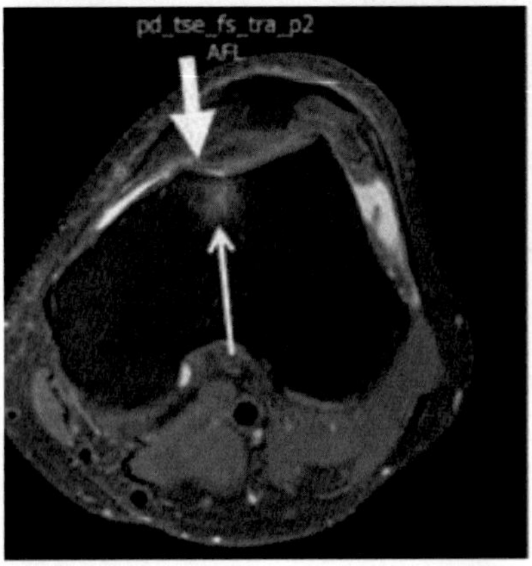

MRI of the knee with cross sectional view

→Injured cartilage and

→bone bruise after an accident

Background

The patellofemoral pain syndrome is one of the most common causes for knee pain and may be present in any age group. As the name says, it describes a pain occurring under or around the kneecap. Contributing factors to this condition are:

- Overuse of the knee articulation (e.g. long downhill jogging, too heavy loading in squat strength training, too many jumps, especially with too deep flexion)
- Shortening of the quadriceps and the hamstrings muscle
- Mal-alignment of the foot-ankle-knee-hip, e.g. pes planovalgus, knee valgus, or internal rotation of the knee and hip
- Insufficient strength of the thigh and hip muscles

Prevention and Treatment Table for Patellofemoral Pain Syndrome

Prevention	Regular stretching or other flexibility exercises to prevent muscle shortening Regular sportsmed exam to recognise any major mal-alignment of foot-ankle-knee-hip and appropriate measures to improve this condition, e.g. specific muscle strengthening to improve alignment if severe and provoking symptoms; eventually insoles/orthosis for a better stance and gait Train hard but smart: not overloading the knee. Omit too heavy loading, too deep knee flexion (omit more than 90°), and too many jumps. And for coaches, control good execution of jumps and strength training with additional weight, and make corrections if necessary
Treatment by Yourself	Usually difficult, as there are many contributing factors. Avoiding movements provoking too much pain. Slight cycling on the flat (or on ergometer with nearly no resistance) with the saddle in a high sitting position for 20min daily is usually helpful. Regular stretching of, especially, quadriceps and hamstrings muscle, but integrate the whole lower limb.

When is a Doctor Needed?	When the pain is affecting daily life or when the symptoms persist for longer than 2–3weeks
Return to Play/ Sports	Depending on the severity. In easy cases, a slight training adaptation for 2–3 weeks whilst treatment is progressing on its way may be sufficient. In more severe cases, a completely altered training program for 6–8 weeks may be necessary to let the knee recover. A well balanced strengthening guided by a physiotherapist seems to be a very promising treatment option.

What Does the Doctor Do?

The doctor takes a history and performs a clinical exam, with a more extensive testing of the knee, stance, gait, and muscle length. Usually diagnosis may be made clinically. In cases with a long history, MRI imaging may be necessary. Sometimes the MRI underestimates the situation, i.e. the patient/athlete has a quite painful condition and the MRI doesn't show too much or is sometimes even normal. This 'little or no finding in MRI but quite severe pain' still confirms the diagnosis as it's typical and it excludes other pathologies.

Treatment-wise, a detailed and individual plan needs to be worked out, as the goal is to eliminate the contributing factors (e.g. mal-alignment, overuse, inappropriate movement pattern, muscle shortening, insufficient muscular control) and support the healing of the usually touched and stressed cartilage with regular but slight exercise (20min of slight knee movement with very low resistance, as cycling flat, high saddle position). Furthermore, active ingredients supporting cartilage such as chondroitinsulfate/glucosaminsulfate, unloading of the knee cap with taping or a brace, and alternative training without stress on the knee cap are beneficial.

Literature

Giles LS et al. Atrophy of the Quadriceps Is Not Isolated to the Vastus Medialis Oblique in Individuals With Patellofemoral Pain. J Orthop Sports Phys Ther. 2015 Aug;45(8):613-9.

Rothermich MA et al. Patellofemoral pain: epidemiology, pathophysiology, and treatment options. Clin Sports Med. 2015 Apr;34(2):313-27

Barton C et al. The 'Best Practice Guide to Conservative Management of Patellofemoral Pain': incorporating level 1 evidence with expert clinical reasoning. Br J Sports Med. 2015 Jul;49(14):923-34

Osteochondrosis Dissecans (OD) of the Knee (Ankle, Elbow) – Rare but Serious

Symptoms

Pain within the knee, usually described as 'deeply inside'. Typically with a sudden onset in later childhood and adolescence, it is often realised in sports, even though not exclusively provoked by sports training or competition.

▶ Figure 1:

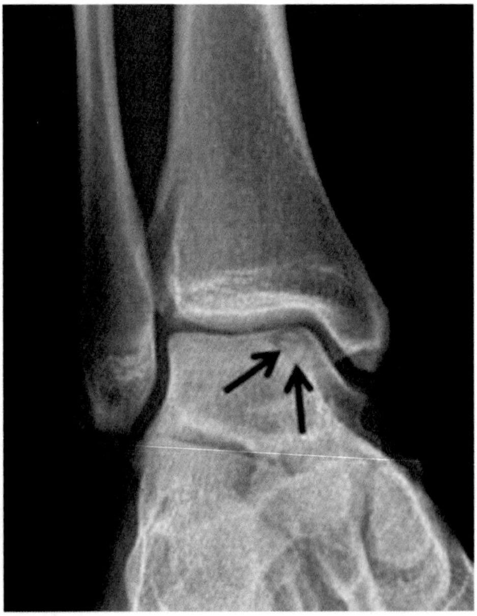

← X-ray of the ankle with osteochondrosis dissecans

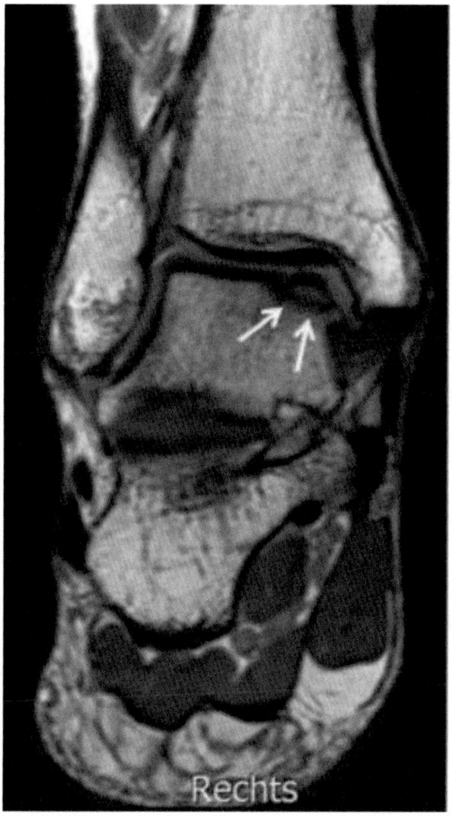

←MRI of the same ankle with osteochondrosis dissecans

Background

In weight-bearing joints—most often in the knee, sometimes the ankle and occasionally in the elbow (in female gymnasts, because of the heavy loading of the elbow joint in this sport)—a usually very localised disconnection of the cartilage from the underlying bone may occur. This is called ostoechondrosis dissecans; a separation or splitting of the cartilage layer from the underlying bone. This ailment may occur in late childhood and adolescence, with or without sports training. Overuse may be one, but not the only, contributing factor. Nevertheless, we observe this condition in youth and adolescent sports and as it is about cartilage, the preservation of a smooth joint surface, and prevention of early onset of osteoarthritis warrant a careful follow-up.

The etiology of the OD disease is not clear and further research is necessary for the better understanding of the disease.

Prevention and Treatment Table for Osteochondrosis Dissecans

Prevention	As etiology is not clear, it is impossible to give good advice for preventive measures.
Treatment by Yourself	Follow the recommendations of your sports medicine physician. It is important to have the patience to let this area of disconnected cartilage get back in good contact with the underlying bone.
When is a Doctor Needed?	Immediately!
Return to Play/ Sports	Usually several months of training adaptation are needed, sometimes a year or more. Quite often, the weight bearing joint articulation may be used only for daily life (and not more) and the sporty activities and the former regular training needs to change completely. It is a really challenging condition!

What Does the Doctor Do?

The doctor takes the history and performs a clinical exam. As usually the clinical findings are sparse, which is very much in contrast to the quite pronounced and irritating pain episodes. Further imaging is needed. If OD is suspected, imaging is usually done with an x-ray and MRI at the same time to have a complete overview.

Treatment is challenging and needs a thorough and well-reflected plan for the following months/year and a lot of patience from all involved parties. There are surgical options, but usually they occur in cases in which the cartilage surface is no longer smooth anymore and where it seems an operative realignment of this loosened cartilage would improve the situation, sometimes with the goal to refix the loosened cartilage, sometimes combined with underlying drilling through the surrounding bone to improve blood flow into the affected zone, sometimes considering a body own transplantation of chondrocytes (i.e. cartilage cells). That said, thorough planning, often an interdisciplinary discussion with an orthopaedic surgeon, and patience are needed to take the right decisions in this disease.

Literature

Richter DL et al. Knee Articular Cartilage Repair and Restoration Techniques: A Review of the Literature. Sports Health. 2016 Mar;8(2):153-60.

Weiss JM et al. The Incidence of Surgery in Osteochondritis Dissecans in Children and Adolescents. Orthop J Sports Med. 2016 Mar 16;4(3):2325967116635515.

Paterno MV et al. Physical therapy management of patients with osteochondritis dissecans: a comprehensive review. Clin Sports Med. 2014 Apr;33(2):353-74.

Swimmer's Shoulder/Thrower's Shoulder/ Impingement of the Shoulder – When the Mechanics Are Impaired

Symptoms

Shoulder pain with overhead movements and activities, usually unilateral, impairing regular training activity. Sometimes pain at night while lying on the injured shoulder.

Onset may be rather gradual in swimmer's shoulder and impingement, whereas thrower's shoulder usually starts abruptly after a bad movement in exercise.

Figure 1: Anatomy of the Shoulder

Figure 1.1: View from the back, view from ahead.
Red: the rotator cuff muscles with the supraspinatus muscle in the narrow passage. Green: ligaments

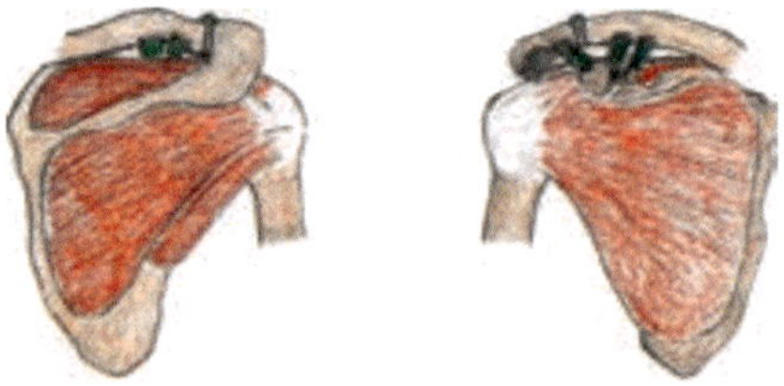

Figure 1.2: Cross sectional view of the shoulder, showing the narrow passage under the acromion

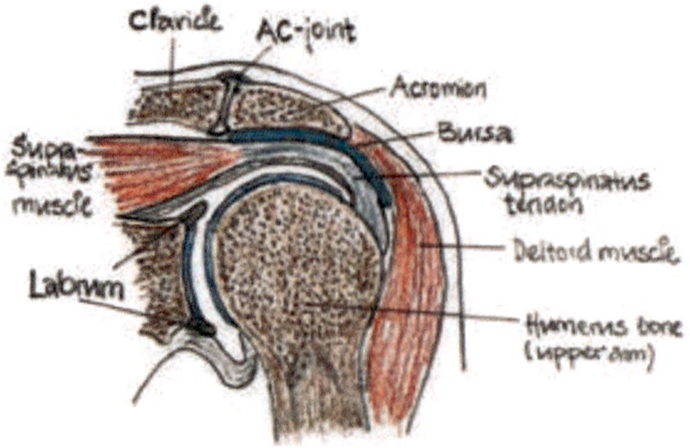

Background

Shoulder impingement: Shoulder impingement describes the conflict of anatomical structures causing discomfort, pain, and impaired movement because of a narrow passage. Often it is an underlying genetically determined condition that causes the space between the head of the humerus (upper end of the upper arm bone) and the acromion (bony roof of the shoulder) and/or the acromio-clavicular joint to be narrow (Figure 1). Sometimes the acromion may even show a distinct hook-shaped pattern narrowing the underlying passage. In sport disciplines with overhead activities, this condition otherwise imperceptible in daily life becomes symptomatic.

Swimmer's shoulder: Athletes with continuous long-lasting overhead activities (like swimmers and kayakers) may develop swimmer's shoulder, an overuse (or training error) injury. Repetitive prolonged use of the shoulder joint and its muscles and tendons in an inappropriate way can damage shoulder structures, mainly the subacromial bursa (bursa underneath the bony roof of the shoulder) and the tendons of the rotator cuff and the biceps muscle. These structures get inflamed and leading to bursitis (inflammation of the bursa) and tendinosis/tendinitis (irritation/inflammation of the tendon). Symptoms are shoulder pain while exercising and pain at night while lying on the shoulder.

Thrower's shoulder: Athletes with brisk overhead activities (like javelin throwers, cricket bowlers, baseball pitchers, but also volleyball and tennis players) may develop thrower's shoulder, an overuse (or training error) injury. Because of repetitive, accelerated, and explosive shoulder movements in elevated arm position, tendons of the rotator cuff get stressed and suffer repetitive minor traumas. This leads to lacerated, often chronically irritated, rotator cuff tendons and to pain while exercising, doing overhead movements, and occasionally pain at night lying on the shoulder.

Prevention and Treatment Table for Swimmer's/ Thrower's/Impingement of the Shoulder

Prevention	For all sports with overhead activities good warming up is a *must*. This includes a general warm-up, warm-up of the shoulder structures, flexibility exercises, and focused strengthening of the shoulder with internal rotation (IR), external rotation (ER), abduction (Abd) to get the shoulder centred. Add some exercises to get the shoulder girdle muscles activated and to achieve good setting of the scapula (shoulder blade). Basic exercises: Internal rotation (IR) 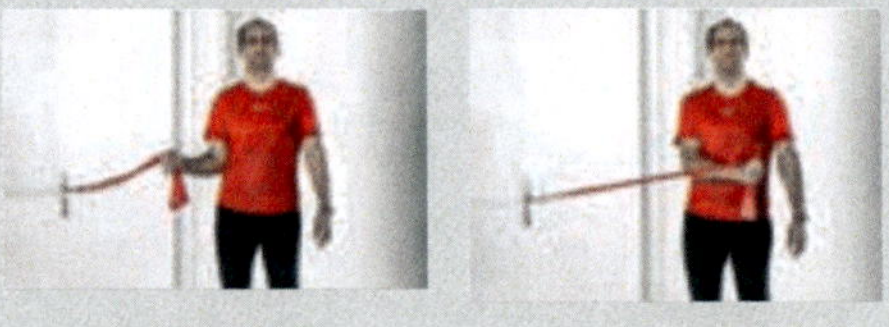 External rotation (ER) 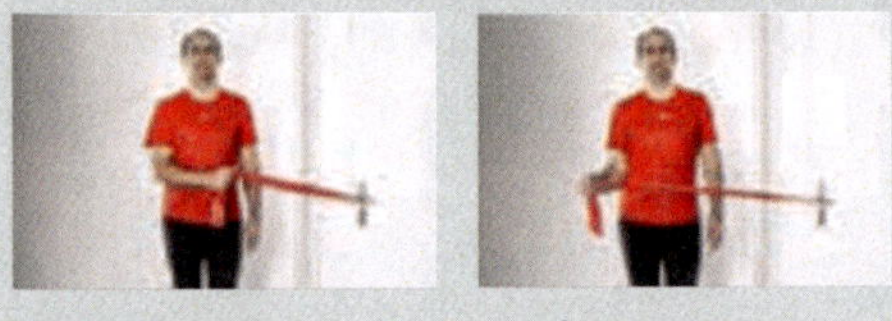 Abduction 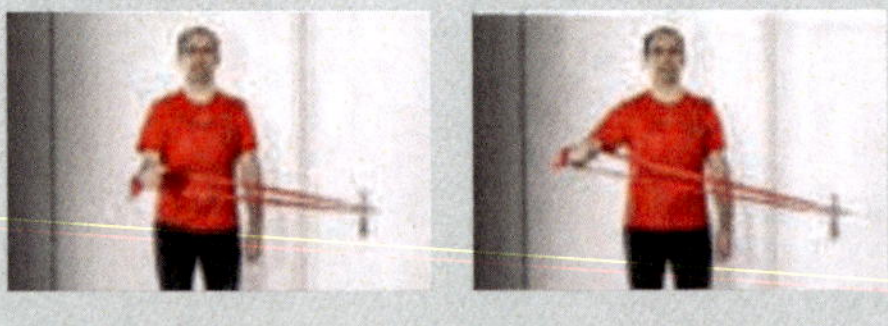 Scapula setting ("Champion-Exercise") 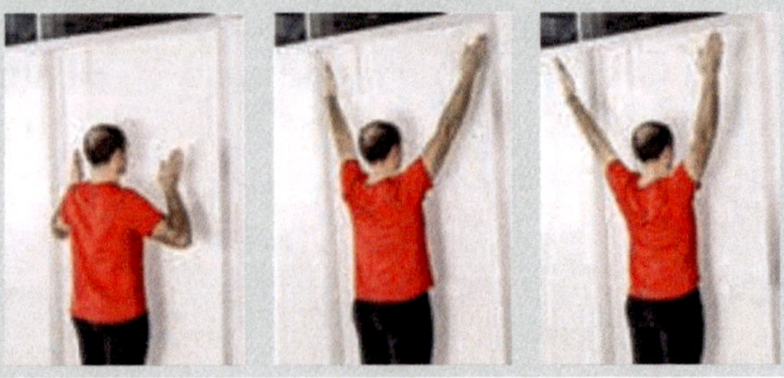

Treatment by Yourself	• A good regime of these shoulder exercises is essential. Perform the exercises regularly. From time to time, do them in front of a mirror and let a sports physiotherapist (or the coach) watch you, as often you're adopting a wrong movement pattern or not respecting the right plane • A frequent training error is the lack of activation of the shoulder blade fixing muscles (as rhomboideus and serratus muscles). Get them activated by proper execution of the exercises (e.g. the cobra exercise, pictured below) 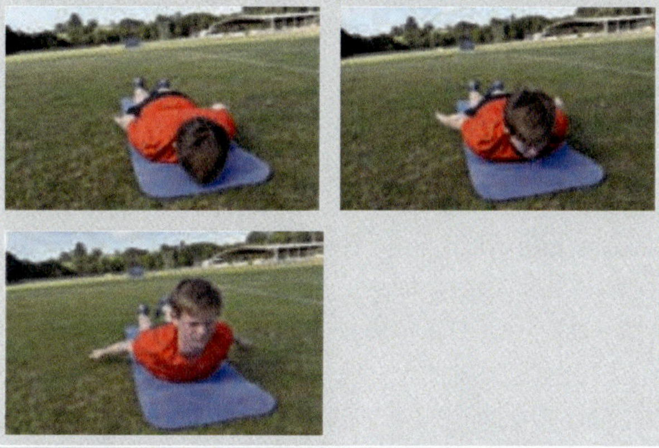
When is a Doctor Needed?	If your shoulder movements remain impaired and symptoms persist for two or three weeks.
Return to Play/Sports	First of all a diagnosis needs to be established. This determines the way to go and the time frame, which has a broad range. In the simplest case, a slight impingement without any structural issues but accompanying trigger points, the RTP may consist of a couple of physio sessions, home exercises (as above), and a slight training reduction. Whereas with a thrower's shoulder, with partial rupture of the rotator cuff tendons, the RTP will last much longer, about 8-12 weeks.

What Does the Doctor Do?

The doctor takes the history and performs a clinical examination. Usually a painful arc in the abduction movement and positive impingement tests are the main findings. Trigger points are frequent and may be clinically diagnosed. X-ray imaging gives an overview of the bony shoulder structures. Depending on your history and the clinical findings, an Arthro-MRI (magnetic resonance imaging with contrast injection) will be performed in case the tendons and the bursa need a closer look. This all leads to a diagnosis and a treatment plan.

Conservative treatment is the usual way to approach all these issues:

Swimmer's shoulder: an inflammatory state and overuse.

Treatment: The reduction of the overuse *must* be addressed, looking at swimming technique, strengthening of the shoulder blade fixing muscles, good-warm up, etc. With bursitis, a cortisone injection may be an option.

Thrower's shoulder: chronically injured tendons because of repetitive minor traumas.

Treatment: Tendon healing. A longer pause with throwing activities is essential, strengthening shoulder blade fixing muscles, good alignment of the shoulder blade on the thoracic cage, and good positioning of the humeral head in the socket with regular home exercises and good warm-up. Furthermore the throwing technique needs a closer look and possibly corrections. After a good healing response, strengthening of the formerly injured tendon is necessary, as this makes the tendon stronger and more robust.

Impingement of the shoulder: is a (too) narrow passage.

Treatment: Optimise smooth shoulder mechanics by home exercises (as above), good warming up, and releasing trigger points. If the passage is too narrow, and conservative treatment doesn't bring any benefit, a surgical approach needs to be discussed.

Literature

Hanratty CE et al. Physical Therapists' Perceptions and Use of Exercise in the Management of Subacromial Shoulder Impingement Syndrome: A Focus Group Study. Phys Ther. 2016 Mar 24. [Epub ahead of print]

Wilk KE, Hooks TR. Rehabilitation of the throwing athlete: where we are in 2014. Clin Sports Med. 2015 Apr;34(2):247-61.

Butler D et al. Sorting swimmers shoulders: An observational study on swimmers that presented to a shoulder surgeon. Int J Shoulder Surg. 2015 Jul-Sep;9(3):90-3.

Batalha N et al. Does a land-based compensatory strength-training programme influences the rotator cuff balance of young competitive swimmers? Eur J Sport Sci. 2015;15(8):764-72.

Batalha N et al. Does a water-training macrocycle really create imbalances in swimmers' shoulder rotator muscles? Eur J Sport Sci. 2015;15(2):167-72.

Wilk KE, Macrina LC. Nonoperative and postoperative rehabilitation for injuries of the throwing shoulder. Sports Med Arthrosc. 2014 Jun;22(2):137-50.

Malliou PC et al. Effective ways of restoring muscular imbalances of the rotator cuff muscle group: a comparative study of various training methods. Br J Sports Med. 2004 Dec;38(6):766-72.

Tennis Elbow/Golfer's Elbow – Overuse of the Outer Respectively Inner Side of the Elbow

Symptoms

Tennis elbow (Epicondylitis humeri lateralis/ulnaris): Painful outer side of the elbow on muscle activation (dorsiflexion of the hand). Local tenderness on the bony prominence at the outer side of the elbow (lateral epicondyle) and just underneath (distal) at the origin of the muscle tendons of the dorsiflexors of the hand.

Golfer's elbow (Epicondylitis humeri medialis/radialis): Painful inner side of the elbow on muscle activation (volar flexion of the hand). Local tenderness on the bony prominence at the inner side of the elbow (medial epicondyle) and just underneath (distal) at the origin of the muscle tendons of the volar flexors of the hand.

Background

The repetitive loading and unloading of the elbow leads to an overuse injury called tennis elbow. Now it's absolutely true that many people have tennis elbow (it is really frequent in the normal population!) and they have never ever played tennis. How's that? The name has been given because, in tennis, beginners with a lot of enthusiasm but a poor technique, especially for the return shot, are more prone to develop this condition. But the same is true for all people making any type of overuse by overloading the dorsiflexion muscles of the forearm, e.g. clerks working on computers, people doing a lot of homework, etc.

What about the golfer's elbow? First of all it's much rarer than the tennis elbow. In golf, it is long putting and chipping that needs a particular volar flexion of the wrist. But again this is also true for swimmers working hard with paddles or other people working hard with their forearm muscles, e.g. a lot of hammering and screwing, etc.

What's happening locally? First of all it's the origin of the muscle tendons at this outer (tennis elbow) or inner (golfer's elbow) condition that are irritated and suffering overuse. This leads acutely to a local inflammation of the proximal tendon and the periost (bone skin) at the origin, provoking pain and local tenderness. At this point this condition would be perfectly treatable. If the overuse with repetitive little traumas continues the tendon-periost link and the tendon suffer microlesions, tiny structural injuries, and interruptions, which take much longer to heal and are more difficult to treat.

Prevention and Treatment Table for Tennis Elbow/ Golfer's Elbow

Prevention	With particular elbow loading movements as the return (backhand shot, i.e. eccentric dorsiflexion) in tennis or the long putting and chipping in golf (volar flexion)—start slow and go slow. Meaning, no abrupt step up of training intensity or excessive increase in training hours. A good warm-up before training and competition, regular flexibility exercises with stretching (daily) and strengthening exercises (once or twice weekly) help in prevention of elbow overuse injuries.
Treatment by Yourself	Local anti-inflammatory treatment, e.g. Voltaren cream. Very effective is a Pasta boli poultice overnight. Stretching exercises of the forearm.
When is a Doctor Needed?	If pain is making daily life uncomfortable and symptoms persist for more than 2–3 weeks.

Return to Play/Sports	Depending on the severity and duration of symptoms. With a short history and immediate treatment, training may be even continued or just slightly adapted. If you wait too long, sometimes a quite long complete training pause is unavoidable, and in advanced stages treatment options aren't that promising, so start treatment early.

What Does the Doctor Do?

The doctor takes the history and performs a clinical exam. Usually diagnosis is then clear and treatment may be started immediately. A local anti-inflammatory treatment, stretching exercises, an elbow brace to unload the tendon, physiotherapy for local treatment, myofascial release, and trigger point therapy with eventually dry needling are usually combined. The training usually needs to be slightly adapted during intensive therapy. If this treatment fails, an imaging (MRI) is usually performed to confirm the diagnosis and more focused myofascial therapy of the neck-shoulder-arm-hand region, focused trigger point therapy with dry needling, and a complete stop of provoking manoeuvres may be the successful treatment approach. When we have to deal with microlesions of the tendon-periost link and the tendon itself, it is understandable that there are only a few treatment options left. *Not* cortisone as, while it prevents an overwhelming inflammatory response, it is not otherwise helping to heal the microlesions. Also surgery is not showing promising results. The best options seem to be either the conservative approach as explained above or PRP injections (platelet rich plasma).

Literature

Coombes BK et al. Management of Lateral Elbow Tendinopathy: One Size Does Not Fit All. J Orthop Sports Phys Ther. 2015 Nov;45(11):938-49.

Knutsen EJ et al. Factors associated with failure of nonoperative treatment in lateral epicondylitis. Am J Sports Med. 2015 Sep;43(9):2133-7.

Thompson C, Visco C. Lateral epicondylosis: emerging management options. Curr Sports Med Rep. 2015 May-Jun;14(3):215-20.

Tyler TF et al. Clinical outcomes of the addition of eccentrics for rehabilitation of previously failed treatments of golfers elbow. Int J Sports Phys Ther. 2014 May;9(3):365-70

Bursitis of the Elbow (or the Knee) – a Red, Hot, Palpable, and Painful Swelling

Symptoms

Pain, distinct and heavy swelling, reddening, and impaired and painful movement to the elbow (or the knee).

Background

Our body is wonderfully organised as it creates, in the subcutaneous tissue, a bursa, in many regions where bony prominences are exposed. This is particularly the case in the kneecap and elbow region, but also over the great trochanter (outside of the hip on the femur bone). Now, this bursa helps to absorb impacts, pressure, and shearing forces. In case of repetitive overuse or a major traumatic injury, it may happen that the bursa reacts to this overwhelming physical stress with an inflammation, the bursitis.

Prevention and Treatment Table for Bursitis of the Knee, Elbow, Great Trochanter (Hip)

Prevention	Prevent repetitive shock and direct impact on these bony prominences, e.g. by wearing an elbow or knee pad for volleyball or handball players.
Treatment by Yourself	Good prevention is essential. Once bursitis is established: in severe cases, see a doctor, as it is a quite massive inflammation. In slight cases, go ahead with local anti-inflammatory treatment, e.g. with a Pasta boli poultice, Voltaren cream.
When is a Doctor Needed?	In all established bursitis cases.

Return to Play/Sports	An established bursitis takes a few days for complete healing, usually a break from sport is indicated, as the bursa shouldn't be re-exposed and the adjacent joint shouldn't be used for some time.

What Does the Doctor Do?

The doctor takes a history and performs a clinical exam to diagnose the disease. Eventually an ultrasound and a diagnostic puncture of the liquid are performed. Treatment consists of local and systemic anti-inflammatory treatment and rest for the concerned limb. If the bursitis is not responding to this treatment within a couple of days, a cortisone injection may be considered to reduce this local overwhelming inflammatory response.

Myofascial Neck-Shoulder-Arm Pain – the Whole Muscle Chain is Painful

Symptoms

Pain in the Neck-Shoulder-Arm region, often unilateral. Mostly radiating from the neck to the shoulder downwards (or vice versa from the shoulder upwards to the neck) often radiating further down into the upper arm. Often combined with an unease and impairment of shoulder movement.

Background

The shoulder joint has the greatest degree of freedom. This brings the advantage of great mobility but also the disadvantage of vulnerability to injury or overuse. In addition, the well-balanced muscle system with the rotator cuff and the shoulder girdle muscles may show muscle hardenings or trigger points. Trigger points in the shoulder region are, for all overhead sports, an extremely frequent condition and it's a must that the sports medicine physician and the treating sports physiotherapist are completely aware of these clinical findings.

Prevention and Treatment Table for Myofascial Neck-Shoulder-Arm Pain

Prevention	• Good warm-up for trainings and competition, especially in overhead sports • Regular stretching flexibility and strengthening exercises for the rotator cuff and the shoulder girdle muscles
Treatment by Yourself	As above.

When is a Doctor Needed?	If symptoms persist.
Return to Play/Sports	Usually no training pause but possibly slight training adaptations necessary, as there are no structural lesions.

What Does the Doctor Do?

The doctor takes the history and performs a clinical exam with particular focus on shoulder movements, strength, muscle hardenings, and trigger points. The clinical diagnosis decides what the treatment consists of, e.g. trigger point therapy, stretching, specific strengthening, and shoulder centring exercises with the sports physiotherapist.

Literature

Gautschi Roland, Manuelle Triggerpunkttherapie: Myofasziale Schmerzen und Funktionsstörungen erkennen, verstehen und behandeln. Verlag: Thieme; Auflage: 3 (13. Juli 2016). ISBN-13: 978-3131474735

Pavkovich R. The use of dry needling for a subject with acute onset of neck pain: a case report. Int J Sports Phys Ther. 2015 Feb;10(1):104-13.Dunning J et al. Dry needling: a literature review with implications for clinical practice guidelines. Phys Ther Rev. 2014 Aug;19(4):252-265.

Hidalgo-Lozano A, Elite swimmers with and without unilateral shoulder pain: mechanical hyperalgesia and active/latent muscle trigger points in neck-shoulder muscles. Scand J Med Sci Sports. 2013 Feb;23(1):66-73.

Scheuermann's Disease – Rounded Thoracic Back, Still Poorly Understood

Symptoms

Rounded back, predominantly in the thoracic part of the vertebral spine (hyperkyphosis of the thoracic spine), often asymptomatic, intermittently provoking midlevel back and neck pain in teenagers. Sometimes combined with hanging shoulders and a bad back posture.

Figure 1: Spine Anatomy

a) normal vertebral spine side view   *b) Scheuermann's disease with hyperkyphosis*

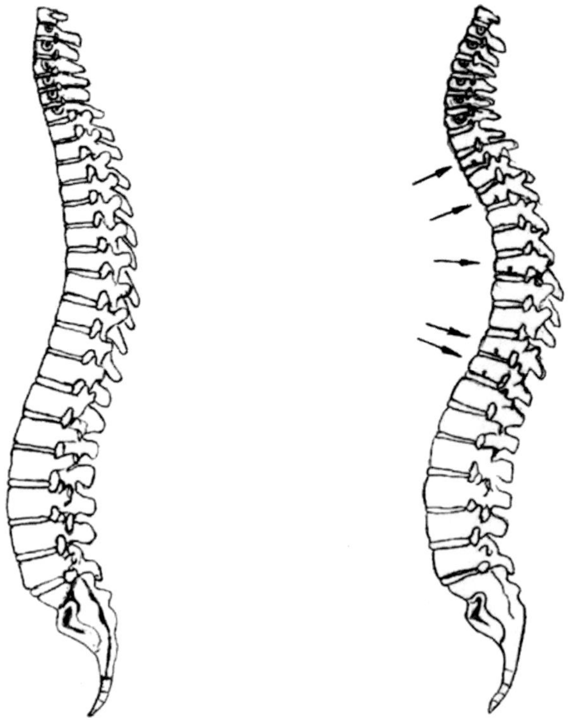

Background

Mr H.W. Scheuermann described a condition where the vertebrae grow unevenly with respect to the sagittal plane, i.e. that the posterior angle is often greater than the anterior. This leads to wedge shaped vertebral bodies and causes a hyperkyphosis of the thoracic spine.

The etiology of the disease is not yet understood and the conditions appear to be multifactorial. While there is no real explanation for what causes Scheuermann's disease, there are good treatment approaches including manual therapy, physiotherapy, and strengthening, and in extreme cases, back braces.

The disease is a self-limiting skeletal disorder of late childhood and adolescence.

Prevention and Treatment Table for Scheuermann's Disease

Prevention	The disease cannot be prevented. But the specific strengthening (good exercise instruction is essential) is your active contribution to prevent pain episodes and hopefully stop the progression of the disease.
Treatment by Yourself	As prevention.
When is a Doctor Needed?	As soon as you observe that your back posture, or the back posture of your athlete/your child, is altering towards a rounded back.
Return to Play/Sports	In many sports no pause needed, but good exercise instruction warranted. In some sports with higher loads on the vertebral spine, however, like gymnastics, judo, wrestling, and others, training needs to be adapted, e.g. no landings in gymnastics, no or only limited randori in judo and fighting in wrestling for 4-6 weeks, until it has settled down, and strengthening shows first benefits.

What Does the Doctor Do?

The doctor takes the history (including sporting activities, back pain episodes, growth in the last few years and months) and performs a clinical exam. X-rays of the vertebral spine are then performed to appreciate the extent of the hyperkyphosis and the possible alterations (wedge-shaped configuration and uneven surface) of the vertebrae. A clinical follow-up on a regular basis, first after three, later after six months is usually scheduled—timing of x-ray exam depends on the evolution of the disease.

Therapy consists of regular strengthening of body core and back muscles. Regular physical activity is highly recommended and also ambitious sports training is usually possible. One thing remains: the focus on core and back strength to be executed twice or three times weekly.

Only in exceptional circumstances is surgery to stabilise the spine deemed necessary.

Good to know: Milan Lucic, NHL hockey player for the Los Angeles Kings; Hunter Pence, professional baseball player for the San Francisco Giants; and Marcel Dettman, leading German techno DJ, have this very condition.

Literature

Wikipedia download 24.2.2016 https://en.wikipedia.org/wiki/Scheuermann%27s_disease

Fotiadis, E et al. 'Scheuermann's disease: Focus on weight and height role'. European Spine Journal 2008, 17(5): 673–8.

Scheuermann, H. W. (1920). 'Kyphosis dorsalis juvenilis '. Ugeskrift for Læger (in Danish) 82: 385–93. Republished as: Scheuermann, H. W. (1977). 'The classic: Kyphosis dorsalis juvenilis'. Clinical orthopaedics and related research 128: 5–7.

Scoliosis of the Vertebral Spine – Strengthening and Physiotherapy Help

Symptoms

Often without any symptoms! Sometimes intermittent back pain due to muscle hardening.

Figure 1: Spine X-rays

1) X-ray Normal vertebral spine frontal view

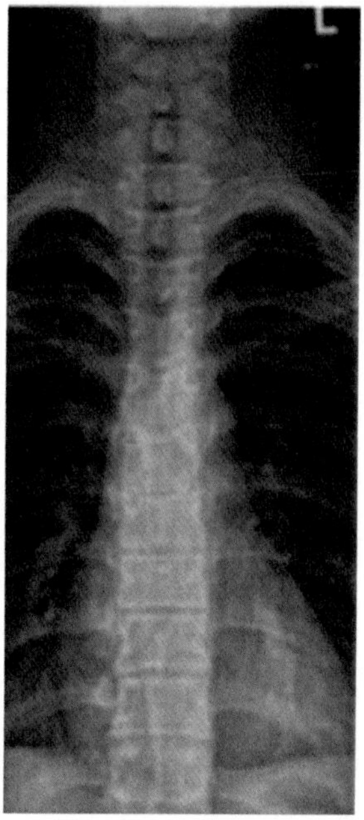

2) X- ray with scoliosis

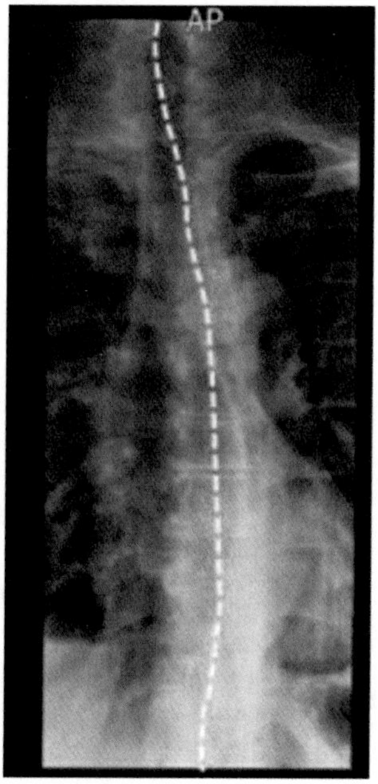

Background

The vertebral spine is composed of 24 free vertebral bodies and the sacrum (+5 adherent vertebral bodies) and has its anatomy with a double S-configuration in the sagittal plane. In the sagittal plane, it forms a lordosis (slight bending backward) in the lumbar and the cervical spine, and a kyphosis (slight bending forward) in the thoracic spine and the sacrum. In the frontal plane, the vertebrae are normally aligned straight.

In case of scoliosis, the vertebral spine goes out of alignment in the frontal plane and forms a curve called 'scoliosis'. The outer side of the curve, the convexity, and the localisation within the vertebral column are giving the name, e.g. a thoraco-lumbar left convex scoliosis.

Slight scoliosis is frequent but doesn't need any treatment or special consideration. Moderate or severe scoliosis is less frequent and needs therapy. Treatment mostly consists of specific strengthening, regular general physical activity, and a follow up.

Prevention and Treatment Table for Scoliosis

Prevention	Regular sporting activity.
Treatment by Yourself	Strengthening exercises as shown by your sports physiotherapist.
When is a Doctor Needed?	For intermediate control, every 6–12months. That said, it doesn't mean that x-rays are always necessary. After a baseline x-ray, the clinical measurement of the scoliosis is, in some cases, sufficient.
Return to Play/Sports	No pause needed. Regular sporting activities and specific strengthening are therapeutic for scoliosis. However you need to discuss with your sports medicine physician whether your scoliosis and high level sporting activities in your sport fit together or what measures need to be taken.

What Does the Doctor Do?

The doctor takes the history and performs the clinical exam. In this exam, a scoliosis will be recognised and can be quantified. This examination is, by the way, an integral part of the regular sportsmed exam. If the scoliosis is deemed important, a baseline x-ray to measure the scoliosis angles (Cobb-angles) precisely is then performed.

Therapy consists usually of specific strengthening, general sporting activity, and a follow-up. Only in very severe cases does therapy with a corset, or even an operation to stabilise the vertebral spine, need to be considered.

Literature

Hasler CC. Back pain during growth. Swiss Med Wkly. 2013 Jan 8;143:w13714. doi: 10.4414/smw.2013.13714

Green BN et al. Is physical activity contraindicated for individuals with scoliosis? A systematic literature review. J Chiropr Med. 2009 Mar;8(1):25-37.

Aebi M. The adult scoliosis. Eur Spine J. 2005 Dec;14(10):925-48.

Myofascial Low Back Pain – When the Gluts, the Lower Back, and the Pelvic Muscle Rebel

Symptoms

Typically unilateral pronounced low back pain in the lumbar region, low back, and on the bottom; sometimes slightly radiating upwards towards the lumbar region, sometimes radiating downwards in the outer thigh. Often, a shift to one side (in the pelvis region) and inability to stand completely straight may be observed.

Background

By far the most frequent etiology for low back pain, in athletes and in the normal population. Myofascial low back pain is for professionals quite easy to diagnose and to treat.

The exact pathophysiology of trigger points it not yet clear (see chapter 'Painful Trigger Points'). Persistent muscular contraction, overuse, trauma, prolonged inactivity, or low tissue oxygenation cause the formation of a taut band within the muscle structure. This structure is particularly tender on palpation and usually shows a typical referred pain pattern for each muscle. As for the lower back and lumbar region glutaeus, quadratus lumborum, and iliacus (lower part of the iliopsoas) muscles are mostly involved to different degrees.

Prevention and Treatment Table for Myofascial Low Back Pain

Prevention	Regular strengthening of your core stability, regular stretching, and other flexibility exercises.
Treatment by Yourself	Stretching and other flexibility exercises for the whole body, but particular for the muscles concerned.
When is a Doctor Needed?	• In unclear low back pain, especially with radiation further down the leg • In case of numbness, and particularly loss of strength, in one of the lower limbs. These are not trigger points but a neuroradicular problem (e.g. disc herniation) may be the cause. A doctor, or an emergency department, should be consulted the same day.
Return to Play/Sports	In case of a myofascial low back pain, the RTP varies: • It may, if treatment started early, allow you to continue your training program and you just need to reduce it slightly for a couple of days. *But* be consistent with the strengthening of your core stability and hip abductors (glutaeus medius and minimus) in this lucky situation • In more severe cases, it may take a couple of weeks to get you back on a competitive level

What Does the Doctor Do?

The doctor takes the history and performs a clinical exam, with focus on the lower back and pelvic region, but also looks at your stance and gait, and the muscle length and possible trigger points around the low back/pelvic region. Depending on the findings, further imaging is neither necessary nor helpful, as trigger points are a clinical finding and cannot be shown with x-ray, CT, or MRI.

Treatment consisting of trigger point therapy may be started immediately and usually needs a couple of sessions with the physiotherapist. Mostly it improves on each intervention but the muscle has a tendency to fall back in the same pattern and rebuild the trigger point so several treatment sessions are necessary. Stretching exercises are part of the treatment plan; after the acute phase has settled, strengthening of the core stability and the hip abductors needs to be addressed. This training will be gradually intensified. It may be a bit provocative at the beginning as challenging the muscle may, in some cases, lead to a short flare up of the same trigger points but it helps to prevent recurrent episodes. In order to really establish good core stability the training program should be performed 4–6 times a week for about 45min and consist of different exercises for either the local and global muscle system (see practical examples in chapter 'Core Stability'). To have a long term and sustainable effect, this strengthening protocol should be continued for about 2–3 month and by then be replaced by a maintenance training session (important!) once or twice a week.

Literature

Gautschi Roland, Manuelle Triggerpunkttherapie: Myofasziale Schmerzen und Funktionsstörungen erkennen, verstehen und behandeln. Verlag: Thieme; Auflage: 3 (13. Juli 2016). ISBN-13: 978-3131474735

Takamoto K et al. Effects of compression at myofascial trigger points in patients with acute low back pain: A randomized controlled trial. Eur J Pain. 2015 Sep;19(8):1186-96.

Pavkovich R. Effectiveness of dry needling, stretching and strengthening to reduce pain and improve function in subjects with chronic lateral hip and thigh pain: a retrospective case series. Int J Sports Phys Ther. 2015 Aug;10(4):540-51

Lumbar Herniated Disc With Neuroradicular Symptoms – Conservative Treatment Mostly Successful

Symptoms

Severe unilateral lower back pain, radiating down the back of the leg. May be combined with numbness or pins and needles in the lower leg or the foot, and sometimes even with a loss of strength in the lower limb. In the latter case, this is a *red flag* and means you must see a doctor the same day!

Figure 1: Herniated Disc

1) MRI lateral view of the lumbar spine with herniated disc

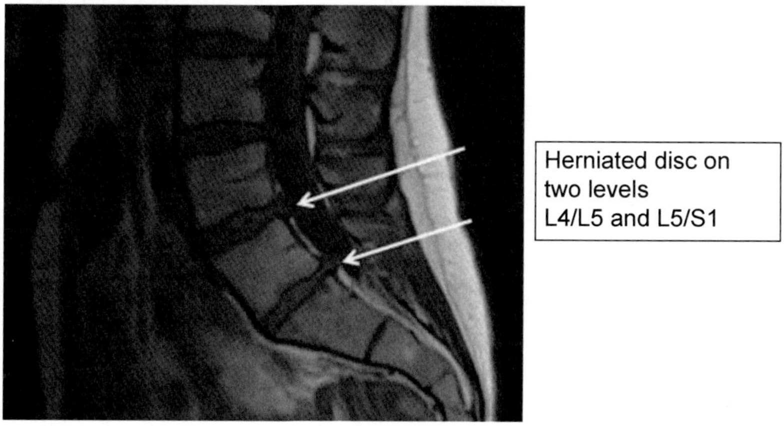

2) MRI cross sectional view of the lumbar spine with herniated disc

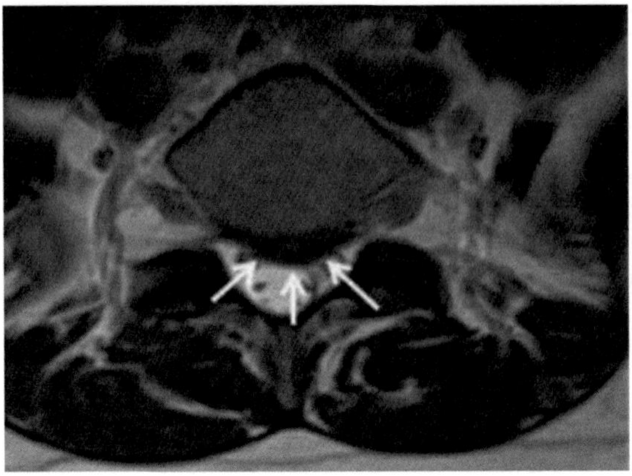

Herniated disc narrowing the passage and putting the nerve root under pressure

Background

A lumbar herniated disc occurs in middle-aged adults and the sports population quite frequently, but the good news is only a very low percentage needs an operation! However, the condition has to be taken seriously. A good and intensive medical and physiotherapy follow up, lifelong strengthening, and good and active back awareness is warranted.

The herniated disc itself is a kind of degeneration of the disc, a rupture of the more rigid ligamentous outer structures of the disc, and a prolapse or herniation of the softer inner disc material (nucleus pulposus). In most cases the herniation doesn't do any harm, as it may happen slightly backwards, where there is largely enough space to accommodate it and it happens unnoticed and without any further symptoms. In some cases, however, when the herniation occurs paramedianly or laterally, it moves to where the nerve root makes its way through the bony opening of the vertebrae (foramen) causing compression and the clinical picture of a herniated disc occurs.

The compression of the nerve leads to the symptoms described above: unilateral severe and radiating pain (usually very specific, according to the nerve root involved following the dermatomas), pins and needles, and some numbness. In more severe cases, loss of reflexes (jerks), further numbness, and gradually increased loss of strength may be experienced.

Lumbar herniated disc is the most frequent location where a herniation of the vertebral column occurs. In other areas, a herniated disc herniation may occur but it is only in the lordosis (forward curve) of the vertebral spine that the herniated disc (which occurs on the inner side of the curve, at the site with the highest pressure) leads to compression of nerve roots serving the lower limb.

Occasionally, herniated disc may be observed in the cervical spine, the other site of lordosis. A cervical herniated disc leads to unilateral neck and shoulder pain radiating in to the arm, numbness, or pins and needles in the forearm or the hand, and sometimes loss of strength—again a *red flag* sign.

Prevention and Treatment Table for Lumbar Herniated Disc

Prevention	Lumber herniated disc is difficult to prevent as it is multifactorial and often there can be a genetic predisposition towards weakness of the tissue and other factors. However disrespect of general recommendations how to lift and bear weight in a healthy way, and overuse of the lower back without respecting basic strengthening of core and back muscles clearly worsen the condition.
Treatment by Yourself	While your discipline and collaboration are appreciated and indispensable in case of a herniated disc, you need professional treatment and advice.
When is a Doctor Needed?	Whenever a lumbar disc herniation is suspected.
Return to Play/Sports	If the diagnosis is confirmed, the professionals involved in your treatment need to establish a treatment plan. First of all, it's about stabilising the condition and reducing the symptoms (i.e. reducing the local pressure to the nerve root). Furthermore, discuss return in your sport with the treating doctors. It may be possible but it is hard work and also needs a lot of patience (RTP rate 78% in basketball, 85% in ice-hockey)

What Does the Doctor Do?

In *red flag* cases with a distinct loss of strength, immediate therapy usually includes systemic cortisone therapy (quite reasonable dose of cortisone tablets to reduce the swelling, usually therapeutic use exemptions announcement to anti-doping agency needed – particularly in cases of a medical emergency), systemic anti-inflammatory drugs (to reduce swelling and inflammation), usually combined with an acid blocker to protect your stomach, and an MR-imaging of the lumbar spine performed the same day. Depending on these findings and the clinical evaluation, further steps may need to be taken. Luckily, in most cases, the body reacts in a positive way to these medications and shows an improvement in the compression signs. Physiotherapy is also started with a focus on unloading the stressed zone, reducing muscle spasms, and creating good body awareness with a good and active back positioning. A local, often CT (computer tomography) guided injection (cortisone) is of additional benefit. Close follow-up in these first days is essential with the patient, the physiotherapist, and the sports medicine physician involved over following days and weeks.

Most cases do not need this immediate approach but a history taking, clinical examination, and, in case of suspicious findings (e.g. numbness, missing reflexes), an MRI within the next few days is appropriate. The treatment approach is less immediate but follows the same lines: reduce the swelling, reduce the pressure, try to keep slightly active (e.g. some walking instead of training), physiotherapy treatment, and close follow up for the next few weeks strengthening for 2–3 months, but with a lifelong horizon. And only in cases of severe compression and a worsening of the loss of strength is an operation needed.

Literature

Minhas S et al. Outcomes After Lumbar Disc Herniation in the National Basketball Association. Sports Health. 2016 Jan-Feb;8(1):43-9.

Nair R et al. Outcomes of Lumbar Discectomy in Elite Athletes: The Need for High-level Evidence. Clin Orthop Relat Res. 2015 Jun;473(6):1971-7.

Schroeder GD et al. Performance-based outcomes after nonoperative treatment, discectomy, and/or fusion for a lumbar disc herniation in National Hockey League athletes.Am J Sports Med. 2013 Nov;41(11):2604-8.

Spondylolysis and Spondylolisthesis – When a Lumbar Vertebral Body Slides, Strengthening is Needed

Symptoms

Localised low back pain, in recurrent episodes, often with sudden onset. Sometimes after a training period with particular loading of the lower back (hyperextension exercises) or repetitive impacts (jumping, landing, running).

Figure 1: X-ray Lateral View of a Vertebral Spine, showing Spondylolysis and Listhesis of L5 on S1

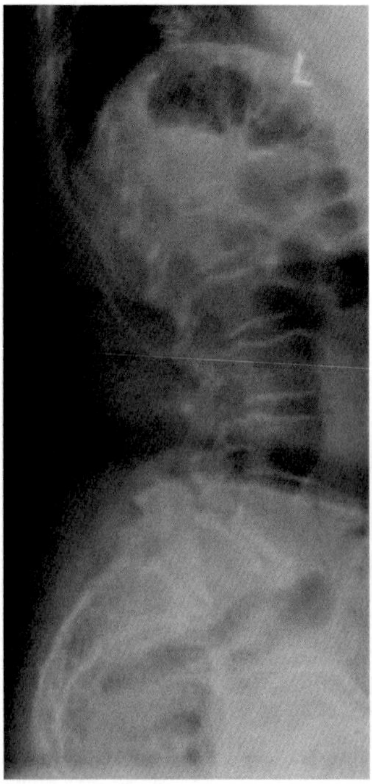

At large: lower part of the lumbar spine featuring the listhesis of L5 on S1

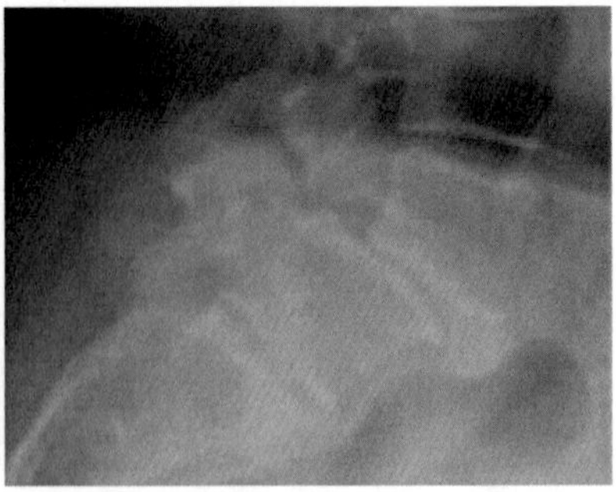

Background

The Latin terms for this condition are as follows:

- *Spondylo:* related to the vertebral bone
- *Lysis:* gap formation respectively local fracture line in the vertebral bow
- *Listhesis:* sliding of one vertebral body on the other

It's a description of either a pre-existing local gap formation respectively an overuse fracture of the vertebral bow (pars interarticularis), usually occurring in the lower lumbar spine (usually vertebra L4 or L5). The etiology is multifactorial and it often remains unclear whether it may be a pre-existing gap, an overuse fracture, or a combination of both. On one hand individual predisposition plays an important role, while on the other hand the growing vertebral spine may due to high loading and repetitive stress cause this condition.

In an asymptomatic, normal population, spondylolysis is found in about 6–12%. In different sports the prevalence (frequency) of this condition is, particularly among young athletes, distinctly increased: female gymnastics, rhythmic gymnastics, figure skating, ice hockey, beach volleyball. Even though the condition leads to a longer period of sometimes quite severe back pain episodes, the treatment pays dividends. While the vertebral bow keeps the fracture line, a pain free stage can be reached and return to normal daily life and to regular sports training is almost always possible. Every situation needs an individual appraisal, especially in cases of a sliding of one of the vertebral bodies.

Prevention and Treatment Table for Spondylolysis/Listhesis

Prevention	No forced repetitive hyperextension exercises, especially not in already tired athletes (as there is insufficient body control, all impact absorbed by passive structures alone).

Treatment by Yourself	Treatment plan according to professional follow-up and recommendations.
When is a Doctor Needed?	If severe low back pain occurs and is not responding to therapy after one or two sessions of physio, you should see a doctor, especially in sport disciplines at risk.
Return to Play/Sports	Once the diagnosis is made, a rehabilitation plan is established. RTP may vary and last up to 8 weeks. In the beginning, leaving out provoking manoeuvres (landing in hyperextended position, hyperextension in general, high impacts with jumps, etc.) and strengthening of core stability and strength endurance of the whole back and trunk muscles are essential. This training program should be started soon, gradually increase in duration and intensity (up to 5–6 sessions a week for 45min for 2–3months). When pain free, at that stage, it may be replaced by a maintenance core strengthening program twice a week 45min lifelong! In general, a return to high level sport is possible.

What Does the Doctor Do?

The doctor takes the history and performs a clinical exam, especially of the lower back, sacroiliacal joint, and pelvis region. The history, the sport discipline, and the localised and focused lumbar pain often worsening on hyperextension are leading to the diagnosis of this condition. X-rays of the lumbar spine are performed. If unclear, additional exams (MRI or CT) are indicated (especially as athletes with persisting episodes of localised low back pain are at higher risk to suffer of this condition).

Literature

Bouras T, Korovessis P. Management of spondylolysis and low-grade spondylolisthesis in fine athletes. A comprehensive review. Eur J Orthop Surg Traumatol. 2015 Jul;25 Suppl 1:167-75

Toueg CW et al. Spondylolisthesis, sacro-pelvic morphology and orientation in young gymnasts. J Spinal Disord Teach. 2015 Jul;28(6) 358-64

Donaldson LD. Spondylolysis in elite junior-level ice hockey players.Sports Health. 2014 Jul;6(4):356-9

Külling FA et al. High prevalence of disc degeneration and spondylolysis in the lumbar spine of professional beach volleyball players. Orthop J Sports Med. 2014 Apr 9; 2(4)

Garet M et al. Nonoperative Treatment in Lumbar Spondylolysis and Spondylolisthesis. A systematic review. Sports Health. 2013 May; 5(3): 225–232.

Haus BM; Micheli LJ. Back pain in the pediatric and adolescent athlete. Clin Sports Med. 2012 Jul;31(3):423-40

Kalichman L et al. Spondylolysis and spondylolisthesis: prevalence and association with low back pain in the adult community-based population. Spine 2009 Jan 15; 34(2): 199–205.

Sacro-Iliac Dysfunction – an Important and Neglected Pelvic Joint

Symptoms

Low back pain, typically unilateral, located in the lumbar region-lower back-pelvic girdle-outer side of the hip. Centre of pain focuses directly above the sacro-iliacal-joint on either side of the sacrum. May have a sudden onset, after a 'bad' movement, but may also appear slowly. It often develops over a long period of time after repeated falls, landings, or dismounts, or severe falls (bike, horse).

Figure 1: Pelvis

1.1) SIJ anatomy and pelvic girdle

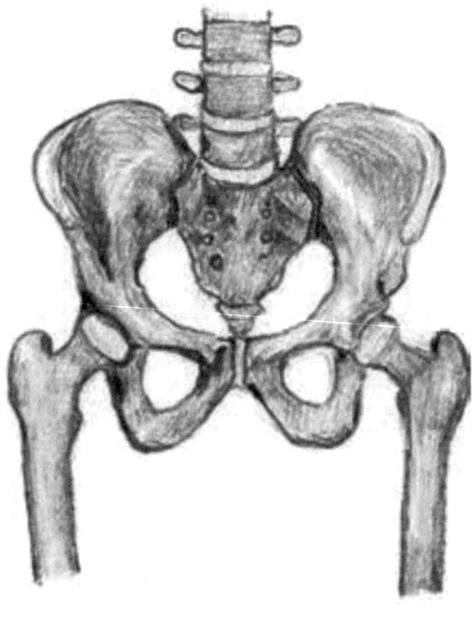

1.2) SIJ nutation/counternutation as movement pattern

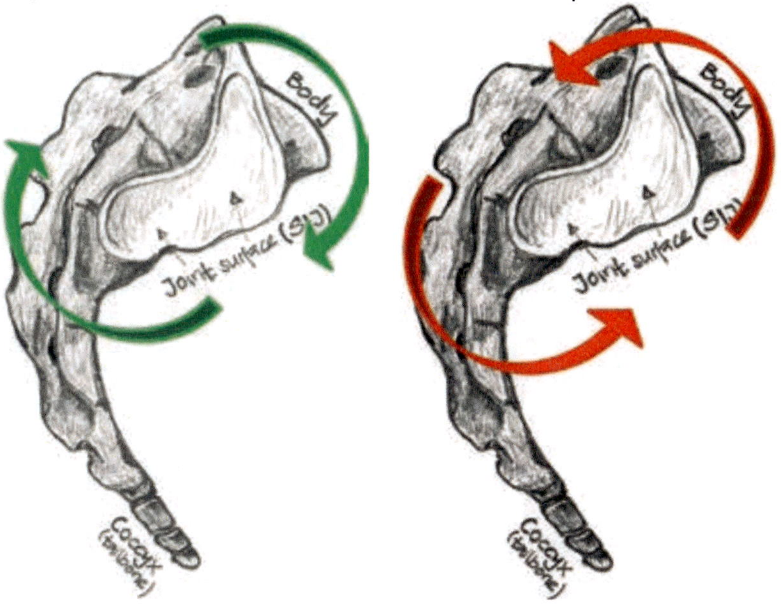

OPTIMAL – Sacral nutation **SUB-OPTIMAL – Sacral counter-nutation**

(nutation/counternutation diagram courtesy AssProf.Dr.med. Manuel Cusi, University of Notre Dame, Sydney)

Background

The sacroiliacal joint (SIJ) is an integral part of the pelvis. It allows only little movements called nutation and counternutation (see Figure 1.2). The pelvis is both origin and insertion of a multitude of muscle tendons important to a well-balanced stance, gait, and locomotion. The SIJ and the bones forming the joint are central to good core control as the corresponding muscles are forming muscle chains crossing simple anatomical boundaries and forming collaborating locomotor systems.

SIJ dysfunction: Describes inappropriate quality of relative motion; the sacrum counternutates when loaded instead of the normal nutation. This is the reason for recurrent muscle tightening, formation of trigger points, because of compensation strategies of the lower back, pelvic girdle, and thigh.

Blocked sacro-iliacal joint: A sudden blocking of the SIJ usually provokes slight twisting with unease in movement, an asymmetry in body posture, and tensing up of core muscles and muscles of the pelvic girdle.

SIJ incompetence: Insufficient control of the pelvic girdle muscles and insufficient core stability leads to the SIJ incompetence pattern with recurrent episodes of low back pain. This condition leads to different compensation strategies including overload of hamstrings, adductors, and hip flexor muscles.

Prevention and Treatment Table for SIJ Dysfunction

Prevention	Regular core stability and back strengthening. All people need this kind of exercises, however it is more important for people involved with sport training and competition, due to all the impacts and power-related activities, to have a more solid and strength endurance trained core. The equation is easy: the higher level athlete you are and the more impacts and shearing forces your sport discipline bears, the better your core stability and your back and trunk muscles need to be.
Treatment by Yourself	See Figure 2: How to Sit Properly and also chapter 'Core Stability'.
When is a Doctor Needed?	In case of recurrent episodes of back pain, think about the SIJ!
Return to Play/ Sports	An episode with a blocked SIJ, low back pain, myofascial findings is treatable, but needs good and close follow-up in the first few days. In this period, training needs to be adapted, possibly even left out for two or three days. Good athlete, coach, physiotherapist, sports medicine physician communication is essential.

Figure 2: How to Sit Properly – Raise Your Body Awareness

1. Sit on your sitting bones (i.e. try to feel the direct contact of the sitting bones to the chair)
2. Close the zip of your trousers, imagine they're a bit tight (i.e. activate your pelvic floor muscles and local core muscles)
3. Let the sun shine on your chest (i.e. open up a bit your upper body, take your shoulder slightly back)

Do this exercise several times a day, hold it for at least 30 seconds, it will help to address SIJ dysfunction and will make you feel better!

What Does the Doctor Do?

The doctor, or physiotherapist, takes the history and performs a clinical exam, almost always revealing typical findings leading to the diagnosis. Immediate therapy with manual therapy (e.g. manipulation, mobility manoeuvres), trigger point therapy, and muscle release techniques is usually started. Depending on the history and severity of symptoms, other modalities may be added.

With recurrent episodes, a more extensive clinical evaluation and an imaging with, for example, SPECT–CT may lead to the diagnosis of SIJ incompetence. The therapy aims to a regain this competence by:

- Building up good core stability by strengthening your core muscles, particularly including pelvic floor, deep abdominal, and deep back muscles
- Acquiring a good (three and four dimensional) awareness of your body, especially of the pelvis and core region – practical exercise in Figure 2.
- Maintaining these capacities by regular training, as a certain vulnerability to recurrent episodes of low back and SIJ pain is evident (see chapter 'Core Stability').

Literature

Cusi MF. Paradigm for assessment and treatment of SIJ mechanical dysfunction. J Bodyw Mov Ther.2010 Apr; 14(2):152-61

Cusi MF, J Saunders et al. Metabolic disturbances identified by SPECT-CT in patients with clinical diagnosis of sacroiliac incompetence. Eur Spine J (2013) 22:1674-1682

Vleeming A et al. The sacroiliac joint: an overview of its anatomy, function and potential clinical implications. J Anat. 2012 Dec;221(6):537-67.

Massoud Arab A et al. The relationship between hamstring length and gluteal muscle strength in individuals with sacroiliac joint dysfunction. J Man Manip Ther. 2011 Feb;19(1):5-10.

Poley RE, Borchers JR. Sacroiliac joint dysfunction: evaluation and treatment. Phys Sportsmed. 2008 Dec;36(1):42-9

Athletic Groin Pain – a Similar Challenge for Athletes and Health Professionals

Symptoms

Pain in the inguinal region, mostly after an acute injury, sometimes with slow diffuse onset, mostly unilateral (just one side), getting worse on physical effort, sometimes with brisk and sharp pain after an involuntary manoeuvre.

Background

Athletic groin pain, whether it be acute or chronic, is a challenge for both the athlete and the treating health professional. A multitude of possible entities may provoke groin pain and, as diagnosis is sometimes complex and treatment long lasting thus requiring the athlete's patience, it will remain tough and challenging (reasoning for a careful and accurate diagnosis, written treatment, and return to play plan).

According to the Doha classification three major subheadings are differentiated:

1) Defined entities for groin pain (as below in Figure 2)
2) Hip related groin pain (as FAI, femoro-acetabular impingement; hip dysplasia)
3) Other causes for hip pain in athletes (nerve entrapment, other medical reason)

The defined entities, by far the most frequent, are further categorised and related to anatomical structures, which help precision in diagnosing and establishing a good return to play plan:

- Adductor related
- Iliopsoas related
- Inguinal related
- Pubic related

Prevention and Treatment Table for Athletic Groin Pain

Prevention	• Good warming-up for trainings and competition for all type of sports is essential! • Sport disciplines that involve sprints, sudden changes of direction, and kicking must be very disciplined, 'aggressive', and very careful in preparing for every single training session • Regular strengthening twice or three times weekly of the leg axis stabilising muscles, including hip adductors and abductors in different sport specific forms (single leg balance, single leg squats, jumps of all sorts and directions, specific strengthening of hip adductors and abductors against gravity) is strongly recommended • Stretching or other flexibility exercises on a daily basis • For recurrent groin pain, x-shaped underpants or neoprene pants seem to help preventing muscular injuries in the groin region • In case of an injury, quickly get professional help and allow enough healing time. It's better investing a few weeks in a first injury than having troubles with a chronic issue and spending 8 months or a year on it.
Treatment by Yourself	Maximise efforts for prevention. Once you have it, seek professional advice.
When is a Doctor Needed?	For acute injury, see (within days) or for recurrent obstinate groin pain.
Return to Play/ Sports	Depends on the severity and the duration of the problem. First of all, an exact diagnosis resulting in treatment and then a return to play plan needs to be established.

Sometimes the season and treatment may continue in parallel (with the clear focus of a proper pause and treatment at the end of the season!). But mostly a break for 4–8 weeks is needed. In this time a detailed return to play plan is essential to be fit and competitive on the day of your return. Often a multimodal treatment, including manual and trigger point therapy of adductor and pelvic girdle muscles, improvement of core stability and awareness, and gradually increased supervised active physical training will be given.

In some cases, as with an inguinal hernia (i.e. herniation of abdominal tissue into the inguinal canal), an operation is clearly the best therapy, with a return to competitive sports within 4–6 weeks.

In case of a *sports hernia* (i.e. painful insufficiency and bulging of the posterior inguinal wall) *and* exclusion of other reasons for groin pain according to different studies, an operation to stabilise the posterior abdominal wall seems to be helpful.

What Does the Doctor Do?

The doctor takes the history and performs a clinical exam. The anamnesis and the clinical examination are very important in this setting, as they indicate on the one hand, the story of the problem (sudden or slow onset, former history, character of pain, pain radiation, former treatment, etc.) and on the other, showing stance, gait, and local findings in the pelvis-hip-groin region as well as manoeuvres enhancing or diminishing pain. Depending on these findings further imaging will be arranged, whether it be x-ray (e.g. overview of the bony structures, pelvis, hip), ultrasound in rest (e.g. structural muscle lesion or scar tissue), dynamic (inguinal hernia or sports hernia with bulging of the posterior inguinal wall), or an MRI (e.g. overuse injury, tendinopathy, other inflammation, etc.). In case of suspected femoro-acetabular impingement (see also corresponding chapter) or intra-articular hip pathology (e.g. labral tear) an arthro-MRI is needed. In unclear cases, diagnostic infiltration may help to differentiate the origin of pain. With these results the diagnosis will be made and a treatment and return-to-play plan established. Again, I recommend it be written as this helps an elite athlete have a very clear protocol where all involved can work from the same page.

Literature

Drew MK et al. Do Australian Football players have sensitive groins? Players with current groin pain exhibit mechanical hyperalgesia of the adductor tendon. J Sci Med Sport. 2016 Jan 7

Yang DC et al. Diagnosis of groin pain associated with sports hernia using dynamic ultrasound and physical examination: A case report. Ann Rehabil Med. 2015 Dec;39(6):1038-41

King E et al. Athletic groin pain: a systematic review and meta-analysis of surgical versus physical therapy rehabilitation outcomes. Br J Sports Med. 2015 Nov;49(22):1447-51.

Mosler AB et al. Which factors differentiate athletes with hip/groin pain from those without? A systematic review with meta-analysis. Br J Sports Med. 2015 Jun;49(12):810.

Weir A et al. Doha agreement meeting on terminology and definitions in groin pain in athletes. Br J Sports Med. 2015 Jun;49(12):768-74.

Crockett M et al. Groin Pain in Athletes: A Review of Diagnosis and Management. Surg Technol Int. 2015 May;26:275-82

Impingement of the Hip: FAI Femoro-Acetabular Impingement – The New Kid on the Block

Symptoms

Hip pain in the groin region, mostly felt 'deep within' (as with everything in medicine, there is no 100%, but, the opposite, a pain of the outer side of the hip is never ever a femoro-acetabular impingement). The pain gets distinctly worse after provoking manoeuvers and after intensive training sessions. It occurs mostly unilaterally, sometimes bilaterally. Even though the femoro-acetabular impingement mostly concerns both hips, only one side is symptomatic and painful at a time.

Figure 1: Normal Hip Anatomy

X-ray normal hip

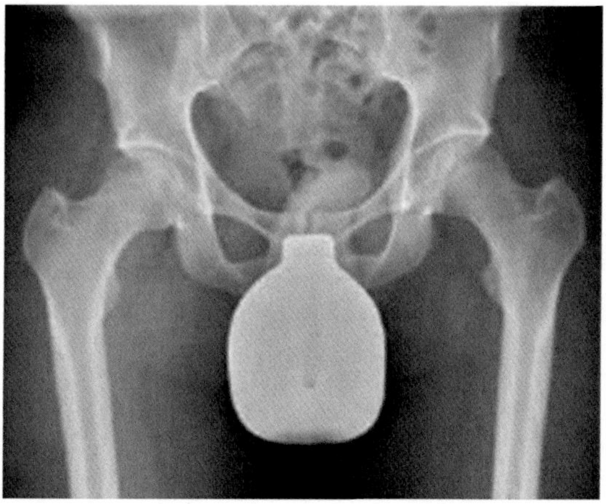

X-ray of the hip and pelvis basically normal

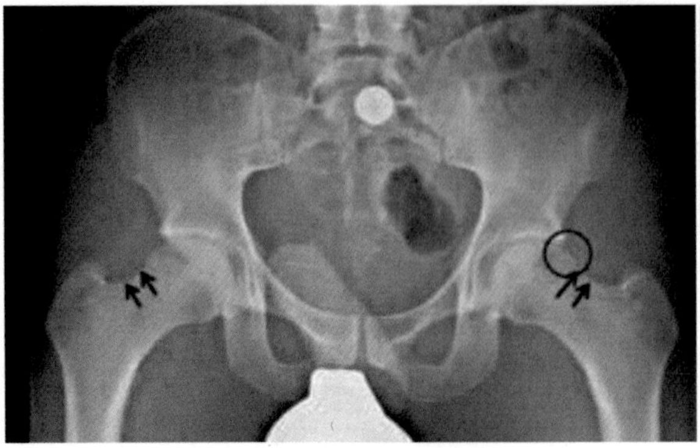

X-ray pelvis: both hips with femoro-acetabular impingement (FAI), mixed type (cam and pincer). Bump (O) and missing offset (←). Sclerosis of the joint socket (roof)

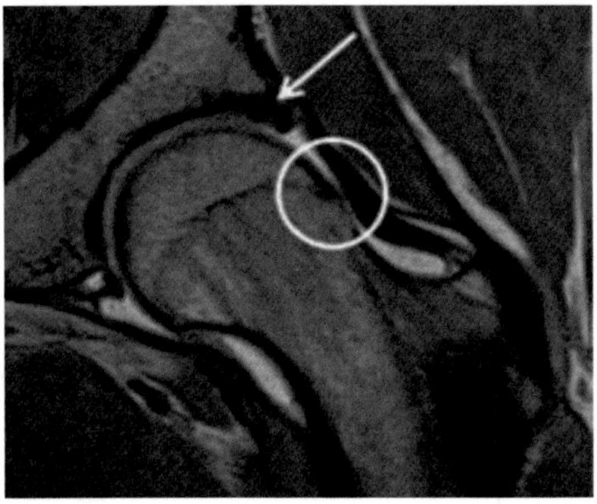

MRI hip with FAI. Bump (O) and pincer formation of the joint socket (←)

Background

The term *'femoro-acetabular impingement'* means a conflict of anatomical structures. In case of the hip impingement, it is about a conflict of the *femoral* head (the ball; uppermost part of the thigh bone) and the *acetabulum* (the joint socket) of the hip. There are two pre-existing configurations, the Cam and Pincer-impingement, differentiated.

Cam-impingement occurs because of a bumpy configuration instead of a nice offset of the femoral shaft, leading to repetitive impacts on the joint labrum, the rim of the acetabulum, and the weight bearing cartilage in the joint socket.

Pincer-impingement occurs because of an excessive overhang of the acetabular coverage, like pincers clamping the femoral head and leading to labral tear, stress to the outer rim of the acetabulum, and incongruent joint movements with secondary stress on the cartilage.

Diagnosis and treatment of femoro-acetabular impingement as diagnosis is still relatively new, but has become the reason for a lot of operations by orthopaedic surgeons.

It is certain, that a heavy femoro-acetabular impingement leads to injuries to the hip cartilage. It is most probable that these severe impingement situations with damaged cartilage will lead to early onset osteoarthritis and that an operation may improve the outcome. However long term data is still not available and questions like, 'Who needs an operation?'; 'Who will benefit from an operation?'; and 'Who will not benefit from an operation?' are not really answered yet.

Observing the high rate of hip impingement operations done now and remembering that twenty years ago it was absolutely *not* an issue and leads to this statement:

'Think twice before operating on a young athlete's hip – Try a conservative treatment first and seek a second opinion done by a (non-operative) sports medicine physician.'

Prevention and Treatment Table of Femoroacetabular Impingement

Prevention	There are two answers: 1. No real prevention possible, as you just have the configuration or you don't. 2. *But, yes,* there are factors recognised as possibly worsening the condition: deep squat jumps and frog hopping, heavy loading, or repetitive jumps out of these two positions. In Ice Hockey sprint exercises on-ice out of this squat position seem to provoke Cam-configuration hips and labral tears of the hip in formerly healthy athletes (Stull et al 2011, Philippon et al 2013).
Treatment by Yourself	Rest, then start with steady and regular exercising without impact and without too much hip flexion (e.g. cycling, deep water running, pull buoy swimming, slight freestyle/crawl and backstroke swimming *but no breaststroke*!)

When is a Doctor Needed?	When the pain impairs your regular training and provokes pain in daily life.
Return to Play/ Sports	Depending on the severity and the diagnosis. A lot of people with the suspected FAI luckily don't have it, but rather myofascial pelvic girdle pain or an adductor muscle problem. Quite a few athletes have slight FAI but a good hip mobility, especially still good internal rotation (IR). They profit from conservative treatment and don't need an operation. A minority has FAI with reduced hip mobility, especially reduced or lacking IR, and often with already injured cartilage. So an operation needs to be planned. The orthopaedic surgeon, the sports medicine physician, and the sport physiotherapist together will prepare a return to play protocol that tries to maintain a good level of general fitness after the operation, alternative training and a gradual loading of the treated hip over 3–4months.

What Does the Doctor Do?

The doctor takes the history and performs a clinical exam, stance and gait, and especially hip mobility and impingement manoeuvre (flexion-adduction-IR). Hip mobility seems to be crucial for both understanding the condition and for indicating further therapy. X-rays of the hip in two projections will give further evidence of the hip anatomy and configuration. If an impingement is suspected with the clinical assessment and the x-rays, an arthro-MRI (MRI with intraarticular contrast injection) is usually performed. This allows assessment of the bone, the cartilage, the labrum of the hip, possible stress zones, but in particular injured zones in the hip cartilage. This imaging, together with the history, the clinical findings, and the profile of the sport discipline, lead to an appreciation of the further treatment plan (see above).

Literature

Loudon JK et al. Conservative management of femoroacetabular impingement (FAI) in the long distance runner. Phys Ther Sport. 2014 May;15(2):82-90.

Wall PD et al. Nonoperative treatment for femoroacetabular impingement: a systematic review of the literature. PM R. 2013 May;5(5):418-26.

Hellman MD et al. Operative treatment of femoroacetabular impingement. Phys Sportsmed. 2014 Sep;42(3):112-9

Wall PD et al. Surgery for treating hip impingement (femoroacetabular impingement).Cochrane Database Syst Rev. 2014 Sep 8;9:CD010796.

Leunig M, Ganz R. The evolution and concepts of joint-preserving surgery of the hip. Bone Joint J. 2014 Jan;96-B(1):5-18.

Philippon MJ. Prevalence of increased alpha angles as a measure of cam-type femoroacetabular impingement in youth ice hockey players. Am J Sports Med. 2013 Jun;41(6):1357-62.

Stull JD et al."At-risk" positioning and hip biomechanics of the Peewee ice hockey sprint start. Am J Sports Med. 2011 Jul;39 Suppl:29S-35S.

Ganz R, Parvizi J, Beck M, Leunig M, Nötzli H, Siebenrock KA. Femoroacetabular impingement: a cause for osteoarthritis of the hip. Clin Orthop Relat Res. 2003 Dec;(417):112-20.

Ito K, Minka MA 2nd, Leunig M, Werlen S, Ganz R. Femoroacetabular impingement and the cam-effect. A MRI-based quantitative anatomical study of the femoral head-neck offset. J Bone Joint Surg Br. 2001 Mar;83(2):171-6

Painful Trigger Points – When the Muscle Hurts!

Symptoms

Painful muscle region, with an impairment of muscle activity. Typical local tenderness, muscle hardening, formation of a taut band structure, and typical and specific referred pain pattern for each muscle.

Background

What's a trigger point?

Etiologic factors for primary trigger point formation include: persistent muscular contraction, strain or overuse, trauma (with surrounding inflammatory reaction), adverse environmental conditions (e.g. cold, heat, etc.), prolonged inactivity and immobility, and low tissue oxygenation. There are also secondary trigger points, i.e. an underlying condition, disease, or injury provoking muscle contraction and overuse leading to a trigger point formation, e.g. myofascial lumbar and leg pain after a successful herniated disc operation. These latter conditions need careful attention and thorough appraisal as there may be an underlying condition your physiotherapist and your doctor should look for.

The formation of a trigger point leads to persistent tightening and sometimes formation of nodules of the muscle fibres. These are mostly invisible, but certainly palpable, as a hardening of the muscle with the formation of a taut band (or nodules) within the muscle structure. Palpating along this taut band structure, an often spindle shaped, more prominent, and more tightened muscle structure may be found. This is called the trigger point. The formation of trigger point often happens in athletes but also in everyday life, so it's not unusual to hear complaints about painful trigger points in the normal population.

Why do we additionally use the term 'myofascial'?

In talking about trigger points, we often use the term 'myofascial', deriving from 'myo', relating to the muscle; and 'fascial', relating to the fascia—the muscle sheath. The muscle and its fascia are an important entity, as the sheath often gives some guidance and shape to the muscle fibres and makes the connection to the adjacent muscles and the neighbouring tissues. In the trigger point treatment, the fascia is included.

Trigger points are a harmless entity and usually easily treatable.

Prevention and Treatment Table for Trigger Points

Prevention	Good warming up, regular stretching and flexibility exercises, and regular strengthening program, self-myofascial release (roll out)—especially for the 'delicate' zones, as shoulder girdle, back and core muscles, pelvis girdle, and hip abductors.
Treatment by Yourself	Local stretching, roll it out, rolling on a tennis ball, etc. Pain, independent of its origin, is a body signal that needs to be taken seriously. As trigger point formation is much more complex than a simple hardened muscle, there needs to be a professional understanding of anatomy, referred pain pattern, muscle chains, and possible underlying conditions and specific strengthening. So seek professional advice and treatment when it comes to trigger point related muscle pain.
When is a Doctor Needed?	When the pain is impairing your training and daily life. Usually the sport physiotherapist is a good person to contact as they will be able to start treatment immediately and give good advice on how to deal with it.

Return to Play/ Sports	Usually no pause needed. However, in severe cases, discuss with the treating sport physiotherapist or sports medicine physician, as there are sometimes heavy and severe trigger point problems, where you need to get to the bottom of it with a longer series of treatment sessions. In a second step the treatment consists of a strengthening and stretching program for this particular muscle group.

What Does the Doctor Do?

After taking the history, the doctor or physiotherapist performs a clinical exam that mostly reveals the muscle hardening, formation of the taut band, and the muscle specific referred pain pattern. The exam includes a general assessment of the movement pattern of the affected body region and often reveals further trigger points and muscle hardening in adjacent and sometimes even antagonistic muscles. *Trigger point treatment* consists of balanced but firm, focused compression directly onto the trigger point itself, manual loosening of the muscle fascia, smoothing of the whole muscle and fascia, and stretching of this muscle.

Instead of manual compression a *dry needling* may be done. In dry needling, the trigger point is treated and released by placing a very thin needle (usually acupuncture needle) into the middle of the trigger point. With dry needling, a muscle twitch response may often be observed.

Once you've started and the pain is distinctly better, the therapist's second step is to ask you to perform *specific strengthening exercises* for the muscle group concerned. This strengthening is usually done for two to three months as it is about preventing a recurrence of this trigger point pain syndrome.

Literature

Gautschi Roland, Manuelle Triggerpunkttherapie: Myofasziale Schmerzen und Funktionsstörungen erkennen, verstehen und behandeln. Verlag: Thieme; Auflage: 3 (13. Juli 2016). ISBN-13: 978-3131474735

Travell, Janet; Simons David; Simons Lois (1999). Myofascial Pain and Dysfunction: The Trigger Point Manual (2 vol. set, 2nd Ed.). USA: Lippincott Williams & Williams. ISBN 0-683-08363-5.

Tough EA et al. Variability of criteria used to diagnose myofascial trigger point pain syndrome—evidence from a review of the literature. Clin J Pain 23 (3): 278–86.

McPartland JM, (June 2004). Travell trigger points--molecular and osteopathic perspectives. Journal of the American Osteopathic Association 104 (6): 244–49.

Alvarez DJ, Rockwell PG. Trigger points: diagnosis and management. Am Fam Physician 2002, 65 (4): 653–60.

Lucas N et al. Reliability of physical examination for diagnosis of myofascial trigger points: a systematic review of the literature. Clin J Pain 2009, 25 (1): 80–9.

Myburgh, C et al. A systematic, critical review of manual palpation for identifying myofascial trigger points: evidence and clinical significance. Arch Phys Med Rehabil. 2008, 89 (6): 1169–76.

Chaitow L; J Walker-DeLaney. Clinical Applications of Neuromuscular Techniques .Vol 2, pg. 20 ff. Churchill Livingstone; 2 edition July 19, 2011

Sport Injuries

Tissue Repair Mechanism and Time Frame – What Does This Mean for Sports?

Symptoms

The disruption of the integrity of skin, mucosal surface, or organ tissue results in the formation of a wound. With the aim of restoring tissue integrity, multiple cellular and extracellular pathways are activated. Four phases of wound healing and tissue repair are differentiated: coagulation, inflammation, proliferation, and tissue remodelling.

Phase /Name	Time Frame	What Happens	How Does It Look Like/Feel Like?
1 Coagulation/ Haemostasis	Immediately (within seconds)	Constriction of blood vessels, formation of a fibrin plug, thrombin activation, platelet activation (crucial in wound healing, release of prostaglanding, leukotrienes, thromboxanes)	*Fresh wound with stopped bleeding*
2 Inflammation	Hours–72h	After the clot formation the *'body's own wound cleaning'* takes place, slowly settling down over 3 days *Neutrophils*, body's own white blood cells, destroy debris and bacteria to prevent infection	*Warm red, swollen early wound*

		Macrophages, larger phagocytic cells, enter the wound, regulate the inflammatory response, and support the formation of granulation tissue	
3 Proliferation	72h–10days	It's the collagen synthetised by fibroblasts providing strength to tissues Angiogenesis (formation of capillaries), the formation of granulation tissue, collagen deposition, epithelialisation, and wound retraction are a further part of the proliferative stage Collagen deposition is maximal by day 5 (Lymphocytes produce an extracellular matrix and regulate the collagen remodelling. Fibroblasts lay down matrix proteins and a different range of collagens)	*Pink, vascular, fibrous tissue,* usually formed underneath the clot
4 Remodelling	10days–2yrs	*Collagens* and *proteins* in the wound *increasingly well organised, eventually regaining structure* similar to the unwounded tissue (collagen type 1 replaced by type 3)	*Scar formation and organisation from red to pink to grey-white,* as vascularity decreases

Factors Influencing Wound Healing and Tissue Repair (in Particular Regard to Sports)

Nutrition

Malnutrition, hypocaloric diet, athletes with bad eating habits, or eating disorders are at a particular risk of having bad wound healing—all are prolonging the inflammation phase, inhibiting fibroblast function, reducing angiogenesis, and impair collagen deposition.

Proteins (delivering amino acids), *carbohydrates* (keeping the metabolism anabolic), *vitamin C* (collagen formation), *vitamin A* (epidermal growth), and *omega 3 fatty acids* (modulating activation pathway, membrane formation) are of particular interest and should be addressed in injured athletes at risk.

Hypoxia

Sufficient oxygen is an essential requirement for a wound to heal (whereas a certain degree of hypoxia facilitates the epithelialisation, i.e. wound closure). *Smoking* clearly causes more wound complications, affects immune system, and impairs collagen deposition.

Infection

A wound infection impairs and prolongs wound healing. Athletes in heavy training periods are more susceptible to any infection due to reduced immune function. Early wound disinfection as well as appropriate wound care is therefore a must in high level athletes.

Immunosuppression

With a reduced immune response, the wound healing processes are delayed and less effective. Patients with HIV, cancer, steroid treatment, or malnutrition have a reduced immune function. High level athletes in strenuous training periods have a lowered immune response too. Particularly in sportsmen and women with low body weight or eating disorders, a reinforcement of an adequate diet should be aimed for.

Medications

The so called *NSAID (non-steroidal anti-inflammatory drugs)* with active substances like ibuprofen, mefenamic acid, diclofenac, etc. were for many years, widely used in the early treatment of any type of injury. With better understanding of the wound healing cascade, we conclude that an anti-inflammatory drug will probably impair the inflammation phase of the wound healing in an acute injury. It should therefore not be used for the first 48–72 hours. If pain is an issue, and a medication needed, paracetamol (just analgesic, no anti-inflammatory action) may be an alternative.

Chronic diseases (e.g. diabetes), older age, and inadequate wound management complete the list of factors negatively influencing wound healing.

Genetics

In some families there is a tendency for overgrowth of scar tissue, extending beyond the wound edges. These are called *keloid scars.* They most commonly occur on shoulders, arms, or upper chest. They may be aesthetically distracting, sometimes they can be itchy and provoke some pain, and unluckily they have a high recurrence rate even after treatment.

Prevention and Treatment Table for Tissue Repair Mechanism/Wound Healing

Prevention	Injuries may happen, that's part of an athlete's life. *But* be ready and do the right things.
Treatment by Yourself	Good and immediate wound disinfection (athlete's little first aid kit) is the right starting point. If the lesion is more severe, look for an appropriate wound care. Allow enough time for wound healing.
When is a Doctor Needed?	As soon as there is a structural lesion in an underlying tissue or a wound of the skin needing stitches. Think about the 6 hours rule if you need stitches (see also chapter 'Skin Injuries')
Return to Play/Sports	Depending on the severity. It's understandable that wound healing is better if you can rest for the first few days. A skin wound with stitches will heal much more nicely if you don't push too hard the first 10–14 days, for example.

Literature

Young A, CE McNaught. The physiology of wound healing. Surgery (Oxford) 10/2011; 29(10):475–479.

Paoloni JA , Milne C , Orchard J , et al . Nonsteroidal anti-infl ammatory drugs in sports medicine: guidelines for practical but sensible use. Br J Sports Med 2009 ; 43 : 863 – 5

Lindaman LM. Bone healing in children. Clin Podiatr Med Surg. 2001 Jan;18(1):97-108

Hunt T et al. Physiology of wound healing. Adv Skin Wound Care. 2000 May-Jun;13(2 Suppl):6-11.

Soft Tissue Injuries in Sports – RICE, PRICE, or POLICE

Symptoms

A soft tissue injury is very common in sport. It may be a simple contusion, a bruise, or even a slight sprain—in all these, there is by definition, no further underlying structural damage.

It usually presents as a tender, slightly swollen, slightly discoloured body site usually allowing activities of daily life and resolving within three to five days.

Background:

Sometimes it's not that easy to differentiate a soft tissue injury from a structural one. In training and competition, a slight injury may not even be noticed (also due to the body's own adrenalin and endorphins released while being active in sports) and, when the organism is cooled down, the pain sensation is much more intense. The indications below may help you to differentiate. If you are uncertain, seek professional advice.

Table 1: Indications to Differentiate a Soft Tissue Injury From a Structural Injury

Soft tissue injury	Structural injury
• Low energy injury • Injury mechanism, usual joint angles respected • No joint effusion • Game could be finished • Weight bearing and walking possible • Slight swelling, slight discolouration • Slight pain	• High energy injury • Mechanism with overly joint movements • Distinct joint effusion • Player needed to be replaced • Weight bearing, walking not possible • Heavy swelling, subcutaneous bleeding • Pain as never before, night pain

As there is no underlying structural damage, treatment is called symptomatic, means reducing the pain and the swelling. The treatment follows the acronyms PRICE or POLICE, see in the following table a comparison of the two propositions.

Table 2: Acronyms PRICE and POLICE for Treatment of a Sports Injury

Acronym	Meaning	Evidence - Comparison	Acronym	Meaning
P	**Protection**	**Protection** prevents further injury at the already vulnerable site and allows a good healing response.	P	**Protection**
R	**Rest** Stop the game, the training, allow some rest, e.g. allow 5–7days.	There is evidence for both: • Immediate **rest** to allow a good initial healing response, just lasting a few days. The signs of the healing response (e.g. pain, swelling, impaired movements) are leading very well through the first days* • **Optimal loading** to allow a functional result, with good common sense and a reasonable observation of the healing response*	OL	**Optimal loading** Start the active re-habilitation as soon as possible, functional treatment approach, e.g. start after 5–7days.
I	**Ice** Bring cold to the injured body site.	**Ice** has an analgetic effect and helps to prevent heavy swelling. Cold water, cooling bandages, crushed ice, cold packs, etc. may be used. Be careful not to burn your skin by applying the frozen cold pack or ice cubes directly, and for too long, onto the skin. Don't use ice sprays anymore, as the ingredients are often problematic, some even toxic, often provoking burning injuries. Use the options above.	I	**Ice** Bring cold to the injured body site.

C	**Compression** Of the injured body site.	**Compression**, e.g. with a bandage (or a cooling bandage), prevents the formation of a bigger subcutaneous haematoma and is mostly comfortable for further transport, etc.	C	**Compres-sion** Of the injured body site.
E	**Elevation** Of the injured limb or body site	**Elevation** will prevent a heavier swelling. This is important for two reasons, the injury leads to swelling (haematoma formation or tissue fluid collection) and lesser use of an injured limb provoking a swelling because of remaining lymphatic fluid.	E	**Elevation** Of the injured limb or body site

* **Common sense is required!** Get professional help and advice by your sports medicine physician and your physiotherapist! You could **rest too long** (for instance, putting an athlete with ankle sprain and band rupture in a cast with crutches for four weeks) and have a poor outcome and lose time. But you could also push too hard and **start loading too early** (for instance, the same athlete, same injury, just giving an orthesis/ankle brace and continue training as before), resulting in insufferable pain, heavy swelling, and poor and insufficient healing of the ruptured ligament.

Prevention and Treatment Table for Soft Tissue Injuries

Prevention	• Good warming up, including sport-specific proprioceptive and strengthening exercises • Appropriate equipment and good training conditions
Treatment by Yourself	See Table 2 above. Whether you use PRICE or POLICE, do it with good common sense.
When is a Doctor Needed?	As soon as a structural lesion is suspected, see Table 1.
Return to Play/ Sports	In case of a simple soft tissue injury, normally no long training pause is needed. In case of a structural injury according to the return to play protocol.

What does the Doctor Do?

The doctor takes the history and performs a clinical exam. If unclear, further imaging may be necessary to exclude a structural injury. The return to play plan will be established according to the diagnosed injury.

Literature

Bleakley CM, P Glasgow, DC Macauley. PRICE Needs Updating, Should We Call The POLICE. Br J Sports Med March 2012, 46(4) 220-21,

Bleakley CM , O'Connor SR , Tully MA , Et Al. Effect Of Accelerated Rehabilitation On Function After Ankle Sprain: Randomised Controlled Trial. BMJ 2010; 340 : C1964

Widman M. "Magic freeze sprays can do deep damage" retrieved 5.6.2016 on http://www.dw.com/en/magic-freeze-sprays-can-do-deep-damage/a-18520903, first published 16.6.2015

Jones MH , Amendola AS. Acute Treatment Of Inversion Ankle Sprains: Immobilization Versus Functional Treatment. Clin Orthop Relat Res 2007 ; 455: 169 – 72 .

Kerkhoffs GM , Rowe BH , Assendelft WJ , Et Al. Immobilisation And Functional Treatment For Acute Lateral Ankle Ligament Injuries In Adults. Cochranedatabase Syst Rev 2002; 3 :CD003762.

Khan KM , Scott A. Mechanotherapy: How Physicaltherapists' Prescription Of Exercise Promotes Tissue Repair. Br J Sports Med 2009; 43 : 247 – 52

Ankle Sprain or Tear – the Most Frequent Sports Injury, Good Management Is Essential

Symptoms

Immediate, local pain, (initial) disability to bear weight on the injured foot, and gradual onset of swelling. In case of a structural injury this swelling may be very pronounced in the days following the injury and take the typical colours of subcutaneous bleeding—purple-blue to green-yellow after a few days.

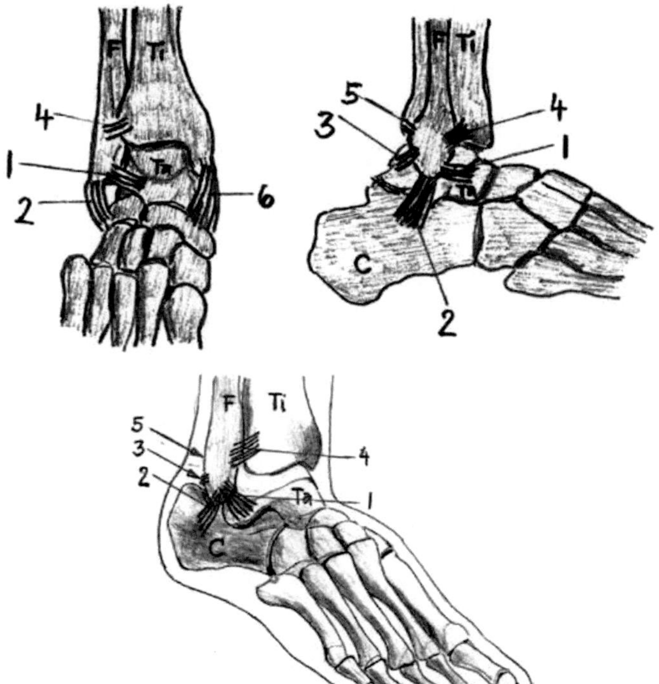

Key:

1. Anterior talofibular ligament
2. Calcaneofibular ligament
3. Posterior talofibular ligament
4. Anterior syndesmosis
5. Posterior syndesmosis
6. Deltoid ligament

C. Calcaneus
Ta. Talus
Ti. Tibia
F. Fibula

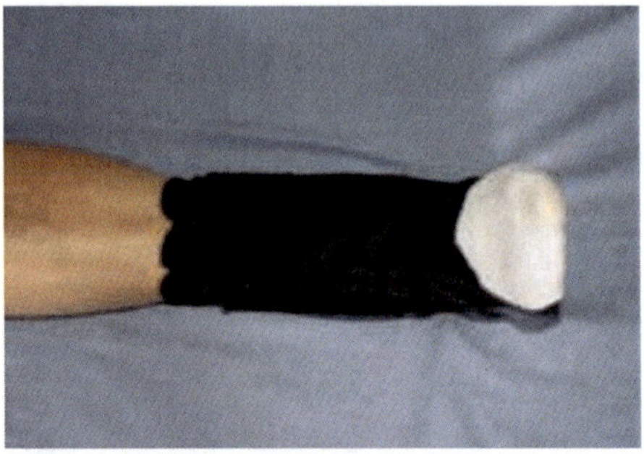

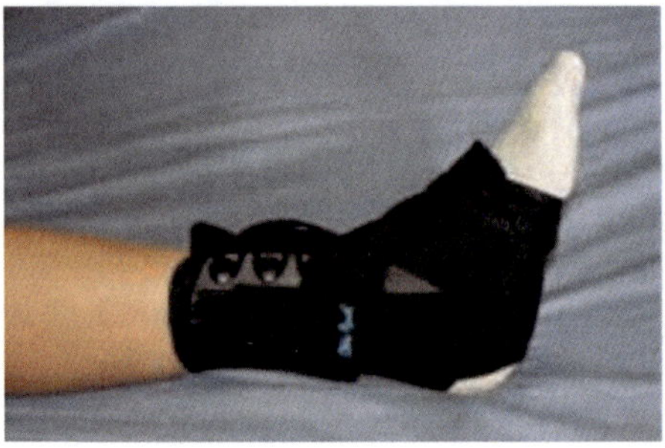

Picture: Ideal orthesis/ankle brace preventing inversion and, equally important, preventing plantarflexion

Background

Ankle sprain or tear is simply the most frequent sport injury. The most often described cause of injury is an inversion-plantarflexion mechanism, leading to high stress on the lateral ligament complex of the ankle with the whole palette of injuries from an simple sprain up to the complete rupture of the whole ligament complex. In high energy accidents, there can also be concomitant injuries to neighbouring anatomical structures (e.g. bone fractures of the ankle, fifth metatarsal, etc.).

Prevention and Treatment Table for Ankle Sprain and Tear

Prevention	• Good warming up, including proprioceptive and strengthening exercises • Good sport shoes and appropriate training conditions (enough light, no obstacles on the pitch, good condition of the pitch, etc.)
Treatment by Yourself	• A mild sprain with no or just slight swelling; no great discolouration and no impairment on gait may be treated by you with PRICE and an elastic bandage • All other conditions need professional treatment
When is a Doctor Needed?	As soon as a structural injury is suspected (e.g. more energy in the misstep, an audible noise during injury, heavier swelling, pain while standing or walking, discolouration, etc.).
Return to Play/ Sports	The healing of the lateral ligament complex takes 6 weeks for initial stabilisation, usually it is the same time to return to sports on a competitive level. But training to be ready for that moment starts much earlier, in the first week after the injury! The individual plan is designed according to the grade of injury, usually leaving out running for 3–4 weeks, jumping and landing for 5–6 weeks, but allowing many other types of training (e.g. with ankle brace on bike one week after the accident, etc.) As shown in the example (Table 1) and in the photos, the orthesis/ankle brace needs to be firm in guiding the ankle and prevent inversion *and* plantarflexion! Sadly there are still quite few really insufficient braces around. Important: The orthesis/ankle brace needs to be worn 24h/7d – especially during the night too. While sleeping our feet would naturally go in a plantarflexed position, thus leading to an insufficient, elongated healing.

What Does the Doctor Do?

The doctor takes the history to understand the injury mechanism, performs a clinical exam to judge the extent of injury. The clinical exam of your sports medicine physician or your sports physiotherapist is relevant in judging the stability of your ankle. Mostly, but not always, x-rays are needed to exclude a fracture or avulsion (the tear of a ligament with its bony insertion). An MRI is needed only if additional injuries are suspected, as it delivers no further information about an acute injury.

After the exact diagnosis, an appropriate treatment plan with the return to sports protocol is established.

Table 1: Example for an Athlete With Complete Rupture of the Anterior Fibulo-Talar and the Fibulo-Calcanear Ligament

Activities	1st week	2nd week	3rd week	4th week	5th week	6th week
Ankle Orthesis	Yes Day And Night	Yes Day And Night	Yes Day And Night	Yes Day And Night	Yes Day/Ev Night	Yes Day/Ev Night
Crutches RICE	Ev 3–7days Yes					
Antiinflammatory therapy Locally	Yes					
Physiotherapy (e.g. initial manoeuvres supporting lymphatic drainage, proprioception, strengthening, etc.)						
Endurance training		Yes				
Strength training						
Running	No	No	No	No		
Team training	No	No	No	No		

Literature

McGovern RP et al. Managing ankle ligament sprains and tears: current opinion. Open Access Journal of Sports Medicine.March 2016 Volume 2016:7; 33—42

Doherty C et al. Recovery From a First-Time Lateral Ankle Sprain and the Predictors of Chronic Ankle Instability: A Prospective Cohort Analysis. Am J Sports Med. 2016 Feb 24. pii: 0363546516628870.

Walls RJ et al. Football injuries of the ankle: A review of injury mechanisms, diagnosis and management. World J Orthop. 2016 Jan 18; 7(1):8-19.

Kobayashi T et al. Intrinsic Risk Factors of Lateral Ankle Sprain: A Systematic Review and Meta-analysis. Sports Health. 2015 Dec 28.

Lievers WB, Adamic PF. Incidence and Severity of Foot and Ankle Injuries in Men's Collegiate American Football. Orthop J Sports Med. 2015 Apr 22; 3(5

McKeon PO. Understanding and treating lateral ankle sprains and their consequences: a constraints-based approach. Sports Med. 2013 Jun;43(6):385-93.

Hubbard TJ, Wikstrom EA. Ankle sprain: pathophysiology, predisposing factors, and management strategies. Open Access J Sports Med. 2010 Jul 16;1:115-22.

Leumann A, R Tsaknis, M Wiewiorski, V Valderrabano. Acute supination trauma of the upper ankle joint – a trifle? http://medicalforum.ch/docs/smf/archiv/de/2008/2008-11/2008-11-126.pdf

Eiff MP, Smith AT, Smith GE. Early mobilization versus immobilization in the treatment of lateral ankle sprains. Am J Sports Med. 1994 Jan-Feb;22(1):83-8.

Non-Structural Muscle Injury – Quick Recovery but Stick to Your RTP

Symptom

Circumscribed well-defined pain and aching in a muscle, onset of pain may be acute (in sport) or gradually increasing with muscle firmness and tension, usually increasing with continued activity. May or may not be painful at rest.

Figure 1: Muscle Structure

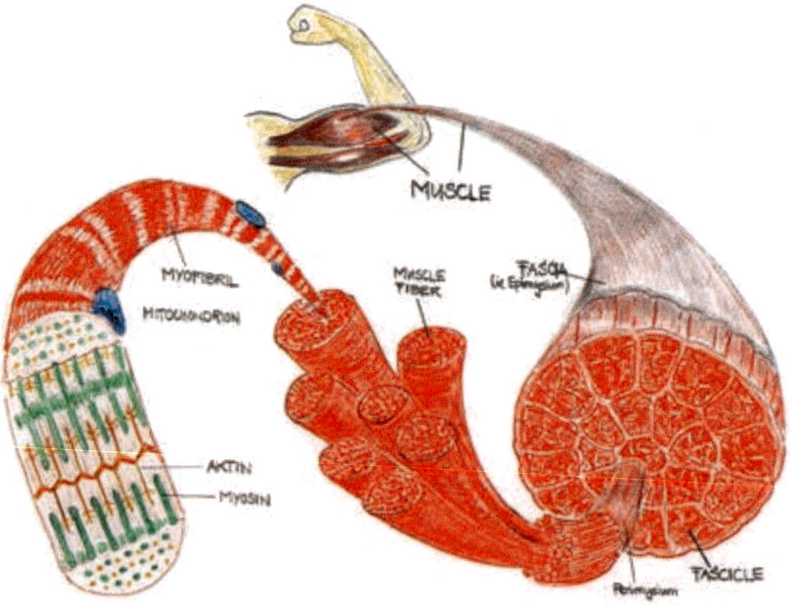

Background

Muscle injuries are frequent in sport. They may be from an indirect (without any external forces, without opponent contact) or direct injury mechanism (with external force, contusion or laceration). The affected muscle may suffer a non-structural or a structural injury. A high percentage of the contusions are non-structural, whereas the indirect trauma mechanism mostly show structural muscle lesions.

On-field sport injuries are often difficult to sort out—which type is it? But this differentiation is important, not yet on-field but directly later, as both need appropriate evaluation, diagnosis, and treatment. Non-structural injuries don't show any structural interruption in the integrity of the muscle and the athlete can normally return to play within 5–10 days, if the RTP plan is properly designed and respected. Whereas structural muscle injuries show this interruption and return to play takes between 6–12 weeks.

The treatment of a muscle injury, non-structural or structural, is almost always conservative and this shows best results. Operative techniques show poor outcomes and are rarely used.

Prevention and Treatment Table for Non-Structural Muscle Injury

Prevention	• Good warming up, integrating sports specific proprioceptive and strengthening exercises. Nordic hamstrings lower-exercise (or other eccentric exercise specifically for hamstrings muscles) • Good management of any muscle disorder, be it non-structural or structural
Treatment by Yourself	PRICE or POLICE are good treatment options, see the corresponding chapter.
When is a Doctor Needed?	In an acute muscle injury, which leads to excessive pain, impaired function, or when a structural muscle injury is suspected.
Return to Play/ Sports	Usually within 5–10 days. Together with your sports medicine physician, physiotherapist, and coach, make a detailed plan for the days ahead. Load gradually, and as you know there is no structural defect, you may increase stepwise and quite quickly, resulting in an early return to sport. Remember: If you don't stick to your RTP, you may easily risk a structural injury!

What Does the Doctor Do?

The doctor takes the history and performs the clinical exam. In muscle injuries, it needs to be emphasised, anamnesis and clinical examination are crucial for a correct evaluation, diagnosis, and treatment plan. In many situations, further imaging with ultrasound, or possibly even MRI, may help rule out a structural muscle injury. It is important to know that there are a few situations where a transient signal alteration in ultrasound and/or MRI may be present *without* any structural lesion. These alterations correspond mostly to interstitial fluid collections (tissue edema) and not to any structural muscle damage.

Literature

Pollock N et al. Time to return to full training is delayed and recurrence rate is higher in intratendinous ('c') acute hamstring injury in elite track and field athletes: clinical application of the British Athletics Muscle Injury Classification. Br J Sports Med. 2016 Mar;50(5):305-10.

Patel A et al. British athletics muscle injury classification: a reliability study for a new grading system. Clin Radiol. 2015 Dec;70(12):1414-20.

Pollock N et al.British athletics muscle injury classification : a new grading system. Br J Sports Med 2014;48: 1347–1351.

Maffulli N et al. Muscle Injuries: A Brief Guide to Classification and Management. Transl Med UniSa. 2014 Sep 1;12:14-8.

Ueblacker P et al. Nonoperative treatment and return to play after complete proximal adductor avulsion in high-performance athletes. Knee Surg Sports Traumatol Arthrosc. 2015 Jun 9.

Ekstrand J, et al. Return to play after thigh muscle injury in elite football players: implementation and validation of the Munich muscle injury classification. Br J Sports Med. 2013 Aug;47(12):769-74.

Tol JL et al. Palpating muscles, massaging the evidence? An editorial relating to 'Terminology and classification of muscle injuries in sport: The Munich consensus statement'. Br J Sports Med. 2013 Apr;47(6):340-1.

Mueller-Wohlfahrt HW et al. Terminology and classification of muscle injuries in sport: the Munich consensus statement. Br J Sports Med. 2013 Apr;47(6):342-50.

Structural Muscle Injury – Lasts Longer

Symptoms

Sharp, needle-like or stabbing pain at time of injury. Often (but not always) athletes experience a 'snap', followed by a sudden onset of localised pain. Possible fall of the athlete while injured.

Illustration 1: Rupture of Muscle Fibre Bundle

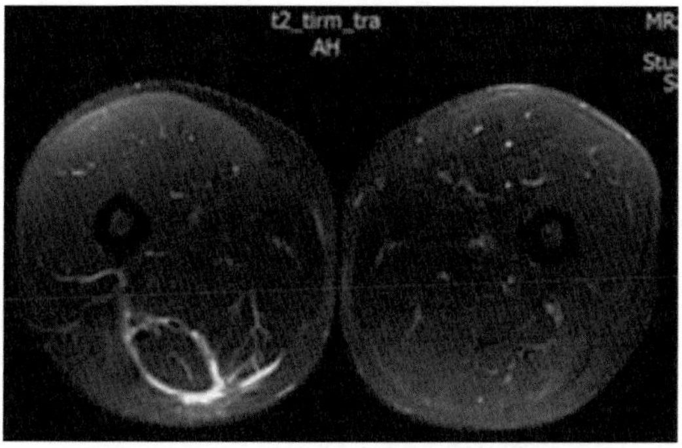

MRI cross sectional view upper thigh with liquid around hamstring muscle

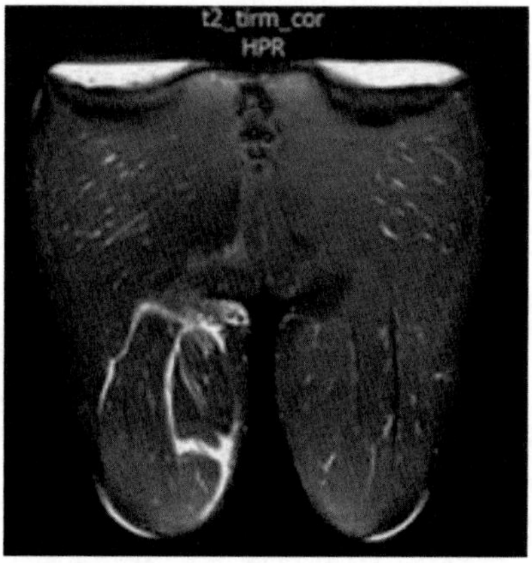

MRI frontal view of bottom/upper thigh with ruptured insertion of the hamstrings muscle

Background

Muscle injuries are very common in sport. In football/soccer, 92% affect the four major muscle groups of the lower limbs: hamstrings 37%, adductors 23%, quadriceps 19%, and calf muscles 13%. Non-contact situations (injury caused by internal forces) account for as much as 96% of all muscle injuries in football/soccer. Whereas contusions or lacerations (caused by external forces like a direct blow from an opponent's knee) are more frequent in contact sports like rugby, American football, and ice-hockey.

Muscles that are frequently involved in injuries are often bi-articular, undergo eccentric contraction, and contain primarily fast-twitch type 2 muscle fibres (e.g. hamstrings, quadriceps, and gastrocnemius). 16% of muscle injuries are re-injuries and associated with a longer absence from competition than the original injury—this underlines the importance of a correct evaluation, diagnosis, and therapy of the initial muscle injury – again patience and a solid RTP are essential!.

Prevention and Treatment Table for Structural Muscle Injury

Prevention	• Good warming up, integrating sports specific proprioceptive and strengthening exercises. Address in particular the muscle groups with the most frequent structural injuries: o Hamstring muscles: Nordic hamstrings lower or other eccentric hamstring exercises o Quadriceps muscles: single leg squats, single leg jumps and controlled landings o Calf muscles: eccentric calf exercises on stairs, possibly with dynamic execution • Good management of any muscle injury, be it non-structural or structural
Treatment by Yourself	A structural muscle injury needs a continuous professional follow-up.

When is a Doctor Needed?	As soon as a structural muscle injury is suspected.
Return to Play/Sports	Depending on the severity the return to play on a competitive level may take: • From 6 weeks, e.g. with a structural partial muscle tear • Up to 12–13 weeks, e.g. with a subtotal muscle tear or complete avulsion of a muscle tendon 5 phases are recommended and characterised by: 1) Acute management (2–3days) PRICE management: *Ice*, moderate stretching as pain allows (to give orientation for the healing response), eventually *rest* in form of crutches (to avoid lengthening of the injured muscle) 2) Post-acute management (3–7days after trauma) POLICE management: including *optimal loading*, tissue drainage supporting measures, compressive bandages (e.g. neopren tube or wrap), muscle stretching, neural mobilisation, and slight isometric exercises 3) Functional rehabilitation and general athletic reconditioning (starting in the first week) When isometric exercises can be performed without pain, concentric activity may be started gradually, only with complete absence of pain, sensorial motor training, general reconditioning respecting the injury site, core stability 4) Athletic reconditioning and specific strength Sport specific rehabilitation, fitness and strength training, already reaching higher levels and aiming to high intensity protocols (without involving the injured body site), exercises gradually involving the injured limb/body site, including slight eccentric exercises 5) Getting ready to return to competition Rehabilitation training with specific strengthening of the injured muscle, in all modalities and angles, gradually increasing volume and intensity. Further including lactacid work and explosive strength of the index muscle, integrating team training, and gradual return to full activity

What Does the Doctor Do?

The doctor takes the history and performs the clinical exam. In muscle injuries anamnesis and clinical examination are crucial for correct evaluation, diagnosis, and decision-making about the appropriate imaging. Ultrasound and mostly also MRI allow the doctor to quantify the extent and exact location of the injured muscle.

Ask your sports medicine physician and your physiotherapist for a detailed six week plan, this allows you to plan your return to sports at your best!

Table 1:

Activities	1st week		2nd week	3rd week	4th week	5th week	6th week
Neopren tube	Yes Day And Night		Yes Day	Yes Day	Yes Day	Yes Day	Yes Day
Crutches PRICE /POLICE	Ev3d	Ev7d					
Stretching (respecting pain)	Start Yes	Yes	Yes	Yes	Yes	Yes	Yes
Physiotherapy (e.g. initial manoeuvres supporting lymphatic drainage, stretching, proprioception, strengthening, etc.)	Yes	Yes	3–5x	3–5x	3–5x	3–5x	3–5x
Endurance training			Yes				
Strength training							
Running	No		No	No	No		
Team training	No		No	No	No		

Literature

Pollock N et al. Time to return to full training is delayed and recurrence rate is higher in intratendinous ('c') acute hamstring injury in elite track and field athletes: clinical application of the British Athletics Muscle Injury Classification. Br J Sports Med. 2016 Mar;50(5):305-10.

Patel A et al. British athletics muscle injury classification: a reliability study for a new grading system. Clin Radiol. 2015 Dec;70(12):1414-20.

Pollock N et al.British athletics muscle injury classification : a new grading system. Br J Sports Med 2014;48: 1347–1351.

Maffulli N et al. Muscle Injuries: A Brief Guide to Classification and Management. Transl Med UniSa. 2014 Sep 1;12:14-8.

Ueblacker P et al. Nonoperative treatment and return to play after complete proximal adductor avulsion in high-performance athletes. Knee Surg Sports Traumatol Arthrosc. 2015 Jun 9.

Ekstrand J, et al. Return to play after thigh muscle injury in elite football players: implementation and validation of the Munich muscle injury classification. Br J Sports Med. 2013 Aug;47(12):769-74.

Tol JL et al. Palpating muscles, massaging the evidence? An editorial relating to 'Terminology and classification of muscle injuries in sport: The Munich consensus statement'. Br J Sports Med. 2013 Apr;47(6):340-1.

Mueller-Wohlfahrt HW et al. Terminology and classification of muscle injuries in sport: the Munich consensus statement. Br J Sports Med. 2013 Apr;47(6):342-50.

Partial or Complete Rupture of a Ligament: Medial Collateral Ligament of the Knee – Treatment Plan and Time Frame

Symptoms

Acute injury to the knee with typically forced inward bending of the knee (valgus stress) with or without contact with an opponent. Distinct pain, mostly superficial swelling, and tenderness on palpation on the inner side of the knee. Impaired movement on the knee, sometimes perceived instability of the knee towards the inner side.

Background

Ligaments are important structures in our body, giving stability to our joints. They consist of very robust and quite rigid tissue, the connective tissue. This tissue contains a solid network of fibres, usually made out of collagen and connective tissue cells. In case of an injury, i.e. partial or complete tear of a ligament, the tissue is able to fix this tear by a specific regeneration process, leading to a scar formation. If sufficient time for this healing response is given, the newly formed ligament is as stable as before the injury (see chapter 'Tissue Repair Mechanism and Time Frame').

Prevention and Treatment Table for a Ruptured Ligament

Prevention	Good strengthening in general and a sport specific warming up with proprioceptive and strengthening exercises in particular are helpful in prevention.
Treatment by Yourself	• In case of a total or partial rupture of a ligament follow the treatment plan of your sports medicine physician and your physiotherapist

	• Respect the healing time of a ligament—6 weeks for initial stability, 12 weeks for a return back to normal
When is a Doctor Needed?	As soon as you feel, or think, a ligament could be ruptured. At least see a doctor if you observe an instability in your ankle, knee, elbow, or shoulder.
Return to Play/Sports	The six weeks healing time to the initial stabilisation and 12 weeks until complete recovery of a totally ruptured ligament give the time frame to plan the return to play. A detailed plan on a six week basis needs to be worked out, as the fitness level may be kept up and a lot of training modalities (without a particular loading) may be started very early, usually in the second week after the accident. With an orthesis on the injured joint to allow a good healing of the injured structure, and formation of solid scar tissue, an optimal loading may be possible.

What Does the Doctor Do?

The doctor takes the history and performs a clinical exam. In case of a complete ligament rupture the diagnosis is usually already clear by now. Sometimes the situation is less clear, i.e. when the patient is not really relaxed; other additional injuries are suspected and initial findings are awaiting additional x-Rays, ultrasound, or MRI, which will confirm or exclude a particular diagnosis.

If a rupture of a ligament, e.g. complete rupture of the medial collateral ligament (MCL) of the knee, is confirmed the treatment plan is established. Many acute injuries with ligament ruptures are treated conservatively, i.e. without surgery. With an MCL rupture, a knee orthesis is adjusted and a treatment plan for the following 6 weeks is established. Usually the orthesis is worn for the whole first 6 weeks. With the start of week 7 the orthesis is still worn for another 6 weeks for sport specific training, but it is discarded for daily life. Six weeks after the initial accidents training close to a competitive level, with the orthesis on (!), is usually possible.

Literature

Bates NA et al. Relative strain in the anterior cruciate ligament and medial collateral ligament during simulated jump landing and sidestep cutting tasks: implications for injury risk. Am J Sports Med. 2015 Sep;43(9):2259-69.

Sankar WN et al. Combined anterior cruciate ligament and medial collateral ligament injuries in adolescents. J Pediatr Orthop. 2006 Nov-Dec;26(6):733-6.

Larsen E et al. Long-term outcome of knee and ankle injuries in elite football. Scand J Med Sci Sports. 1999 Oct;9(5):285-9.

ACL (Anterior Cruciate Ligament) Rupture – When the Central Knee Ligament Goes

Symptoms

After an acute injury with a distortion, a twisting or hyperextension of the knee, the athlete observes a sore knee, usually with a quite distinct swelling within hours. Sometimes the acute trauma may be combined with an audible noise and a giving way when the anterior cruciate ligament (ACL) tears. With the rupture of the ACL, the onset of the 'giving way' feeling is one of the leading symptoms.

Figure 1: MRI lateral view of the knee

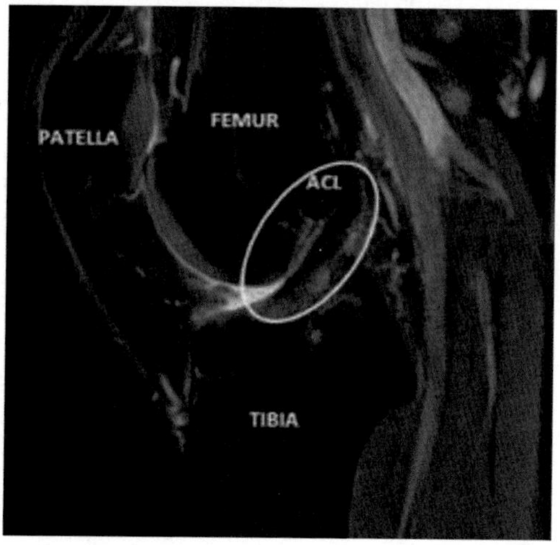

MRI knee: Anterior cruciate ligament normal and fully intact

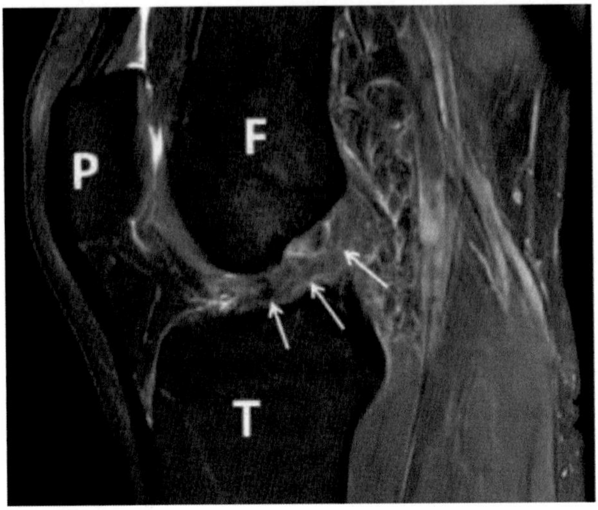

MRI ruptured ACL

P Patella, F Femur, T Tibia

Background

The anterior (ACL) and the posterior cruciate ligament (PCL) are important central stabilisers of the knee. At a first glimpse, one could assume the knee is just a simple hinge joint, but with this view we miss the importance of the knee for both sports and daily life. The knee offers, on the one hand, more mobility in the flexed state as rotational movement and sideward bending are possible. On the other hand, it secures stability mainly by the central ligament pillar, formed by the anterior and posterior cruciate ligament, limiting mainly translation but also excessive sideward, rotational, and extensional movements. In addition, there is the active muscle control that plays an important role in knee stability.

The rupture of the anterior cruciate ligament is the most frequent severe injury in many popular sports, e.g. soccer, rugby alpine skiing. It is often associated with additional lesions in the knee joint, e.g. meniscus tear, capsular lesions, cartilage lesions, additional ligaments lesions like the medial collateral ligament. These additional lesions influence the choice of therapy.

Prevention and Treatment Table for ACL Rupture

Prevention	Good muscular control helps in the prevention of injury to the lower limb in general and to the ACL in particular. Several good studies show that warming up, including specific strengthening and proprioception exercises is essential and protects the ACL!
Treatment by Yourself	If the ACL is ruptured consultation with your sports medicine physician and physiotherapist is needed to ensure appropriate decision making.
When is a Doctor Needed?	As soon as you observe an injury mechanism as described above or if you feel these giving way mechanisms in your knee.
Return to Play/Sports	Extremely important discussion: • For many sports (e.g. ball sports, alpine skiing, martial arts) an operative reconstruction of the ACL is a must, as these sports need this particular control of stability of translational knee movements. The return to sports at a competitive level usually takes 6 months. In alpine skiing (with the increased specific technical skills and the external forces), it takes up to 9 months • Interestingly, in other sports, like road cycling and swimming, an operative reconstruction of the ACL is not necessary and certainly not indicated throughout the running season, as muscle control mechanisms may completely compensate the lack of the ACL • In the latter case, or where an operation is only done at a later stage, a proper rehabilitation process with professional instruction of the co-contraction concept (i.e. simultaneous contraction of quadriceps and hamstrings muscle), regular strengthening of quadriceps and hamstrings muscles (e.g. 3–4 times per week), and gradual sport specific loading exercises over a time period of 2–3months is highly recommended • If other knee structures (e.g. a medial collateral ligament or a meniscus) are also torn, this enters into consideration and influences the treatment plan bringing it closer to the operative approach

What Does the Doctor Do?

The doctor takes the history and performs the clinical exam. Any distinct swelling (i.e. effusion of the knee joint) and the translational instability, as examined in the clinical investigation, often reveal the diagnosis. If an ACL rupture is suspected, an MRI is performed to confirm the diagnosis and to exclude additional injuries to other knee structures. Knowledge from the clinical situation, the MRI results, and the requirements of the sport discipline influence a final decision about the precise treatment plan.

Literature

Schneider J. Early surgery for menisco-ligamental injuries in elite athletes. Unfallchirurg. 2014 Jan;117(1):19-23.

LaBella CR et al. Anterior cruciate ligament injuries: diagnosis, treatment, and prevention. Pediatrics. 2014 May;133(5):e1437-50.

Ardern CL et al. Return-to-sport outcomes at 2 to 7 years after anterior cruciate ligament reconstruction surgery. Am J Sports Med. 2012 Jan;40(1):41-8.

Shah VM et al. Return to play after anterior cruciate ligament reconstruction in National Football League athletes. Am J Sports Med. 2010 Nov; 38(11):2233-9.

Meniscal Tear – When the Knee Suddenly Hurts

Symptoms

Sudden onset of sharp knee pain located on either the medial (inner side) or lateral (outer side) of the joint, often after combined movement of knee flexion and rotation. Pain usually lasts for some seconds (sometimes minutes) until there is complete pain relief.

Sometimes a meniscal tear may impair knee movements up to complete blocking of knee flexion and extension. This is typically with a bucket-handle type of tear (see below).

Background

The meniscus is a fibro-cartilaginous anatomical structure within the knee with a double semilunar shape and works as an attenuator and shock-absorber and flexible stabiliser of the knee. Its shock-absorbing function is essential for the sustainability and longevity of the knee cartilage and prevention of osteoarthritis. The meniscus also contributes to the stability of the knee.

In some injuries the meniscus may tear. In flexion-rotation manoeuvres, a longer flap of its fibrocartilaginous matrix may be caught and pinched between femur and tibia causing pain. This flap may become bigger and bigger, and the pinching eventually harm the cartilage surface. The therapy of choice in acute meniscal tears consists is arthroscopic treatment—a minor operation (keyhole operation)—to remove this injured flap and a leave as much as possible of the still intact non-injured meniscus.

In young athletes with peripheral lesions of the meniscus, a suture is an interesting option as there is no meniscal material removed and complete recovery seems possible. In this case the rehabilitation and return to play process usually take longer but are worthwhile because the more meniscus is removed, the higher is the risk of posttraumatic osteoarthritis (i.e. degenerative deterioration of the knee).

Also in acute injuries, some meniscal tear do not need an operation, e.g. most of the posterior located lesions (only symptomatic in very deep and loaded knee flexion) and strictly horizontally oriented meniscal tears, as an operation doesn't seem to be better than a conservative treatment.

A particular case is the bucket-handle type of meniscal tear (see picture). Due to the shape of this lesion, the knee may be completely blocked or experience distinct movement limitation because of the displaced bucket-handle bit of the meniscus. The bucket-handle lesion needs an operation to remove the ruptured piece of meniscus.

Recent studies show that in a degenerative meniscal tear (i.e. 'wear and tear' lesions of the meniscus in the older/master athlete) surgery or conservative therapy are showing equal results, even in case of mechanical symptoms (Sihvonen 2013; 2016). This means, that in these older/master athletes a conservative approach may be tried, and if symptoms persist after 6 months, a surgical approach should be considered.

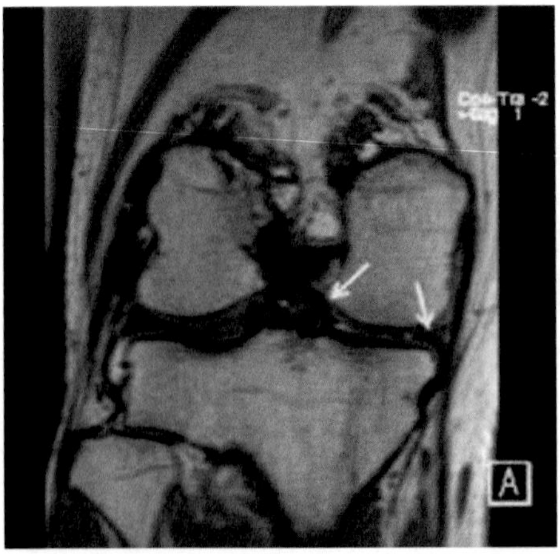

MRI of the right knee. Bucket-handle meniscus tear on the inner side whereas the outer meniscus is fine (nicely shaped blade triangle)

Prevention and Treatment Table for Meniscal Tear

Prevention	Good warming up, proprioceptive exercises, and regular strengthening of the lower extremity muscles (especially quadriceps and hamstrings muscle) are preventative.
Treatment by Yourself	In case of an acute meniscal tear with a flap in the weight bearing zone (anterior and middle part), there are usually no self treatment options. Discuss the issue with your sportsmed physician and your physiotherapist.
When is a Doctor Needed?	If an acute meniscal tear is suspected.
Return to Play/ Sports	RTP depends on the size and location of the lesion. After the removal of a small flap, slight training can be started within 2 weeks and complete return to competitive sports may be possible within 4 weeks. For a sutured meniscus RTP takes 8–10 weeks, with crutches for the first 4–5 weeks.

What Does the Doctor Do?

The doctor takes the history and performs a clinical exam. The history and the exam (with particular meniscal tests) usually reveal whether a meniscal tear is probable or not. If a tear is suspected, a MRI is usually also performed to confirm the diagnosis and analyse the type and size of the lesion. MRI are nowadays quite accurate in diagnosing meniscal lesion, but there are still a couple of 'signal alterations' visible in the MRI that are due to stress (e.g. shearing forces on the meniscus) but do not correspond to any structural lesion in the meniscus.

Literature

Phelan N et al. A systematic review and meta-analysis of the diagnostic accuracy of MRI for suspected ACL and meniscal tears of the knee. Knee Surg Sports Traumatol Arthrosc. 2015 Nov 27. [Epub ahead of print]

Snoeker BA et al. Risk factors for meniscal tears: a systematic review including meta-analysis. J Orthop Sports Phys Ther. 2013 Jun;43(6):352-67

Giuliani JR et al. Treatment of meniscal injuries in young athletes. J Knee Surg. 2011 Jun;24(2):93-100.

Sihvonen R et al. Mechanical Symptoms and Arthroscopic Partial Meniscectomy in Patients With Degenerative Meniscus Tear: A Secondary Analysis of a Randomized Trial. Ann Intern Med. 2016 Apr 5;164(7):449-55.

Sihvonen R et al. Arthroscopic partial meniscectomy versus sham surgery for a degenerative meniscal tear. N Engl J Med. 2013 Dec 26;369(26):2515-24.

Shoulder Dislocation – Careful Attention to Prevent Repetition

Symptoms

Usually after a fall, a collision with an opponent or an obstacle, or another major impact on the shoulder, the joint may be dislocated. There is sudden onset of pain, movement impairment (the athlete tries to protect the shoulder by stabilising the injured side with the other arm), and sometimes visible, and mostly palpable, dislocation of the humeral head (bone of the upper arm) out of the shoulder joint.

Figure 1: Shoulder X-ray: (courtesy Dr. med. Beat Stauber, Radiology Sonnenhof Hospital Berne)

Normal: ap projection	*Dislocated left shoulder:*

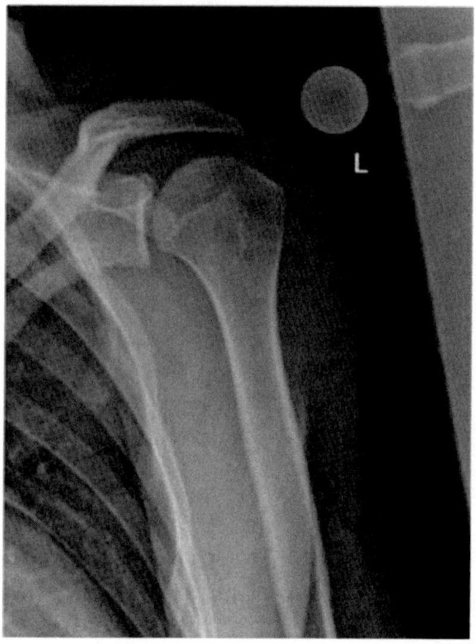

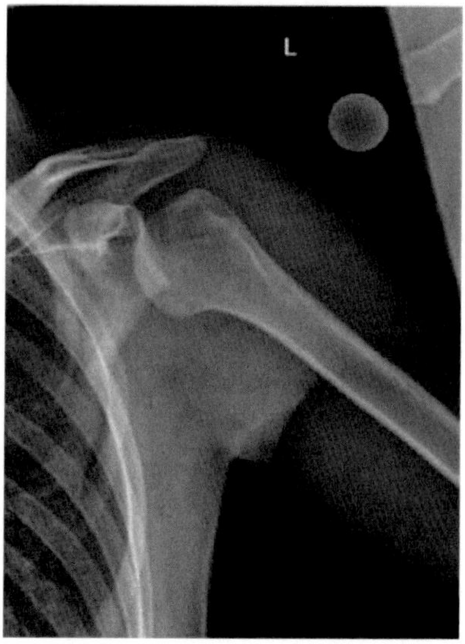

Dislocation at large:

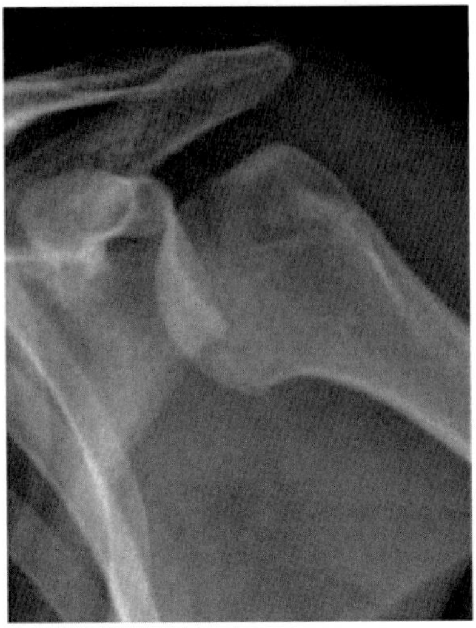

Background

The shoulder joint has a quite small and shallow socket. To improve joint stability, but still allow a wide range of movement, the labrum (i.e. fibro-cartilaginous lip) enlarges this articular surface and keeps the ball in the socket. In major trauma, predispositional factors may influence a dislocation. Predispositional factors are:

- Age (people under 40yrs are more prone to this injury)
- Gender (males more often than females)
- Hypermobility (hyperlaxity of the ligaments and shoulder capsule)
- Genetics
- Sports specific demands, particularly those of overhead or collision sports
- Earlier shoulder dislocation
- Pathological factors on first shoulder dislocation such as Hill-Sach's lesions (i.e. impression in the humeral head while dislocated) or bony Bankart lesions (i.e. partial fracture of the lower part of the socket)

Prevention and Treatment Table for Shoulder Dislocation

Prevention	• For primary prevention: Good warm-up, strengthening of the upper body and shoulder girdle muscles • Secondary prevention (after the first event): Good strengthening is highly important and must be taken seriously, as it does prevent recurrent shoulder dislocation in the future.
Treatment by Yourself	• In acute shoulder dislocation, you should immediately look for professional help • We emphasise secondary prevention with shoulder strengthening as the most important contribution in prevention of a further event
When is a Doctor Needed?	Acute shoulder dislocation is an emergency (however not life-threatening), so call for professional help or go to an emergency department.
Return to Play/Sports	The RTP protocol is based on a thorough initial diagnosis and treatment plan. • In *uncomplicated shoulder dislocation*, the RTP protocol may start immediately, with a renouncement of overhead activities and rotational manoeuvres for the first couple of weeks. Usually a 6–8 week protocol with a focused and continuous building up of strength, an improvement of intra- and inter-muscular coordination of the shoulder girdle and rotator cuff muscles, and a good scapula setting are essential • In *shoulder dislocations with further structural damage*, especially with bony lesions of the socket, and/or labrum lesions, an early operation seems to be beneficial. The RTP is established according to the injury pattern and may therefore vary

What Does the Doctor Do?

A shoulder luxation is not life-threatening but needs to be considered as an emergency as it is usually painful and the reduction of the dislocated joint should be done within a reasonable time frame. So the doctor takes a very brief history (e.g. trauma mechanism and possible earlier shoulder dislocations) and performs a clinical exam. After administration of analgesics, x-rays are taken (if available within reasonable time) to exclude a fracture and confirm diagnosis. Thereafter the reduction is performed, which is quite often challenging because of muscle spasms and may need anaesthesia. Thorough appreciation and further imaging is essential to recognise the full extent of the damaged structures—labrum intact; bony socket intact; humeral head without impression; rotator cuff muscles intact—with this information the diagnosis may be made and a treatment plan established. In recurrent dislocations, sport orthopaedic assessment is advised. Possibly, surgical reconstruction (arthroscopic or open technique) is necessary.

Literature

Funk L. Treatment of glenohumeral instability in rugby players. Knee Surg Sports Traumatol Arthrosc. 2016 Feb;24(2):430-9

Hutchinson M, B McCormack. Predicting recurrent shoulder instability.Br J Sports Med 2015;49:14 911-912

Olds M et al. Risk factors which predispose first-time traumatic anterior shoulder dislocations to recurrent instability in adults: a systematic review and meta-analysis. Br J Sports Med doi:10.1136/bjsports-2014-094342

Dickens JF et al. Return to play and recurrent instability after in-season anterior shoulder instability: a prospective multicenter study. Am J Sports Med. 2014 Dec;42(12):2842-50.

AC-Contusion/AC-Dislocation/Acromio-Clavicular Joint Separation – When You Fall on Your Shoulder

Symptoms

Acute shoulder pain after a fall on the shoulder or after a collision. Swelling and tenderness of the outer upper edge (i.e. AC joint region), sometimes with a visible elevation of the clavicle. Typically sharp pain sensation with cross over movements of the arm or when rolling over in bed (putting the AC joint under stress).

Figure 1: AC Joint, AC-Dislocation

Figure 1.1: AC joint posterior view (with ligaments)

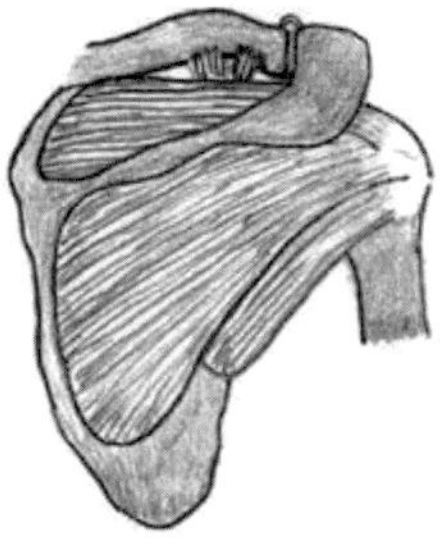

Figure 1.2: AC joint frontal

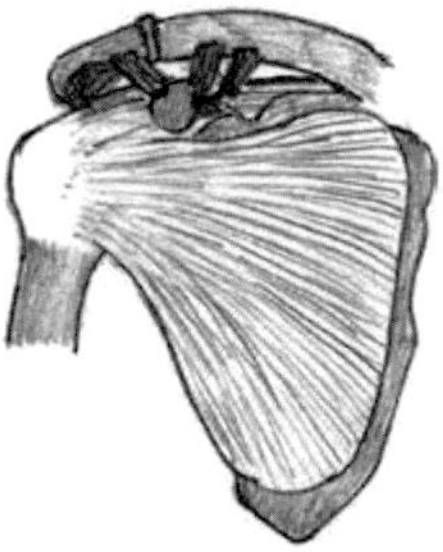

Figure 1.3: X-rays with additional weights showing a raised stand of the clavicle in case of an AC dislocation grade II

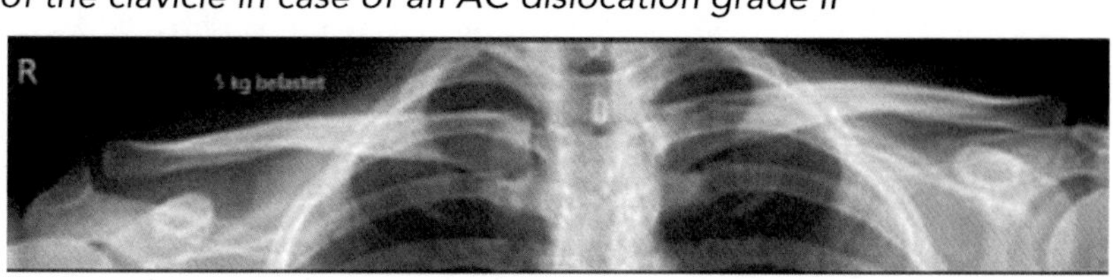

X-ray panoramic view with AC dislocation Grade II on the right

Background

AC-joint is the acromio-clavicular joint—A from the acromion (i.e. bony part of the shoulder blade) and C from the clavicle (i.e. collar bone). The clavicle is central in guiding the scapula (shoulder blade) on the thoracic cage and keeping it in at a constant distance. The AC joint, with its ligaments, is the direct link between clavicle and shoulder and secures and positions the shoulder together with the scapula fixing muscles. Therefore the AC joint is central in linking the shoulder to the body and in stabilising the shoulder in a balanced way.

After an injury to the AC joint, any further stress to the joint and the ligaments is painful. In a structural injury (partial or complete rupture of ligaments of the AC joint) it may take a couple of weeks until to settle down and start to heal before the desired strengthening program of the shoulder may be intensified. With AC dislocation grades II and III a certain hypermobility of the AC joint will remain, but experience and studies show that in these still minor degrees injuries conservative treatment is clearly better than an operation.

Higher grade injuries (grade IV, V, VI) need a thorough examination, interdisciplinary discussion, and decision-making with an experienced orthopaedic surgeon, as the outcome very much depends on the severity and extent of the injury.

Prevention and Treatment Table for AC-Contusion/AC-Dislocation

Prevention	Good warming up, with particular focus on the shoulder, for overhead and contact sports.
Treatment by Yourself	Once the diagnosis is given, put your effort into doing home exercises as shown by professionals and be patient, as it usually takes a couple of weeks to settle down.
When is a Doctor Needed?	As soon as you suffer a hit to your shoulder that impacts its movements for a couple of days.

Return to Play/ Sports	Simple AC contusion and AC dislocation grade I, II, and III are all treated conservatively. Depending on the severity of the injury, the trauma mechanism and the requirements of your sports discipline, RTP will vary: • In AC contusion and AC dislocation grade I, a RTP under guidance of the physiotherapist may take 1–3 weeks • AC dislocations grade II and III take distinctly longer to enable good strengthening of the shoulder girdle. Overhead activities are integrated in the RTP and gradually intensified. It may take 10–12 weeks to reach complete recovery and to perform on a competitive level in overhead or collision sports

What Does the Doctor Do?

The doctor takes the history and performs a clinical exam with particular focus on shoulder movements. Typically cross-over movements and overhead manoeuvres cause particularly sharp pain, as the shoulder is under axial pressure and the AC-joint stressed and painful.

Usually x-rays will be used to see the bony structures and exclude a fracture of the collar bone (clavicle) and the shoulder blade. In most frequently observed acromioclavicular joint separations grade I, II or III, a conservative management plan will be proposed.

Literature

Cook JB et al. Surgical management of acromioclavicular dislocations. Clin Sports Med. 2014 Oct;33(4):721-37.

Doyscher R et al. Acute and overuse injuries of the shoulder in sports. Orthopade. 2014 Mar;43(3):202-8.

Reid D et al. Acromioclavicular joint separations grades I-III: a review of the literature and development of best practice guidelines. Sports Med. 2012 Aug 1;42(8):681-96.

Rotator Cuff Injury of the Shoulder – Acute vs Overuse

Symptoms

Mostly sharp, but sometimes dull, shoulder pain with overhead activity or pain while directly lying on the concerned shoulder. There are difficulties getting dressed (e.g. getting into a t-shirt or a jacket) as the range of motion of the shoulder is typically limited with particular weakness in the abduction of the arm.

Figure 1: Shoulder Anatomy with Rotator Cuff Muscles

1.1) Shoulder anatomy frontal view

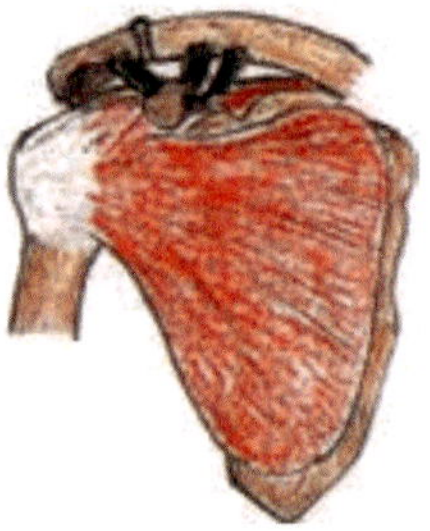

1.2) shoulder anatomy view from the back

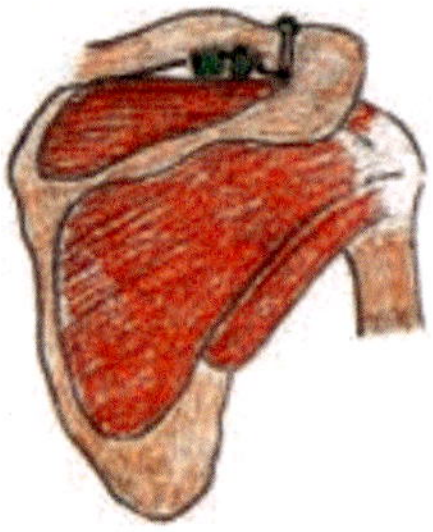

1.3) Cross sectional view of the shoulder

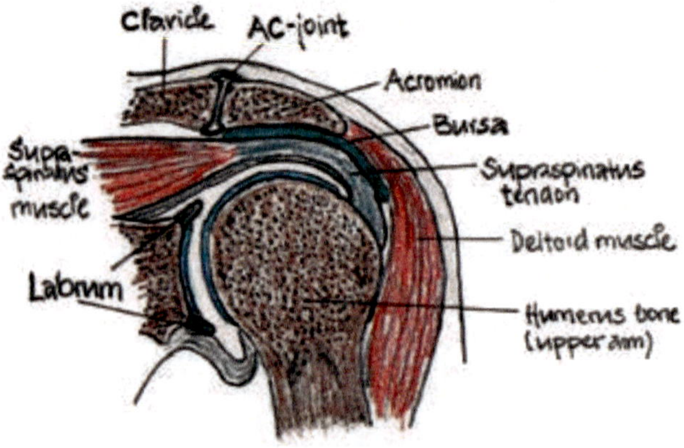

Background

The shoulder joint has a fantastic range of motion because of its particular anatomy and the rotator cuff muscles and tendons. The rotator cuff is a muscle-tendon system, functionally wrapping the articular capsule, and by ideal positioning of the tendon insertions, allowing a multitude of shoulder movements (see Figure 1). This results in both a well-balanced shoulder stability and an impressive range of motion in all directions: internal rotation (IR); external rotation (ER); abduction; adduction and flexion-extension. Thus we readily understand the importance of the integrity of the rotator cuff and the good-functioning of all of its parts.

The history of an incident, typically a collision or a fall (e.g. tackling in rugby or fall in a gravity sport) leads us to suspect an *acute* rotator cuff injury. Whereas recurrent and continuous exposure of the shoulder in overhead activities (e.g. throwing disciplines, but also repetitive minor traumas) may lead to *overuse* of the rotator cuff (for the latter see also chapter 'Swimmer's and Thrower's Shoulder').

With the heavy trauma of the *acute* injury we often face *partial or sometimes full-thickness ruptures* of one or several tendons of the rotator cuff. With *overuse* injuries we mostly face structurally minor to moderate injuries, but quite often *recurrent and therapeutically challenging tendinopathies.*

Prevention and Treatment Table for Rotator Cuff Injuries

Prevention	• Warming up of the shoulder in overhead and collision sports is essential! • If the shoulder seems to be your weak point, particular attention to specific strengthening of the rotator cuff and shoulder girdle muscles is warranted
Treatment by Yourself	See the basic shoulder warm-up program with four exercises: • As shown in the chapter Swimmer's shoulder/ Thrower shoulder

When is a Doctor Needed?	As soon as you suspect a structural injury of the rotator cuff.
Return to Play/Sports	Depends on the severity of the injury: • For a slight tendinopathy without structural lesion: physiotherapy, home exercises, and a slight training reduction will do the job • In most other cases, omitting overhead activities and shoulder collisions (for team and contact sports) for a couple of weeks combined with close physiotherapeutically guided shoulder rehabilitation is the most promising way • In case of a minor partial rupture of the rotator cuff: treatment is usually conservative but RTP will take 6–8 weeks • In complete ruptures, a thorough interdisciplinary assessment together with an experienced orthopaedic surgeon is recommended in order to make a good decision about further treatment (operative reconstruction vs non-operative). In such cases, RTP is prolonged and will take 12 weeks and more.

What Does the Doctor Do?

The doctor takes the history and performs a clinical exam, with particular focus on shoulder movement and possible limitations. X-rays give basic information about the bony shoulder structure, but don't give further information about tendons and muscles. In case of a suspected structural lesion of the rotator cuff, an arthro-MRI (magnetic resonance imaging with contrast injection into the joint) allows recognition of possible small tears in the rotator cuff and excludes or confirms other possible pathologies.

Literature

McElwany MD et al. Rotator cuff repair: published evidence on factors associated with repair integrity and clinical outcome. Am J Sports Med. 2015 Feb;43(2):491-500

Desjardins-Charbonneau A et al. The efficacy of manual therapy for rotator cuff tendinopathy: a systematic review and meta-analysis. J Orthop Sports Phys Ther. 2015 May;45(5):330-50

Shaffer B, Huttmann D. Rotator cuff tears in the throwing athlete. Sports Med Arthroscop. 2014 Jun;22(2):101-9

Concussion – Respect Your Head (and Your Opponent's)

As concussion is a well-studied medical condition and a multitude of publications is found, we base the chapter very much on official definitions and guidelines.

Symptoms

'A concussion is a disturbance in brain function caused by a direct or indirect force to the head. It results in a variety of non-specific signs and/or symptoms (some examples listed below) and most often does not involve loss of consciousness.

Concussion should be suspected in the presence of any one or more of the following:

- Symptoms (e.g. headache), or
- Physical signs (e.g. unsteadiness), or
- Impaired brain function (e.g. confusion), or
- Abnormal behaviour (e.g. change in personality).'

(SCAT 3 Questionnaire- What is a concussion? Br J Sports Med)

Figure 1: Concussion – Hammer on to Your Laptop – How Does This Feel?

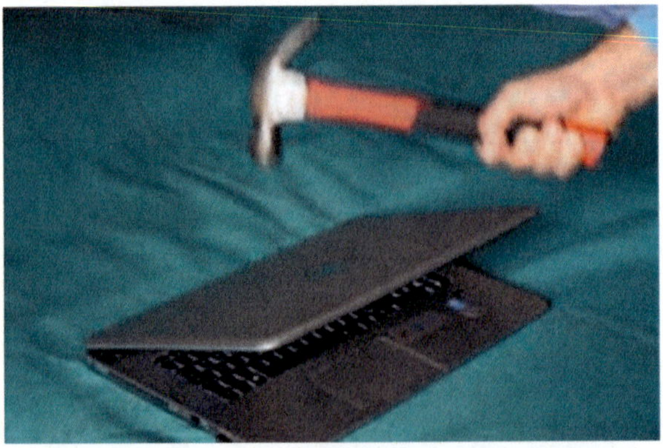

Background

'A concussion is a type of brain injury. It's the most minor form. Technically, a concussion is a short loss of normal brain function in response to a head injury. But people often use it to describe any minor injury to the head or brain. Concussions are a common type of sports injury. You can also have one if you suffer a blow to the head or hit your head after a fall.

Symptoms of a concussion may not start right away; they may start days or weeks after the injury. Symptoms may include a headache or neck pain. You may also have nausea, ringing in your ears, dizziness, or tiredness. You may feel dazed or not your normal self for several days or weeks after the injury. Consult your health care professional if any of your symptoms get worse, or if you have more serious symptoms such as:

- Seizures
- Trouble walking or sleeping
- Weakness, numbness, or decreased coordination
- Repeated vomiting or nausea
- Confusion
- Slurred speech

> *Doctors use a neurologic exam and imaging tests to diagnose a concussion. Most people recover fully after a concussion, but it can take some time. Rest is very important after a concussion because it helps the brain to heal.'*
>
> (Concussion definition. U.S. National Library of Medicine)

Prevention and Treatment Table for Concussion

Prevention	Some sports are more prone to concussion than others (e.g. rugby, ice hockey, American football) and luckily there is an increasing awareness of the concussion, specifically in the named sports. So concerted efforts of sport officials, medical commissions, coaches, and players are being undertaken to make the sport safer, by for instance: • Adaptations of rules of the game (e.g. strict penalising in soccer if elbows are used against an opponent's head)

	• Promotion among players and coaches to respect the opponent's head (e.g. respect my head, sihf.ch) • Heavy penalties for offences involving the opponent's head • Further research Despite these remarkable efforts the sports specific risks of concussion remain.
Treatment by Yourself	• If you think you have an acute concussion, or you notice symptoms as described above, seek professional medical advice • Rest is very important after a concussion because it helps the brain to recover
When is a Doctor Needed?	If a concussion is suspected.
Return to Play/Sports	If the diagnosis of a concussion is established, many sport disciplines have a specific return to play protocol that guides you back to training and competition. These protocols are established to protect you, your head, and your brain, as long-term complications from this one event *and* the impact of a second possible impact leading to more severe consequences must be avoided. The protocol simply allows you a safe return to sport. As a rule of thumb, and to give you a rough idea of the milestones: • 24–48h complete rest • No training, just walking • One week no vigorous effort, no competition, just making your way slowly back into training

What Does the Doctor Do?

The doctor takes the history and performs a clinical, neurological exam. The latter is fundamental for further decisions, possible further imaging and the treatment plan. Often an early diagnosis on the field or on the pitch directly during a game is required. This is sometimes challenging. Specific diagnostic tools and questionnaires are of additional help.

Literature

Pfister T et al. The incidence of concussion in youth sports: a systematic review and meta-analysis. Br J Sports Med. 2016 Mar;50(5):292-7.

McNamee MJ, Partridge B, Anderson L. Concussion Ethics and Sports Medicine. Clin Sports Med. 2016 Apr;35(2):257-67.

Sharp DJ, Jenkins PO. Concussion is confusing us all. Pract Neurol. 2015 Jun;15(3):172-86.

McCrory P et al. Consensus statement on concussion in sport: the 4th International Conference on Concussion in Sport held in Zurich, November 2012. Br J Sports Med. 2013 Apr;47(5):250-8.

SCAT 3 Questionnaire- What is a concussion? Br J Sports Med download 1.3.16 http://bjsm.bmj.com/content/47/5/259.full.pdf

Concussion definition. U.S.NationalLibrary of Medicine, download online 1.3.16 https://www.nlm.nih.gov/medlineplus/concussion.html

Skin

Skin Structure and Function – How to Deal With Dry Skin in Sports

Our skin is the body surface being in contact with the elements of nature: we feel the heat and the cold, the dry air and the water, the warm breeze and the icy snowstorm. What we are maybe a little less aware of is that our skin is a body organ. Good examples are:

- *Blood flow to the skin (thermoregulation):* Huge in a hot environment and minimal in cold conditions, so blood vessels to the skin are fully open and working at their maximum in the heat, and restricted to a minimum in cold temperatures (important physiological phenomenon when it comes to pre-cooling before and cooling therapy after efforts)
- *Barrier function of the skin to prevent infections (defence system):* Important that this barrier system is intact
- *Body surface exposed to the sun (radiation damages):* In countries like Australia, at the age of 70 years, 2 out of 3 suffer from skin cancer

The surface of the skin has a very thin slightly fat film that protects the skin (no drying out, intact barrier against fungi and bacteria) and keeps it elastic and smooth. The skin has as slightly acid pH of 5, which helps to further protect it from many germs.

In daily training and competition our skin is exposed to a multitude of things, and naturally these exposures vary with the sports discipline: gymnasts (hands rubbed with magnesia holding bars, rings, pommel horse, etc. with a firm grip) differ from swimmers (being 2–3 times a day for several hours in the water), and sailors (on open water exposed to the wind, water and sun, the latter reflected by the water) differ from road cyclists (exposed to all kind of weather and air conditions, especially sunlight, heat or cold, rain or even snow). So you, as an athlete and a coach, know best, what particular exposures you have in your discipline.

Common in all sports is sweating, the exposure to hot and cold, and the need for a shower, often more than once a day. Is there any harm with that? To remove the possible dirt of the training and to wash away the sweat after the effort we take a shower and there's nothing wrong with it. But it's in the repetition of taking this shower where we find the problem: we are not only removing the dirt and sweat but also this slight protective film we have on the skin. And we also change the skin's pH (pH skin 5 /pH water 7). As we mostly use a shower gel to clean our body, things are even more pronounced, as these gels, like all soaps, are bases or base detergents. While they are so good for washing and cleaning, they also have a highly alkaline pH (pH 9–11), which is bad for the skin as they remove all of this protective film and change the pH of the skin completely to alkaline. That's also the explanation for the observation that many athletes have really dry skin. The result is that they have a 'sandpaper' skin, with a dry surface, sometimes itching, sometimes cracking, and last but not least a skin which is prone to cause further problems (see chapter 'Atopic Dermatitis'). Table 1 gives some advice about what to do to treat dry skin.

Table 1: What to Do When You Have Dry Skin in Sport?

- Re-think your shower habits—instead of three a day, one or two will do it
- Don't use the mostly advertised shower gels, but use pH balanced products instead (having a pH of 5.5, very close to the skin pH)
- Use the pH balanced gel sparsely. If you shower twice a day, use once just plain water
- Possibly use a moisturiser or body lotion (strictly without fragrance) to cover the touched body sites

Table 2: What's the pH?

pH: Is a value indicating in numbers from 1–14 the acid-base-scale. It indicates in fact the amount of hydrogen ions (H^+) in a negative logarithmic scale ($pH = -\log(H^+)$), i.e. the lower the number the more acid it is. Some examples are directly drawn into scale:

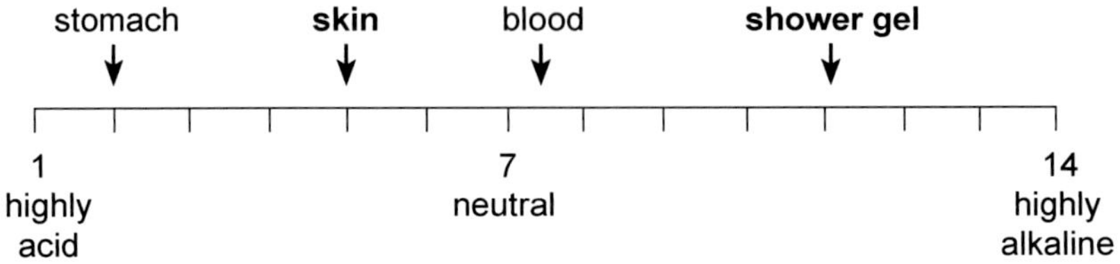

Different parts of our body have different pH values:

skin pH 5; water ph 7; shower gel pH 9–12; blood pH 7.35–7.45; stomach pH 1–4; vagina pH 4

Atopic Dermatitis – 20% of All Athletes Concerned!

Symptoms

Very dry skin, often itching, sandpaper-like, predominantly on shins, hollow of the knee (popliteal fossa), hollow of the elbow (cubital fossa), behind the ears, and around the eyes. Forming thin crusts, sometimes crackling, often scaling. If going further, dry, plaque-like reddish skin thickenings (as an eczema), and after scratching sometimes excoriated and slight bleeding may occur.

Background

About 20–30% of the population has an atopic dermatitis, also called neurodermitis. Among athletes studies confirm a percentage of 20%. So it's extremely frequent and widespread. The illness is characterised by a reduced resistance of the skin to alkaline substances—the skin is more sensitive to many things, but especially soap (and water). As discussed earlier (see chapter 'Skin Structure and Function') our skin is the protecting surface of our body. Once the fine natural fat film on the surface is washed away, we first feel unwell and it gets itchy. We will start to rub and to scratch; badly enough and we begin making things worse. By the scratching there's a short comfort but the skin structure will be damaged and this results in an inflammation (reddish, warm skin). Eventually the skin loses its protective barrier function. This opens the door to all kind of infections, discomfort, and itching continues and the vicious cycle turns unfortunately around (Figure 2). This explains partially the given names of this disease: 'dermatitis' means inflammation of the skin, 'a-topic' means not at the right place. The neurodermitis term should emphasise the skin inflammation related to this vicious cycle of feeling unwell: itching, scratching, getting more inflamed, etc. But it is a bit of an unlucky name, as it makes you think of a 'neuro thing' (i.e. related to nerve structures), which is not the case.

The predisposition to have this illness is genetic, the manifestation may vary—sometimes not being present for years and suddenly appearing. Usually it is getting better after childhood and adolescence. It is more frequent in families with hay fever and bronchial asthma.

Figure 1: Vicious cycle of Atopic Dermatitis

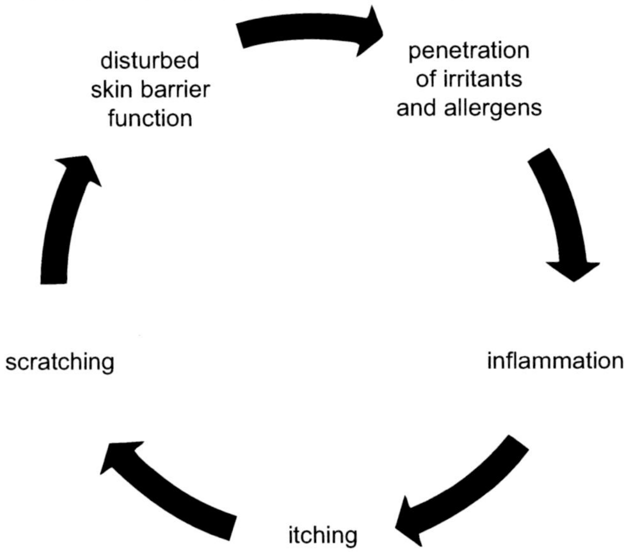

Prevention and Treatment Table for Atopic Dermatitis/Neurodermitis

Prevention	• If you have Atopic dermatitis, follow skin care proceedings for dry skin to limit or even prevent flare-ups, e.g. not shower too much, sparsely use of pH balanced (pH 5.5) shower gel, etc. • Cut your fingernails short (helps to prevent scratching injuries). If skin itches, rub with your fingertips, it will give a similar relief, but harms less

	• It is important to regularly put fragrance-free moisturiser on, especially on the itchy parts
Treatment by Yourself	See above. Have a moisturiser ready anytime (e.g. in your training bag), especially for winter season and for the touched body sites. If it gets worse, give the skin back its natural film back by using a body oil (almond oil) or a thick cream or ointment (it is important that this is fragrance-free).
When is a Doctor Needed?	In severe cases.
Return to Play/Sports	Usually no pause needed.

What Does the Doctor Do?

The doctor confirms the diagnosis by the history and clinical observation; if uncertain, possibly a skin biopsy and patch tests will be carried out for further allergy testing. Concerning treatment, other options will be added: corticosteroid creams of different strength, Gr I to IV (Gr I being very low in corticosteroid action, Gr IV the strongest); oil bathes or other good ointments saving corticosteroids as pimecrolismus ointment (Protopic) or tacrolismus cream (Elidel). To reduce the itching, antihistamine as tablet or drops may be used. If the accompanying skin infection is severe, antibiotics may be needed.

Literature

Macucci F et al. Asthma and allergy in young athletes in Siena Province. Preliminary results. J Sports Med Phys Fitness. 2007 Sep;47(3):351-5. Clin J Sport Med. 2006 Sep;16(5):401-5.

Katelaris CH et al. Patterns of allergic reactivity and disease in Olympic athletes. Clin J Sport Med. 2006 Sep;16(5):401-5

Interdigital Mycosis of the Feet, Other Skin Infections – Watch Your Feet

Symptoms

It's itching, scaling, flaking, and sometimes blistering, in between and around the toes.

Background

Actually a foot mycosis is nothing to really worry about, but important enough to recognise and to treat properly as it may be the entry port for another infection. Foot mycosis is frequent, in normal population as well as among athletes. It's medically called tinea pedis (tinea = fungi; pedis = of the foot). It's so common among the sports community that some doctors call it 'athlete's foot', which, I must say, is a bad name—as if all athletes would have a foot mycosis all the time.

Parasitic fungi are easily transmitted in moist communal areas where people go barefoot, such as around swimming pools, or shower or locker rooms, and require a warm and moist environment like the inside of a sport shoe to incubate and grow.

Prevention and Treatment Table for Interdigital Mycosis of the Feet

Prevention	Watch your feet! They deserve a dry climate: • Dry your feet and your toes with your own clean towel • Put dry socks on • Let your sport shoes dry after training • Possibly wear thongs in communal moist areas

Treatment by Yourself	Treat a foot mycosis properly, as it may otherwise be an entry port for a more serious infection.
When is a Doctor Needed?	If you don't have this antimycotic cream and if it's an established mycosis.
Return to Play/Sports	Usually no pause needed. In severe cases, however, particularly with an eczema or additional bacterial superinfection (because of delayed treatment mostly), a longer time out of 10 or 14 days will be necessary, until the infection is treated.

What Does the Doctor Do?

The doctor shortly takes the history and looks at your feet and toes to confirm the diagnosis. Treatment with antimycotic cream, twice daily a thin layer on all touched areas, especially in between the toes. Wash hands, and very important, continue treatment for two more days after the lesions have disappeared, as fungi live longer than you think. If the skin is inflamed, treatment is combined (antimycotic and slight corticosteroid) to address the inflammatory response.

Prevent other skin infections—*don't* have an 'entry port'. As an elite athlete, your immune system is a bit reduced (see 'Prevention of infectious diseases in sports '), so prevent further infections and don't allow your feet to become an entry port and you catch a more severe skin infection crawling up your leg. Therefore disinfect any abrasion or wound properly (small first aid kit) and in case of a foot mycosis start treatment early and finish it to the end!

Literature

Ashack KA et al. Skin infections among US high school athletes: A national survey. J Am Acad Dermatol. 2016 Apr;74(4):679-684.

Purim KS et al. Fungal infection of the feet in soccer players and non-athlete individuals. Rev Iberoam Micol. 2005 Mar;22(1):34-8.

Lacroix C et al. Tinea pedis in European marathon runners. J Eur Acad Dermatol Venereol. 2002 Mar;16(2):139-42.

Sun Protection – Simply a Must, Like Brushing Your Teeth

Sunlight does a lot of good things to us human beings: allows life on earth, gives daily rhythm, supports good mood, and as research of the last few years has shown, is essential for the forming of active Vitamin D3 in our skin. On the other hand, sunlight and, in particular ultraviolet rays (UV), may also seriously damage our skin. Acute overdose leads to sunburns and chronic (or in repetitive sunburns) leads to skin cancer.

Three types of UV rays are differentiated:(4)

1. **Type A (UVA)** are present throughout the whole day, long wave (315–400nm), not absorbed by the ozone layer. UVA is used in solariums. In the past UVA was considered less harmful, but today it is well known that it contributes to skin cancer by indirect DNA damage (DNA: acronym for deoxyribo nucleic acid and stands for the genetic information in each body cell)
2. **Type B (UVB)** mainly present from 11am to 3pm, medium wave (280–315nm), mostly absorbed by the ozone layer. UVB may directly cause DNA damage as it penetrates the skin quite deeply. Overexposure to UVB leads to sunburn but also some forms of skin cancer
3. **Type C (UVC)** not reaching the earth surface, as absorbed by the ozone layer and atmosphere, short wave (100–280nm)

All bands of UV radiation damage collagen fibres and accelerate aging of the skin. We further know that the number of sunburns does mirror the direct damage of DNA by ultraviolet.(4)

Figure 1: Ultraviolet Radiation and Environmental Factors:[3]

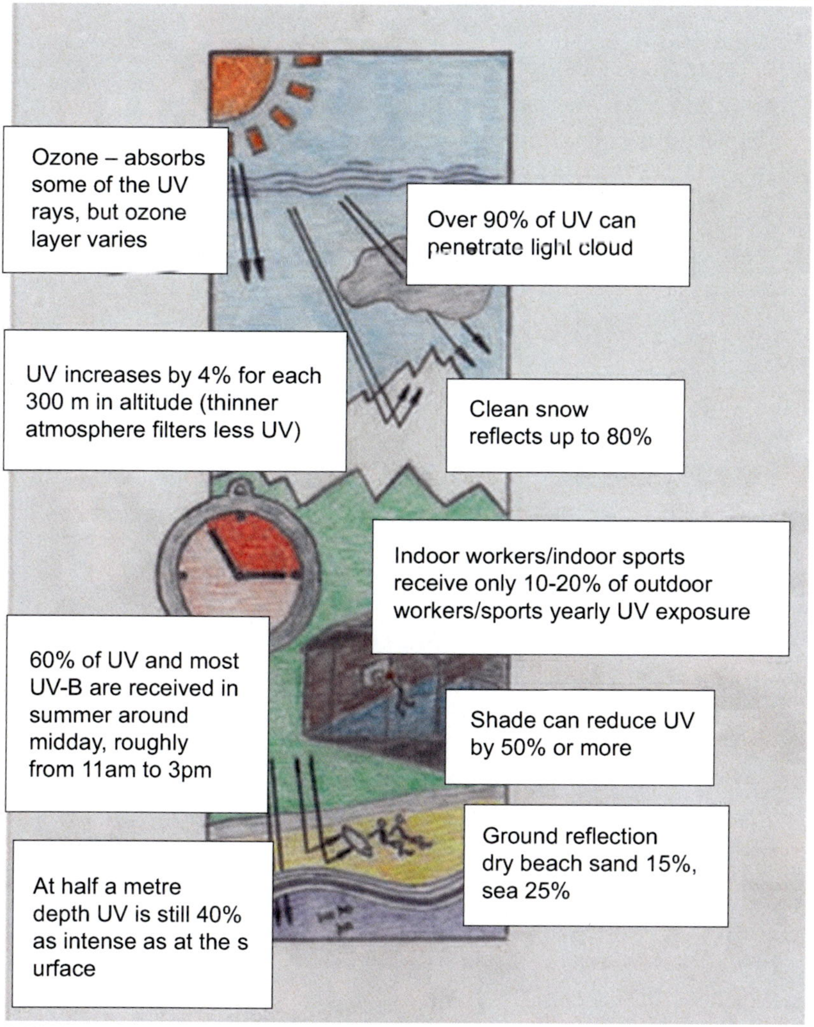

Our skin does adapt to the sunlight by forming more melanin, leading to darker skin pigmentation. This is an adaptational mechanism, protecting our skin, but it is slow (takes days and weeks to adapt). To prevent sunburn we need sun protection measures and good common sense, as ultraviolet is also responsible for the formation of the bone-strengthening and otherwise important Vitamin D. First studies are showing that people exaggerating sun protection measures may have Vitamin D3 deficiency.

How much sunlight is needed to support the formation of Vitamin D3?

Experts propose during summer time 15–20minutes of incidental sun exposure to the face, arms, and hands. In countries with a lot of sunshine and an elevated risk of skin cancer, e.g. Australia, South Africa, Mediterranean countries, sun protection measures are essential (and clearly precede the thoughts of skin forming melanin or Vitamin D3 metabolism).

What's your skin type?

It is important to know how sun sensitive your skin is. For that purpose, skin types have been described, Type I being the most sensitive with no pigmentation answer after sun exposure and Type VI being the less sensitive.(5)(6)(7)

Table 1: Fitzpatrick Scale for Skin Types(5)(6)(7)

Type	Burns	Tans	Skin Colour; Hair; Eyes; Other
I	Always	Never	Pale white; blond or red hair; blue eyes; freckles
II	Usually	Minimally	White, fair; blond or red hair; blue, green, or hazel eyes
III	Sometimes Mild	Uniformly	Cream white, fair; any hair or eye colour
IV	Rarely	Always Well	Moderate brown
V	Very Rarely	Very Easily	Dark brown
VI	Never	Never	Deeply pigmented dark brown to darkest brown

There are unfortunately people with sun sensitive skin. This is a genetic trait and there's no other way than to cope with it. Athletes with skin Type I or II need to be much more careful with their sun exposure and need to follow sun protection recommendation more thoroughly than others. That said, all outdoor sports need sun protection—as an outdoor athlete, you are simply more exposed than the normal population!

Table 2: Sun Protection in Sports—What to Do

Slogan	Meaning	In Sports
Slip	Slip on a shirt	Closed t-shirt. When training in the mid of the day is inevitable, wear UV protective clothing!
Slop	Slop on sunscreen	All over, especially on exposed body parts and 'sun terraces' (ears, nose, cheeks, neck, upper arms, legs). Even use titanium dioxide or zinc oxide products
Slap	Slap on a hat	Wear a hat, or a cap with a neck flap
Seek	Seek shade	Train in the shade as much as possible, or in the morning and later afternoon
Slide	Slide on sunglasses	Wear sport glasses (sports, laterally closed sunglasses)

This important and successful health campaign was launched by the Cancer Council Australia in the 1980s, changing the general public's sun protection attitudes and behaviour. In 2007, the slogan was updated to 'Slip, Slop, Slap, *Seek, Slide*' to reflect the importance of seeking shade and wearing (laterally closed) sunglasses.

Table 3: Survey Results of 'Physical Activity, Sun Exposure, and the Sporting Exposure and the Sporting Involvements of Young Involvements of Young Queensland Adults'[2]

'Slip, Slop, Slap – childhood 'inoculation' with sun protection habits?'
'There is the perception that because young adults have been exposed to sun protection campaigns during their schooling years that sun protection is internalised and is as much of a habit as brushing teeth. This is often not the case. Sun-protective behaviours are influenced strongly by attributes of the current environments in which sports take place, and by normative factors.'

'Sport-specific practicalities must always be considered'
'There is no 'one size fits all sports' for sun protection. While there will always be some general recommendations that can be made, sport-specific policies, resources, rules and incentives will often be necessary.'

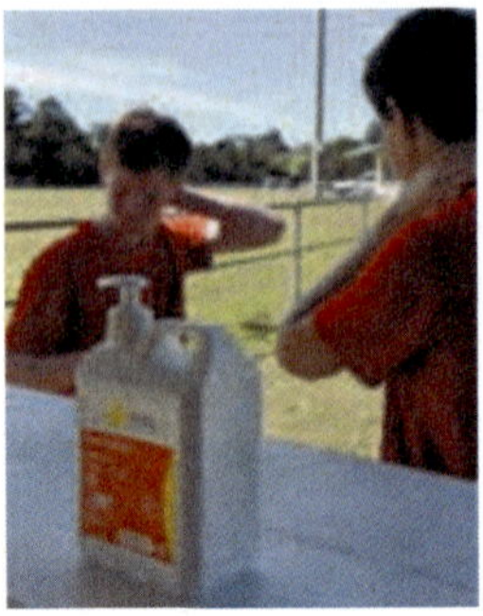

Sunscreen and Sun Protecting Factor (SPF)

What does the SPF 30 on a sunscreen mean? Imagine that your skin starts to burn after 15min full sun exposure, a sunscreen with sun protection factor 30 means that it protects for 30 x 15min, meaning 450min. So one application per day will do it? No. Experts recommend reapplying every second hour, especially if you are swimming or sweating a lot, like in sports. So reapplying is more important than having a really high SPF.

Blockers and absorbers in sunscreens[4][8]

Sunscreen may contain either **organic chemical absorbers** (like avobenzone, oxybenzone, or octyl methoxycinnamate) or **inorganic physical blockers** (like titanium dioxide and zinc oxide).

Chemical absorbers work by absorbing UV radiation. They can be further differentiated by the type of radiation they absorb, UVA, or UVB, or both.

Physical blockers work by reflecting or blocking completely UV radiation and they are easily recognisable by the whitening appearance. At present both type of sun protection seem safe and efficient.[4][8] Physical blockers are possibly slightly superior as they completely block UV radiation before entering the skin and cause less frequently rashes in skin sensitive persons.

What to do when you got sunburnt and the sport event goes on?

For the ongoing event: seek shade, wear UV protective long sleeve rashers, and put physical blockers (titanium oxice or zinc oxide) on.

For the treatment, follow the recommendation of the Skin Cancer Foundation (9):

- **Cool it down:** get out of the sun, take a cold shower shortly or jump in a cool pool. You may use cool compresses regularly plunged in icy water (but don't put ice cubes directly on your skin)
- **Moisturise:** use a gentle moisturiser (if available, fragrance-free) to keep the skin moist, repeat it after a couple of hours for 2–3 days. Sometimes you get moisturiser with aloe vera (see below)
- **Decrease inflammation:** aloe vera is considered safe and seems beneficial. Alternatively or additionally, an over-the-counter cortisone cream (class I, weak) may help reducing the inflammation
- **Stay out of the sun:** wear loose, breathable clothes
- **Drink enough:** the sunburn and skin inflammation draws fluid to the skin. Drink enough, including some sports drinks containing electrolytes
- **Seek a doctor:** if a larger skin area shows severe blistering

Literature

(1) 'Preventing Skin cancer' retrieved on the Cancer Council Australia website online 15.4.2016: http://www.cancer.org.au/preventing-cancer/sun-protection/preventing-skin-cancer/

(2) Physical Activity, Sun Exposure and the Sporting Exposure and the Sporting Involvements of Young Involvements of Young Queensland Adults. Cancer Research Centre, School of Population Health, the University of Queensland. November 2004 – April 2006 retrieved online 15.4.2016 http://www.uq.edu.au/cprc/docs/PASS-Final-Report.pdf

(3) 'Ultraviolet radiation and health' retrieved 15.4.2016 on the WHO website http://www.who.int/uv/uv_and_health/en/

(4) Ultraviolet on Wikipedia website retrieved 28.4.2016 https://en.wikipedia.org/wiki/Ultraviolet

(5) Fitzpatrick, T.B. The validity and practicality of sun-reactive skin types I through VI. Archives of Dermatology 1988, 124 (6): 869–871

(6) Fitzpatrick, T. B. Ultraviolet-induced pigmentary changes: Benefits and hazards. Therapeutic Photomedicine, Karger, vol. 15 of 'Current Problems in Dermatology ', 1986: 25-38

(7) 'Fitzpatrick scale' retrieved online on Wikipedia 15.4.2016: https://en.wikipedia.org/wiki/Fitzpatrick_scale

(8) Chemical vs Physical? Which type of sunscreen is best? in WallStreetJournal retrieved 28.4.16 http://www.wsj.com/articles/chemical-vs-physical-which-type-of-sunscreen-is-best-1402354797

(9) 5 ways to treat a sunburn Website of the Skin Cancer foundation, retrieved online 5.6.2016 http://www.skincancer.org/prevention/sunburn/five-ways-to-treat-a-sunburn

Insect Protection While Travelling as an Athlete – About Mosquitoes, Ticks, and Other Bugs

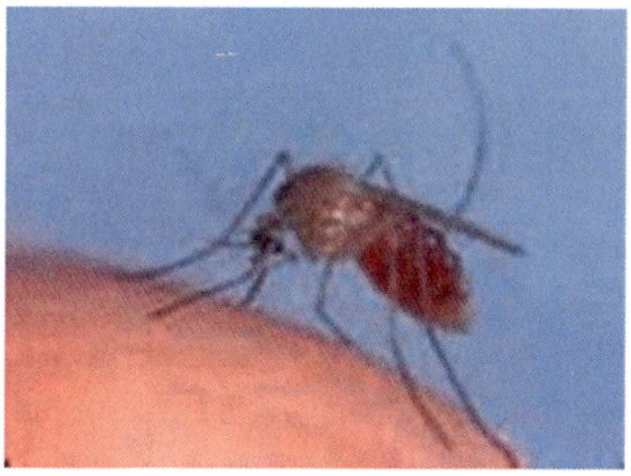

The best policy is to get informed about the countries you are travelling to. Usually you may find really good information on travel websites, such as:

- in English: Website of the Centers of Disease Control and Prevention, Traveler's Health: http://www.cdc.gov/travel
- in German and French: Travel Website of the Expert Committee of the Swiss Universities and the Swiss Tropical and Public Health Institute: www.safetravel.ch

As general recommendations, you optimise the protection against mosquitoes and ticks and the risk of diseases they transmit by doing the following (slightly adapted version of the Centers for Disease Control and Prevention):

- Wear a long-sleeved shirt, long pants, and socks
- Treat clothing with permethrin or purchase pre-treated clothing. Permethrin-treated clothing will retain repellent activity through multiple washes
- Repellents used on skin can also be applied to clothing but provide shorter duration of protection (same duration as on skin) and must be reapplied after laundering
- Apply lotion, liquid, or spray repellent to exposed skin. Products containing the following active ingredients typically provide reasonably long-lasting protection:
    - o *DEET* (chemical name: N,N-diethyl-m-tolua-mide or N,N-diethyl-3-methyl-benzamide)

- o *Picaridin* (chemical name: 2-(2-hydroxyethyl)-1-piperidinecarboxylic acid 1-methylpropyl ester)
- o *Oil of lemon eucalyptus (OLE)*
- o *PMD* (chemical name: para-menthane-3,8-diol), the synthesised version of OLE
- o *IR3535* (chemical name: 3-[N-butyl-N-acetyl]-aminopropionic acid, ethyl ester)

For mosquitoes:

- Use common sense. Reapply repellents as protection wanes and mosquitoes start to bite
- Use bed nets. Bed nets are most effective when they are treated with a pyrethroid insecticide

For ticks:

- If you're an athlete regularly practising training or competition activities in forests (orienteer, mountain biking, etc.), where tick borne encephalitis is endemic (viral disease, endemic to most European countries), vaccinations are strongly recommended
- Check yourself daily (your entire body), remove attached ticks promptly, and disinfect the site
- To remove the tick, use flat tweezers (anatomical), catch the tick, and pull it slowly but firmly straight backwards (perpendicular to the skin)
- If you observe an outspreading slightly purple coloured reddening of the skin (Erythema chronicum migrans) around the zone of the former tick bite, see a doctor. You have possibly a Lyme borreliosis (bacteria) and need antibiotic treatment (see Photo 1)

Photo 1: Lyme Borreliosis With Erythema Chronicum Migrans After Tick Bite
(courtesy Dr Lorenz Boehlen, FMH Dermatology, Berne)

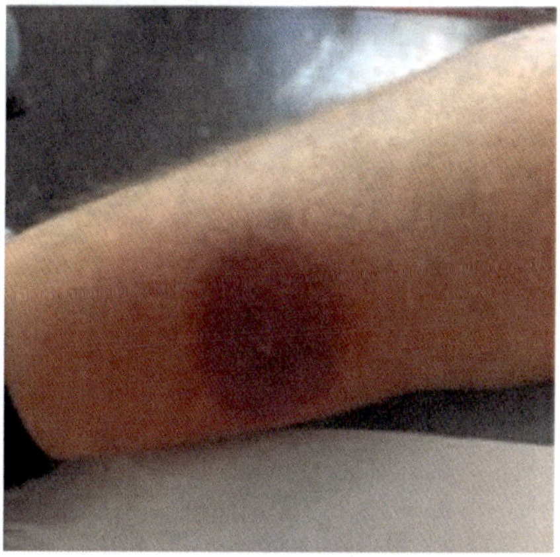

Literature

'Protection against Mosquitos, Ticks & other arthropods' retrieved on the Website of the Centre of Disease Control 15.4.2016 http://www.cdc.gov/travel/yellowbook/2016/the-pre-travel-consultation/protection-against-mosquitoes-ticks-other-arthropods

Tick borne encephalitis on Baxter Website, retrieved online 5.6.2016 http://www.baxter.com.sg/press_room/factsheets/vaccines/tick-borne_encephalitis.html

Skin Injuries – Management of a Simple Bruise to an Open Wound

Superficial Bruise

Symptoms

The skin is only superficially bruised. There is usually a slight bleeding.

Prevention	Wear the usual protectors, where appropriate. In bike sports, wear gloves (often forgotten).
Treatment by Yourself	Clean the wound with plain tap water, then disinfect. When sport continues, put a plaster dressing on to prevent contamination and to protect other players. Re-do wound care after training/competition.
When is a Doctor Needed?	No need!
Return to Play/ Sports	Immediately.

Deep Abrasion

Symptoms

Due to a high movement energy in sports, which is in case of a sport trauma decelerated to zero, the skin may suffer a more important injury in form of a deep abrasion. This leads a larger wound and a more profound but diffuse bleeding, as the whole epidermis and often also the dermis is abraded.

Depending on the injured surface and the depth of the wound it takes often weeks until the skin is nicely regenerated.

Prevention	• Wearing protectors, if appropriate, for elbows and knees • Wearing long sleeves • Being careful in slippery curves with gravel
Treatment by Yourself	• A thoroughly made inspection and wound cleaning are essential as quite often small bits of gravel, dirt, or wood may be stuck and hidden in the deep wound. Disinfect the wound properly • In case of a deep abrasion, a treatment with an antiseptic cream (e.g. Flammazine) is appropriate, as it keeps the wound clean and helps the skin to regenerate a bit quicker. Change the dressing initially daily with a thin cream layer covered by a gauze. Healing time may take several days to two weeks. When the wound is getting smaller (usually new rose coloured skin growing in), a treatment change to disinfection once daily and a plaster dressing may be appropriate
When is a Doctor Needed?	Usually no need if appropriate treatment has started.
Return to Play/ Sports	Depending on the location and severity: Often no pause needed but in severe cases up to 10–14 days.

Bad Blisters

Symptoms

A simple blister is actually not worthwhile describing, really badly healing or inflamed blisters warrant more attention.

A blister occurs where too much mechanical energy is applied on our skin. It often appears after having changed something (e.g. new training shoes, wet and sandy training conditions, intensive work with the hands to grip sports equipment, etc.).

Prevention	• Get used to new training shoes, stepwise possibly • Take a pair of used training shoes with you to be able to change
Treatment by Yourself	• If it's a small blister, disinfectant and a plaster dressing is fine • If the blister is still intact, best thing is to leave it as it is, as it's closed and sterile • If it's a really large one, disturbing, skin possibly already open, leave the skin on, you may possibly open the blister in one corner to be able to disinfect it properly. Use iodine to dry out the skin and kill the microbes • If the region is already quite inflamed then it is time for an iodine bath. Put the touched body site for 10min in an iodine bath (plastic bowl with tap water and iodine solution, as much as is needed to give it the colour of a dark black tea). Then let the skin air-dry and repeat this treatment 5–6 times per day
When is a Doctor Needed?	Not needed.
Return to Play/ Sports	Immediately. In very severe cases, according to the progress of treatment.

Burning Injuries

Symptoms

Slight burning injuries (usually Grade I) may happen by accidentally rubbing your skin on a synthetic sport surface. Other burning injuries happen usually by contact to fire, a very hot surface, or a hot liquid. Three grades are differentiated:

- *Grade I:* Reddening of the skin, often persisting, feeling as it is still burning
- *Grade II:* Blister formation on the contact site with the hot surface or hot liquid. Uncomfortable, burning pain

- *Grade III:* Skin destruction with white-greyish sometimes black skin rags. Sometimes painful, sometimes no pain anymore (nerve endings damaged)

Prevention	Be careful with fire, hot water, and hot surfaces.
Treatment by Yourself	• *Immediate cooling under cold tap water!* • When a blister appears and it's not disturbing, leave it like that. If it's open or disturbing, open it slightly in one corner but leave the blister skin on, as it may still help to protect. Use disinfectant and a gauze dressing • If it's a bigger surface, in Grade II, a treatment with an antiseptic cream (e.g. Flammazine) is recommended
When is a Doctor Needed?	A burning injury, Grade II, seriously touching the face or covering a large surface (an entire arm, a large part of the leg), and any Grade III burning injuries should be treated by a doctor.
Return to Play/ Sports	• Grade I and II: if not too large in size, immediately • Severe Grade II (big surface) and Grade III: according to the treating doctor.

Cutting Wound

Symptoms

If the trauma is more severe and there are cutting surfaces or heavy shearing forces involved, a cutting wound may result. The skin lays open; sometimes visible in the bleeding wound is fat tissue (subcutaneous fat tissue) or other underlying structures.

Prevention	• Where protectors and helmet, wherever appropriate and indicated • Wear a mouthguard
Treatment by Yourself	You may perform a first wound cleaning and disinfection, cover the wound region with a slight gauze dressing for the transport to the next doctor.

When is a Doctor Needed?	Within 6 hours! A cutting wound needs stitches, so you need to see a doctor or an emergency department of a hospital. To allow primary good wound healing and prevent bacterial infection, the wound needs to be closed within the time frame of six hours. Often a rappel injection to prevent tetanus is also performed.
Return to Play/ Sports	• In 'usual' wounds without any concomitant injury, in particular without any head injury, without concussion, a return into competition the same day may be possible • In doubtful cases (large and dirt wounds, possible additional injury) and with a head injury or a concussion, RTP according to the treating doctor (certainly not the same day)

Literature

Yanturali S et al. Injury and illness among athletes during a multi-day elite cycling road race. Phys Sportsmed. 2015 Nov;43(4):348-54.

Eye

Burning Eye/Redness of the Eye – Good Tips for Self-Management

Symptoms

After travelling, exposure to a lot of sun, exposure to wind, carrying dust, or a whole day indoors with the air-conditioning on high, we may suffer burning and redness of the eye/s. If you wear contact lenses, this may even be more pronounced

Prevention and Treatment Table for Burning Eye/ Redness of the Eye

Prevention	Wear sunglasses that are laterally closed. In snow sports, on glaciers, close to or on water surfaces, it's a must, as sunlight is reflected in these conditions If you wear contact lenses, rinse and clean them regularly, especially when it's dusty. Always take your glasses with you when travelling. For long journeys, wearing glasses may be more comfortable
Treatment by Yourself	Seek the shade, stay indoors Wash your eyes and calm them with black tea. Prepare a fresh black tea (let it steep for 8–10min to let the tanning agents come out into the water), and let it cool. Plunge a tissue in the black tea and put it on your eyes for 5–10min. You may repeat that three to four times a day. The tanning agents of the black tea are astringent and sooth the irritated eye

	Control for a foreign body – ask another person to check your eyes.
When is a Doctor Needed?	Usually no need.
Return to Play/Sports	Immediately

Conjunctivitis – When the Eye Really Matters

Symptoms

Conjunctivitis is an inflammation of the outer part of the eye, so it's easily recognisable by a reddening, itching, and swelling of one or both eyes. It often provokes tears. Often there's also a sometimes transparent, sometimes yellow, discharge around the eye.

Background

The conjunctiva is a mucous membrane covering the eyeball and the inner layer of the eyelid. It produces some mucus and tear fluid (distinctly less than the lacrimal gland) and has a function of immunosurveillance, as it is an outer membrane of the body (see Figure 1).

Figure 1: Conjunctiva and Eye, Cross Sectional View

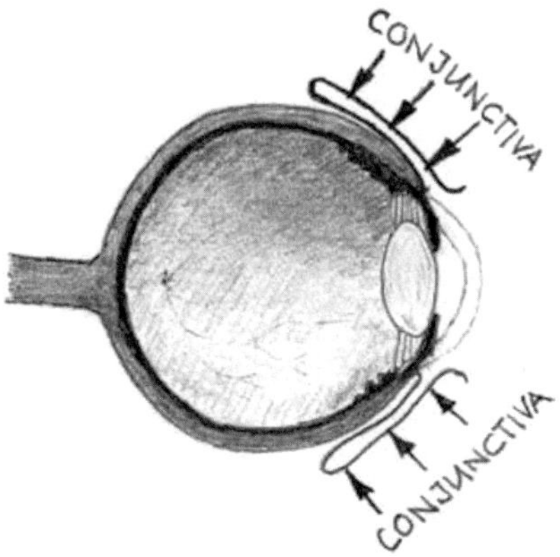

There are three main known origin of conjunctivitis. Table 1 may help to differentiate:

Table 1:

	Symptoms/ clinical picture	History	Itching	Contagious
Viral (most frequent)	Quite variable	After travelling or contact with many people, swimming pools	No, but burning	Highly contagious
Allergic (very frequent)	Always both eyes, itching red eyes, watery discharge	Allergy against pollen known, seasonal	Yes, strongly	Not contagious
Bacterial (less frequent)	Mattering and adherence of the eyelid on waking, often yellow discharge	Never had it before. After travelling or contact with many people	No, but burning	Highly contagious! See a doctor
Other reasons (rare)	Variable	Variable	Variable	Seek a doctor if not resolved after 4–6 days

Prevention and Treatment Table for Conjunctivitis

Prevention	• If you're prone to catching conjunctivitis, wear sunglasses in demanding situations for your eyes • If you wear contact lenses, always take your glasses with you when travelling
Treatment by Yourself	• Seek the shade, stay indoors • Wash your eyes and calm them with black tea. Prepare a fresh black tea (let it steep for 8–10min, to let the tanning agents come out in the tea water), and let it cool. Plunge a tissue in the black tea and put it on your eyes

	for 5–10min. You may repeat that three to four times a day. The tanning agents of the black tea are astringent and calm the irritated eye • Use Visine (tetrahydrozoline, boric acid) eye drops 4–5 times daily, as they contain an astringent and disinfectant agent. In case of an allergic conjunctivitis use Spersallerg (antazolin/tetryzolin) 4–5 times daily as they contain an antihistaminic and astringent agent • Don't wear any contact lenses while suffering a conjunctivitis. With hard lenses, clean them thoroughly. With soft lenses, put them in the rubbish bin and wash again your hands thoroughly.
When is a Doctor Needed?	If the conjunctivitis is severe, possibly of bacterial origin, or not getting any better after 3–4 days, you should see a doctor.
Return to Play/ Sports	• *Be aware* viral and bacterial conjunctivitis are contagious. With a viral or bacterial conjunctivitis, it is recommended you stay off the team so other team members are not infected • In slight cases, and individual sports, an immediate return is possible • In severe cases, according to the progress of treatment: individual training on a lower level is often possible, team training or competition needs to be discussed with the treating doctor

What Does the Doctor Do?

The doctor confirms the diagnosis. Depending on the probable diagnosis, a swab test (to determine the type of bacteria) may (or may not) be taken and treatment with appropriate eye drops is started immediately. Application of black tea swabs may give some comfort. Very strict hygiene with repeated washing of your hands, especially after having touched your eyes, is essential. Treatment propositions:

- Viral conjunctivitis: eye drops, like Visine
- Bacterial conjunctivitis: antibiotic eye drops 4–5times daily as long as necessary, usually 2 days longer as symptoms are persistent
- Allergic conjunctivitis: anti-allergy eye drops, like Spersallerg; possibly even antihistamine tablets

Literature

Alfonso SA et al. Conjunctivitis. Prim Care. 2015 Sep;42(3):325-45.

Eye Injury – Eyesight is Priceless

Most eye injuries in sports are preventable. The type of injury may vary from a slight bruise to a catastrophic loss of vision of one eye.

Symptoms

Tenderness, swelling, bruising, bleeding, blurred or double vision, and possibly loss of vision. The patient sometimes has a spasm of the eyelid and cannot open the eye.

Background

Sport disciplines resulting in eye injuries vary from country to country. In the USA, the most prevalent eye injuries are observed in basketball, water sports, baseball, and racquet sports.[(1)] In Scandinavian countries, it's soccer, floorball, bandy, and squash.[(2)] In Canada, it's ice hockey.[(3)]

The trauma may be caused by a ball, a puck, a racquet, a finger, a fist, or something else. Depending on the cause there may be different types of injury:

- Cuts or scrapes to the eyelid
- Cuts or scrapes to the inner eye, e.g. cornea
- Blunt traumas
- Penetrating trauma

The first situation is one of the most frequently encountered, and is harmless, just needing disinfectant and some rest. The three others and in any case of unclear eye injury, a medical doctor needs to be contacted quite quickly, but depending on the injury, immediate ophthalmological care may be needed.

To prevent eye injuries, rules have been adapted (high stick rules and wearing of certified face protectors in juniors' ice hockey). The availability of certified eye protectors is important in reducing eye injuries in racquet sports, field hockey, and floorball.

Illustration 1: Eye Protector In Floorball (Courtesy of Matthias Hofbauer, Swiss National Floorball Player)

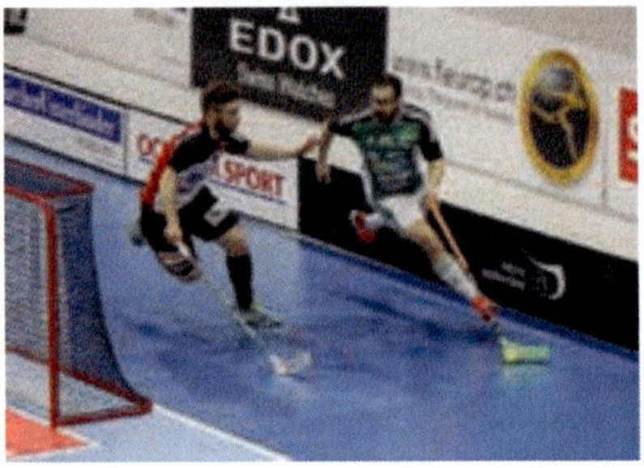

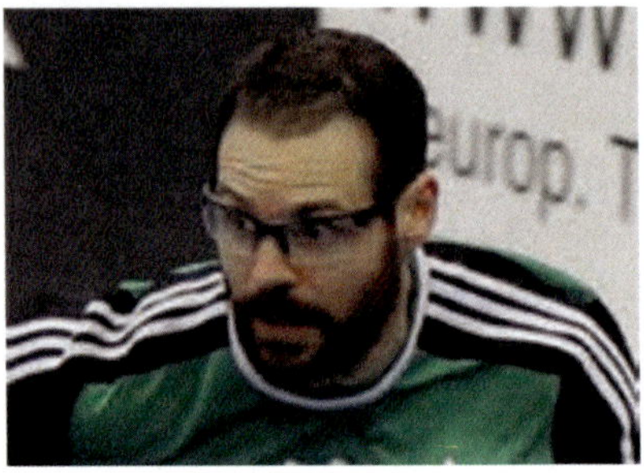

Prevention and Treatment Table for Eye Injuries

Prevention (also see Links below)	• Wearing appropriate eye protectors (contact lenses offer no protection, and ordinary glasses do not provide adequate protection) • Functionally one-eyed people should wear appropriate eye protectors. Coaches and health professionals should motivate one-eyed people to follow this recommendation
Treatment by Yourself (also see Links below)	Slight bruises and scrapes to the eyelid, with intact vision, may be self-treated. For all other type of eye injuries, you need to see a doctor the same day and, in some cases, immediately. In more serious situations: • Do not examine the eye further and do not remove any foreign object with force. If available and appropriate, gently rinse the eye with some saline to remove dirt • Do not use any creams or drops before medical assessment • Pad the eye by putting a sterile dressing (e.g. gauze pad) on the eye and fix it gently with tape or bandage, without applying too much pressure

	• Consult a medical practitioner, an ophthalmologist, or the emergency department of the nearest hospital
When is a Doctor Needed?	As above, as well as in any doubtful situation.
Return to Sports/Play	According to the severity. Be careful. Even in slight cases, with just a scratch on the eyelid, during competition, if doubtful, sit out of the game.

What Does the Doctor Do?

The medical treatment depends on the severity of the injury and needs to be individually discussed. As eye injuries need to be taken extremely seriously, you must follow the medical advices concerning return to play.

Literature

(1) Rodriguez J, AM Lavina and A Agarwal. Prevention and Treatment of Common Eye Injuries in Sports J. Am Fam Physician. 2003 Apr 1;67(7):1481-1488. http://www.aafp.org/afp/2003/0401/p1481.html

(2) Drolsum L. Eye injuries in sports. Scand J Med Sci Sports 1999: 9: 53-56, http://www.sportmedicine.ru/articles/eye_injuries_in_sports.pdf

(3) Pashby T. Eye injuries in sports. Journal of Ophthalmic Nursing & Technology [1989, 8(3):99-101], http://europepmc.org/abstract/med/2724346

Links

There are two valuable factsheets on the topic available online, one from FIMS (International Sports medicine Federation) and the other from Sports medicine Australia:

- http://www.fims.org/files/5214/2056/2358/PS6-Eye-Injuries-and-Eye-Protection-in-Sports.pdf
- http://sma.org.au/resources-advice/injury-fact-sheets/eye-injuries/

Nearsightedness, Farsightedness, Contact Lenses in Sports – What to Look For

There's not much to say about common eye illnesses and sport. Wearing ordinary glasses or contact lenses does not impair sport performance, but having full vision is certainly an advantage in almost all sports. That's why vision is regularly tested in the annual sportsmed exam. It may also be helpful to be aware of a few things, which may make life a bit easier:

Depending on your sport discipline you may prefer contact lenses instead of ordinary glasses:

- In rugby, soccer, or martial arts, as glasses may be broken or the cause of injuries
- In racquet and other ball sports, roller-skating, or ice skating, as your field of vision may be impaired by glasses
- In water sports, like swimming, sailing, or surfboarding, as contact lenses bring a huge advantage not impairing the vision like glasses would

Tips for contact lenses in sport:

- Put lenses in at least 30min before competition or usual daily training (ideally to adapt the balance of lacrimation)
- After longer training or competition, take the lenses out, as the metabolism of the cornea is raised (the eye layer directly underneath the contact lens) and recovers better without coverage by the lens
- With water sports and sport disciplines close to sand or with possible dust exposure, soft contact lenses may be beneficial
- In sport disciplines related to dehydration and/or with an airstream, e.g. running, cycling, it may be profitable to use form-stable, hard contact lenses, and to further protect the eye from the airstream with sunglasses

- Don't keep contact lenses in your eyes for too long, respect the recommendations of the manufacturer and your optician/ optometrist
- Thorough care of contact lenses is essential (take enough cleaning solution with you while travelling)
- When long-distance travelling, always take a pair of glasses and spare lenses with you (in case you lose them or of a conjunctivitis, which is more frequent in time of travel)

Tips for glasses in sports:

- Check your glasses with your optician/optometrist for an optimal fit
- Wear a retainer or strap in sports
- Possibly consider sport glasses or corrective swimming goggles

Literature

Komori Y et al. The use of contact lenses during water-polo play: a 20-year study of Japanese college players. J Sports Sci. 2013;31(6):607-11.

Schnell D, Khaireddin R. Corneal metabolism with contact lenses in competitive sports. Ophthalmologe. 2013 Jun;110(6):502-10.

Ear, Nose, Throat

Common Cold – More Frequent in Athletes Than in the Normal Population

Symptoms

Discomfort, slight headache, sore throat, sneezing, running nose, eventually slight rise in body temperature

Background

Why is the common cold described again under the Ear, Nose, Throat chapter? It is because the nose-throat region is the entry point for this viral infection. A recent study has, for the first time, shown that the term *'catching a cold'* is quite right, for this is what happens when we get a virus infection. With cooler temperatures, the mucosal surfaces of the nose are cooler and less well-supplied with blood, resulting in a diminished local antiviral immune response. This enables the replication of the common cold virus (rhinovirus) and a start for the infection.

Prevention and Treatment Table for Common Cold (Most Often Rhinovirus Infection)

Prevention	• See the chapter 'Prevention of Infectious Illnesses in Sport' and follow these recommendations to face the 'open window' situation athletes have. • Most important recommendation: Don't catch a cold! What does this mean? o Wear appropriate training suits and change wet and moist clothes after training.

	o In winter, wear a cap, warm underwear, and gloves. o Eat a well-balanced diet, drink enough, look for enough sleep, and general recovery.
Treatment by Yourself	So called symptomatic treatment. Drink a lot of freshly made tea (lime tree) with pure honey. Echinacea has proven to be effective against viruses, rinse your mouth with echinacea syrup or drops, or suck echinacea tablets before swallowing them (e.g. Echinamed, 3 x 3 tbl daily).
When is a Doctor Needed?	Usually not needed. If it is not getting any better after 4 days, see a doctor. If additional symptoms (e.g. high fever, severe headache, nearly fainting) are present then see a doctor the same day.
Return to Play/Sports	• With fever (i.e. elevated temperature) usually axillary temperature >37°C, ear (tympanal) or mouth temperature (enoral) >37.5°C: *NO sport!* This is very important, as elevated temperature indicates a still active illness, so while doing sport you will spread the germs and make things worse. Training with fever could be fatal, as it may induce a deadly heart rhythm anomaly. • When temperature is fine, you are getting better, *'start slow, go slow'*. You may start with slight aerobic or warming up exercises, e.g. 30min or even just 2 x 15min extensive at a very low pace or a general warming up and some flexibility exercises. Then try then to come back into regular training within 7–10 days by slightly adding to the training load.

Literature

Human rhinovirus induced cytokine/chemokine responses in human airway epithelial and immune cells.Rajan D, McCracken CE, Kopleman HB, Kyu SY, Lee FE, Lu X, Anderson LJ.PLoS One. 2014; 9(12):e114322. Epub 2014 Dec 12.,http://www.ncbi.nlm.nih.gov/pubmed/25500821

Swimmer's Ear (External Otitis) – an Annoying Ear Pain

Symptoms

Ear pain, on one side typically, stinging, often with some hearing impairment, not getting any better. Stinging pain while pressing firmly on the tragus (i.e. ear cartilage, which forms a kind of lid of the ear entrance) or while pressing the ear cartilage firmly forward from the back of the ear.

Figure 1:

1.1 Normal external ear

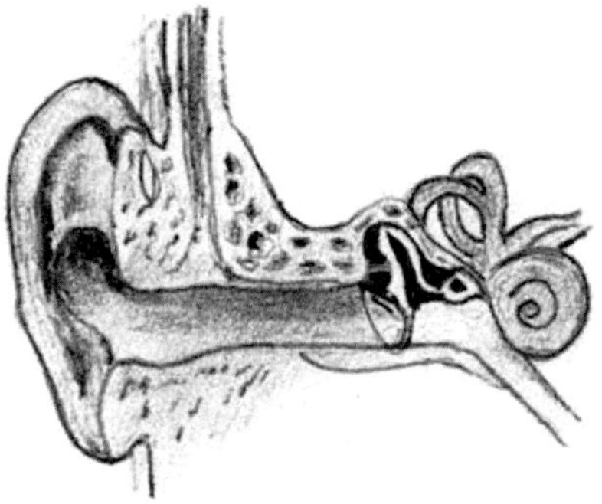

1.2. External otitis /Swimmer's ear

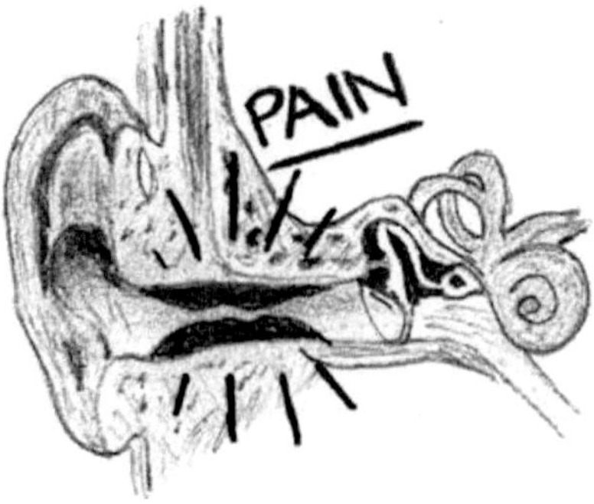

Background

An often encountered outer ear infection, typically in water sports athletes, like swimmers and divers. It is a mostly bacterial infection of the ear canal with pain, reddening, swelling, narrowing of the canal, and sometimes hearing impairment.

Prevention and Treatment Table for Swimmer's Ear (External Otitis)

Prevention	• Important to dry the ear region (and the hairs) after training and shower, especially in winter. Let the ear dry out. Only use headphones when the ear is completely dry! • Wear a cap in winter • Possibly use ear plugs for prevention
Treatment by Yourself	If you are prone to Swimmer's ear, application of the following mixture is helpful: • Twice a week 3 drops of almond oil and 1 drop of Desomedine (disinfectant eye drop). Yes, eye drops! Because it is a very gentle disinfectant, it is perfect for regular use, and is an over the counter product • Alternatively use 'diver's eardrops', but be careful with them, as the active ingredients are often quite strong and vary a lot
When is a Doctor Needed?	Usually a quick check is needed, as the doctor needs to look into the ear to check canal and eardrum. You also need antibiotic eardrops, to be applied 5x 3–4 drops daily for 5–6days (normally one or two days longer than symptoms last). A quick second check after 4–5days to see if the treatment was effective allows a decision on a return to water training.

Return to Play/ Sports	Normally the athlete is not severely ill but the ear is affected by a bacterial infection and often really painful. Training in the water will immerse the site of infection, and to swim lap after lap with an aching ear drives you mad! To use an earplug isn't an option either, as it is quite painful and creates an ideal moist climate for further spreading bacteria and inviting other germs, so allow 3–4 days without water contact. Aerobic exercises at land and flexibility training may be continued, slight strengthening exercises are possible after the 3rd or 4th day. Once the infection is resolved, go back to previous training.

What Does the Doctor Do?

Confirms the diagnosis; excludes that it is possibly an infection of the middle ear (medial otitis, very frequent in childhood, much less prevalent in adolescence or in adults) and gives ear drops containing the required antibiotic treatment.

Literature

Hajioff D, MacKeith S. Otitis externa. BMJ Clin Evid. 2015 Jun 15;2015. pii: 0510.

Wrestler's Ear – How to Prevent 'Cauliflower Ear'

Symptoms

Usually painless, but really visible swelling of the ear-shell. Due to shearing forces after contact between the ear and the ground or an opponent.

Background

The swelling is caused by bleeding underneath the skin of the ear, lifting the skin and showing a kind of bubbly swelling. It is not painful and is sterile, so there is no infection. The blood beneath the skin will be influenced by our body, become hard, and remain like that. If it remains like that, ears look quite prominent and are called 'cauliflower' ear. It's up to you whether this bothers you or not, but the ear will not have its fine, well-shaped form with curves and hollows but a firm, solid, and a slightly clumsy aspect.

Prevention and Treatment Table for Wrestler's Ear

Prevention	If Wrestler's/ Rugby/Judo ear is a possibility for you, wearing of a soft training helmet may possibly help (as used in rugby/soccer goal-keepers).
Treatment by Yourself	Don't try to treat yourself, as it must be done in a sterile way. And being honest, no one can do this on himself in a clean and appropriate way. Check with your sports medicine physician or somebody else on the medical team.

When is a Doctor Needed?	Even if it's not harmful, the sports medicine physician is the doctor to see.
Return to Play/ Sports	Immediately. Wear a slight compression bandage around your head for training in the first few days. For 3–4 days, training sequences with possible shearing forces to the ear should be avoided to let it heal well.

What Does the Doctor Do?

The doctor puts a sterile needle in, sucks the blood out, and puts a compression bandage on. Frequently this must be repeated the next day, as it fills up again.

Literature

Mudry A, Pirsig W Auricular hematoma and cauliflower deformation of the ear: from art to medicine. Otol Neurotol. 2009 Jan;30(1):116-20.

Schuller DE et al. Auricular injury and the use of headgear in wrestlers. Arch Otolaryngol Head Neck Surg. 1989 Jun;115(6):714-7.

Allergic Rhino-Sinusitis – When the Nose Is Dripping

Symptoms

Running nose, abundant secretions in the upper airways, sometimes descending through the back of the throat (postnasal drip) provoking coughing and impaired respiration through the nose.

Background

An allergy is an excessive body reaction to an external antigen like plant pollen, dust, or domestic mites (the latter is very frequent and often unknown!). Its appearance is mostly seasonal and presents as an inflammation of mostly the ear-nose-throat region (allergic rhino-sinusitis), often the conjunctives (allergic conjunctivitis), and occasionally the lungs (allergic asthma). You may already know about your allergy to pollen, mites, etc. with reaction of the eyes (slight irritation, conjunctivitis) and possibly the nose (rhinitis). An allergy is more likely if somebody in your family suffers from allergic illnesses ('positive family history' or you have an allergic history in the past).

Prevention and Treatment Table for Allergic Rhino-Sinusitis

Prevention	See treatment
Treatment by Yourself	• Once you know the diagnosis, follow the instructions of your sports medicine physician or GP. • For a pollen allergy, a reduction of the irritating stimulus is often helpful: o Washing your hair in the evening with plain water (to rinse the pollens out)

	o Rinsing your nose with saline in the evening (to rinse the pollens and clean the mucosal surfaces in the nose) o Wearing sunglasses during the day • For a mite allergy, the so called 'encasing' procedures are very effective. This means to encase pillow, blanket, and mattress in a mite dust tight cover. Also, reduce dust catchers at home (long hair carpets, big curtains, etc.). Ask your doctor, they will know more about it.
When is a Doctor Needed?	To have a correct diagnosis the doctor is needed.
Return to Play/ Sports	No need for a pause.

What Does the Doctor Do?

The doctor confirms the diagnosis by taking the history, clinical examination, and allergy testing. The most frequent and easy testing is the skin-prick test. Around 20 drops containing typical irritating stimuli (different pollen, domestic mites, etc.) are applied to the skin to look for a possible allergic reaction to this particular allergen. Additional blood testing may be performed. According to the diagnosis, treatment will be started. Besides the recommendations above, it consists of an anti-inflammatory and antihistaminic nose spray (different formulas available, just antihistamine, just cortisone, or containing both). In more severe cases, you should go for the combined one, as cortisone heads off the overwhelming allergic reaction and gives a protective effect and antihistamine helps to diminish it. If this is still inadequate, systemic antihistamine treatment as tablets may also be used.

Desensitisation treatment is an interesting option as it addresses the excessive allergic reaction: the body's immune system is trained to accept the former allergen (i.e. desensitise) by presenting very little doses of it. This treatment seems to be really effective but usually takes three years and needs to be started out of the allergen season. Talk to your doctor about it.

Literature

Dijkstra HP, Robson-Ansley P . The prevalence and current opinion of treatment of allergic rhinitis in elite athletes. Curr Opin Allergy Clin Immunol. 2011 Apr;11(2):103-8.

Alaranta A et al. Allergic rhinitis and pharmacological management in elite athletes. Med Sci Sports Exerc. 2005 May;37(5):707-11.

Sinusitis – Painful Pressure Within the Head

Symptoms

Acute Sinusitis: Severe headache, focused mostly on the affected region, the sinus involved. Local tenderness. Feeling really ill, possibly elevated temperature or fever (not compulsory). Possibly impaired respiration through the nose, possibly pus discharge in nasal secretions.

Chronic Sinusitis: Variable, possibly a lighter headache than in the acute form. Possibly more nasal secretions, possibly with pus discharge, possibly impaired respiration through the nose. But no fever, not feeling ill, but just 'out of sorts'. Often an impairment of performance. A hidden and undiscovered chronic sinusitis may be a reason for impaired performance (see also chapter 'Unclear Fatigue in Sports').

Background

Sinuses are bony cavities with a mucous membrane inside our head that are formed during our growth, mainly in childhood, and are usually fully established by the age of 12–14years. You have several sinuses: two frontal, two maxillary, a central one (sphenoidal), and several smaller ones up in the nose (the ethmoidal cells, see Figure 1). All connect with the nose, but the opening from a sinus towards the nose is already small and in case of inflammation it's even narrower or closed. As soon as the aeriation and a fluid exchange from a sinus to the nose is impaired, problems may start. And this happens quite often.

Luckily our body balances that out for a long time, but if the connection remains closed, and some bacteria rest in a sinus, sinusitis (i.e. inflammation) appears. We differentiate acute from chronic sinusitis, but both are not good for sport performance. Additionally sinusitis, whether acute or chronic, bears the risk of postnasal drip—the dropping or running down of pus, bacteria, and secretions in the back of our throat leading to coughing and infection of the lower airways, bronchitis, or even pneumonia.

Figure 1: Sinus in the Head – Frontal and Side View

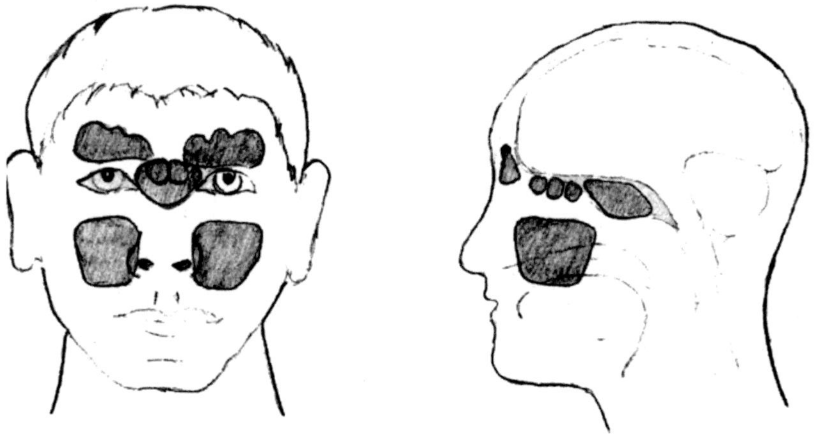

Figure 2: Acute Sinusitis – Frontal and Side View

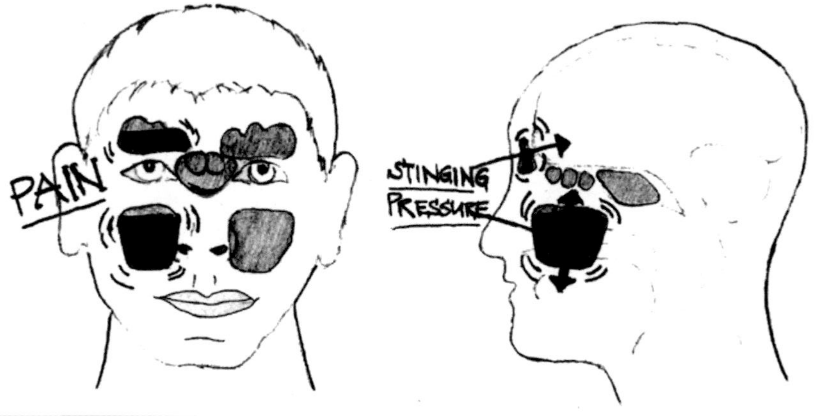

Figure 3: Chronic Sinusitis – Frontal and Side View

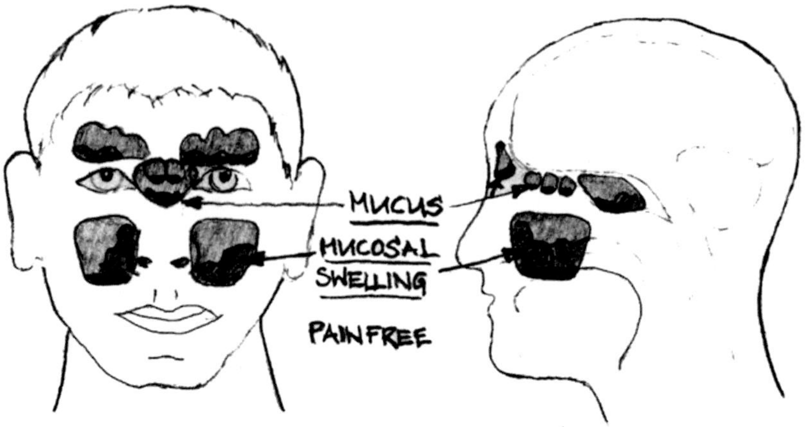

Prevention and Treatment Table for Sinusitis/Acute and Chronic

Prevention	If you are prone to suffer sinusitis, rinsing the nose with saline solution may be helpful. If it happens all the time, you need to see an ENT (ear, nose, throat) specialist to discuss whether the connection ways possibly need an enlargement.
Treatment by Yourself	As prevention. In some cases, early rinsing of the nose with saline nose drops for five days (Otrivin© 3x/d) and anti-inflammatory herbal drug (Gelodurat 3x/d or Sinupret 3x/d) have proven effective in preventing more severe acute sinusitis.
When is a Doctor Needed?	• In both cases. o In acute sinusitis, see a doctor, as you will feel really ill o In chronic sinusitis, it's more of a suspicion, as explained above

Return to Play/ Sports	Treatment needs to be initiated as soon as possible. • In acute sinusitis, the athlete is really ill, usually has fever, and needs antibiotics. Recovery needs to respect this • In chronic sinusitis, training may, in case of an antibiotic treatment, be reduced for a time, and then adapted to previous plans after that

What Does the Doctor Do?

The doctor confirms the diagnosis with history, clinical examination, possibly x-rays, or CT scan. In established acute sinusitis, antibiotic treatment for 10 days is usually started, together with nose drops for 5 days (to reduce the swelling of mucous membranes and open the sinuses), and rinsing saline solution to get all the dirt, bacteria, and discharge out. Rinsing the nose must be continued and after a few days, a nose spray with corticosteroids is started for two months to really reduce swelling of the mucous membranes and re-open the passage ways between the sinuses to the nose.

In chronic sinusitis, antibiotic treatment may or may not be initiated. Nose drops (5 days), rinsing with saline, and the nose spray containing cortisone (2 months) are essential in this situation.

Pharyngitis/Angina Tonsillaris – a Sore Throat and Difficulties Swallowing

Symptoms

Sore throat and difficulties in swallowing. Feeling as if the throat is burning. Possibly enlarged lymph nodes along the throat and underneath the chin. You may possibly recognise a reddening of the internal throat in the mirror.

Figure 1: Drawing of the Defence Ring in Our Throat

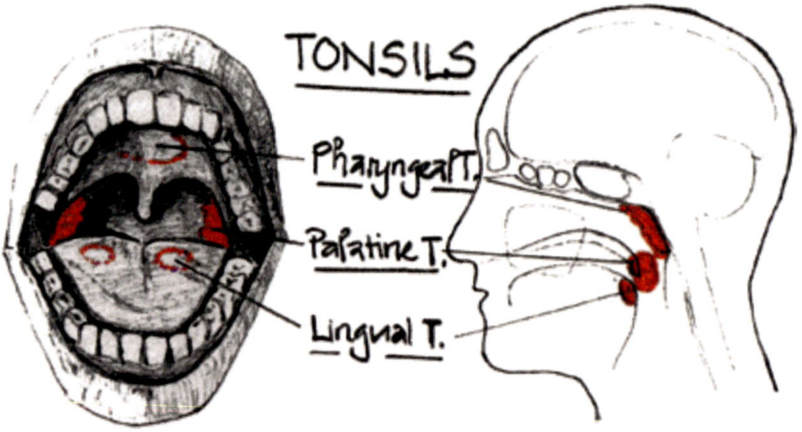

Background

Pharyngitis describes an inflammation of the pharynx (upper back part of our throat). There are several glands that help us to defend ourselves against all kind of microbes (see Figure 1). Most frequently pharyngitis is *viral*, with a general reddening and a sore throat. This means a virus has hooked onto the mucosal surfaces of the throat causing the inflammation. It may involve other nearby parts of this defence ring, in particular the tonsils (or tonsillary glands). These may well be involved in a viral infection, which hurts and leads to swelling, but will disappear with symptomatic treatment. This needs to be differentiated from *bacterial infection of the tonsils* (*tonsillitis* or angina tonsillaris).

Prevention and Treatment Table for Pharyngitis /Tonsillitis

Prevention	• See extensive preventive measures in chapter 'Prevention of Infectious Diseases': o Wash your hands regularly o Use your own drinking bottle, etc.
Treatment by Yourself	As above.
When is a Doctor Needed?	In case of suspected tonsillitis or a pharyngitis with fever.
Return to Play/ Sports	• With simple viral pharyngitis, without fever, slight aerobic exercise may be possible, if unsure check with your doctor • With *fever*, strictly no training! • In case of tonsillitis and antibiotic treatment, a pause for a few days will help to recover. *Less is more* in these situations

What Does the Doctor Do?

The doctor confirms the diagnosis by taking the history, clinical examination, and a swab test for particular bacteria (scarlet fever, streptococcal group A infection) to determine whether antibiotic treatment or supportive care is indicated. In case of scarlet fever, antibiotics need to be taken for usually 10 days to prevent long term health problems.

What about surgery if tonsillitis occurs regularly?

In earlier days, ENT and paediatric doctors readily sent kids with their first episode of tonsillitis, or just slightly enlarged tonsils, for an operation to remove the tonsils. Luckily these times have gone. It is widely accepted that our defence ring in the throat is important. Operations are now only indicated when the tonsillitis becomes a frequently repeated illness. As a rule of thumb: as long as your tonsils maintain normal shape, and you don't need antibiotic treatment more than 2–3 times a year, you shouldn't consider an operation.

Respiratory System/Lungs

Upper and Lower Respiratory Tract Infections – Deep Coughing and Grisly Discharge

Symptoms

Coughing and difficulties in breathing, particularly in the cold and under effort.

In **upper** respiratory tract infections, secretions from the nose and the not very frequent sputum are usually transparent or a bit yellow.

In **lower** respiratory tract infection, however, coughing usually produces sputum (expectoration), mostly coloured, transparent-grey-yellow-green-brown, in this order, indicating the severity of the illness. Transparent is the least severe while the green-brown indicates severe infection, which can eventually lead to pneumonia.

Figure 1: Upper and Lower Respiratory System, Cross Section

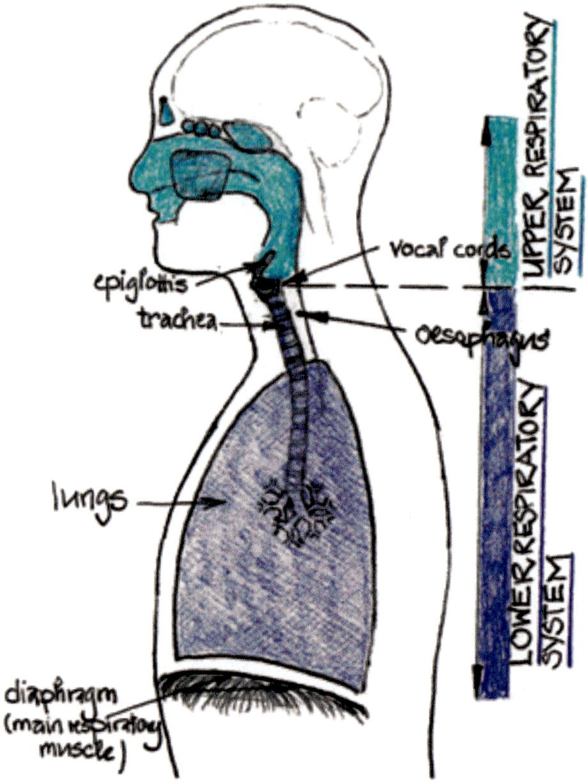

Background

In Figure 1 you see our respiratory system. Colours show the upper and the lower airways.

- *Upper airways:* Nose with sinuses, mouth, upper part of the throat, down to the larynx and vocal cords
- *Lower airways:* From the vocal cords back down, trachea (main airway in the lungs), bronchii (airway branches) to the alveoles (smallest units in the lungs, where gas exchange takes place)

It is important to remind ourselves of the connection of both systems and the quite frequent situation of the *postnasal drip*, i.e. the inflammation in an upper part of the airways (nose, eventually sinuses), the production of secretions, and the dripping down of these secretions into lower areas of the airways, thus spreading the inflammation and infection further, down into the bronchii and the lungs.

Prevention and Treatment Table for Upper and Lower Respiratory Tract Infection

Prevention	• As for the common cold. See also chapter 'Prevention of Infectious Diseases In Sports'. Please take these measures seriously, especially if you are prone to catch respiratory infections • Be conservative and stay away from others when you have an infection of the lower airways • Competing with active bronchitis is not good for you! It takes a long time to cure it. Your competition calendar is filled with events but you will definitely delay healing, will prolong the irritation of the airways, and make you cough for weeks and months if you compete. You may also be causing serious harm to your respiratory system. It is, by the way, one of the possible explanations why endurance sportsmen and women are so often touched by airway illnesses, in particular exercise-induced asthma
Treatment by Yourself	Follow the recommendations of your sports medicine physician.
When is a Doctor Needed?	• Coughing, sneezing, running nose, and slightly elevated temperature don't need a doctor • If it gets more severe, with symptoms such as never-ending coughing, sputum coloured (as described above), fever, see a doctor

Return to Play/ Sports	Depends completely on the severity of the illness. • In light cases, it's possible just a slight training reduction • In really severe cases, up to cessation of training for a week or ten days • With fever, NO sports! This doesn't mean that if I have no fever, I may perform. NO, please read thoroughly the prevention chapter about the high frequency of airway diseases in endurance sports. The missed healing time of these infections is a serious issue, not only in general but for you very personally too.

What Does the Doctor Do?

The doctor confirms the diagnosis by history, clinical exam, possibly lung function testing, possibly blood exam, possibly chest x-ray. Therapy aims for treating the infection and inflammatory response with these secretions. It consists in rinsing the nose with saline to clean it and wash away the discharges, down swelling of the mucosal surfaces in upper and lower airways with nosedrops (e.g. Otrivin), natural products, e.g. Gelodurat 3x1/d; Sinupret 3x1/d; try to liquefy the secretions with Acetylcystein 600mg x1/d. In infection of the lower airways, with fever or suspected beginning of pneumonia, an antibiotic treatment for 7–10days may be started.

Literature

Svendsen IS et al. Training-related and competition-related risk factors for respiratory tract and gastrointestinal infections in elite cross-country skiers. Br J Sports Med. 2016 Mar 3. pii: bjsports-2015-095398.

Gleeson M, Pyne DB. Respiratory inflammation and infections in high-performance athletes. Immunol Cell Biol. 2016 Feb;94(2):124-31

Mårtensson S et al. High Training Volumes are Associated with a Low Number of Self-Reported Sick Days in Elite Endurance Athletes. J Sports Sci Med. 2014 Dec 1;13(4):929-33.

Hausswirth C et al. Evidence of disturbed sleep and increased illness in overreached endurance athletes. Med Sci Sports Exerc. 2014;46(5):1036-45

Exercise Induced Asthma – Frequent in Endurance Sport, but Check Your Diagnosis

Symptoms

We would expect people with EIA (exercise induced asthma) to exhibit the asthma specific symptoms like shortness of breath, wheezing, and elevated respiratory rate. They may be present, but much more likely symptoms are: coughing attacks after physical efforts, delayed recovery after intensive trainings and competitions, and decreased stamina, all symptoms typically worsening in cold air.

Figure 1: Ultrastructure of the Lungs and the Alveoli with the Gas Exchange (courtesy Prof Dr Ewald Weibel, Institute of Anatomy, University of Berne)

1.1 Resin cast of the lung airways and lung circulation

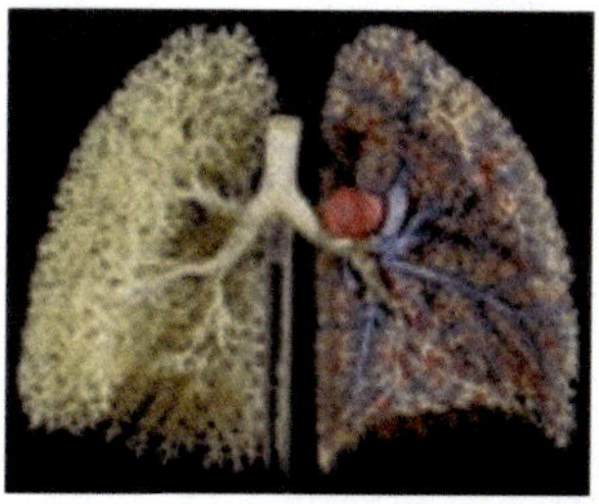

1.2 Lung ultrastructure – bronchi and alveoli

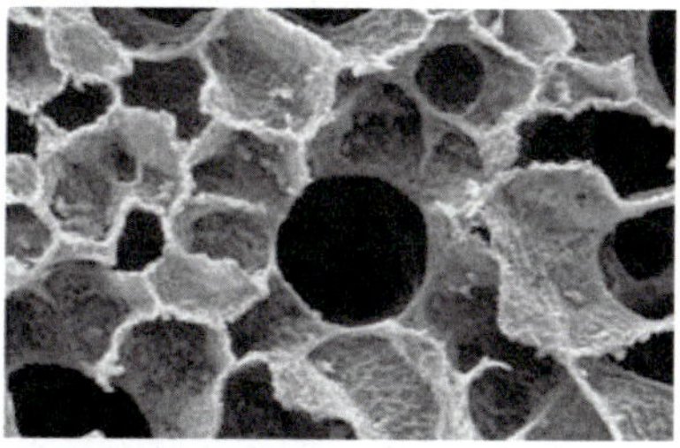

1.3 finest layer of alveoli with visible erythrocytes in the capillaries

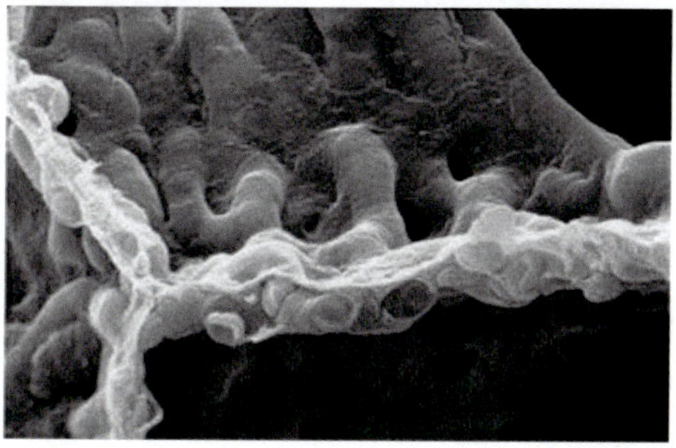

1.4 electronmicroscopic picture of the gas exchange lung capillary, thin layer to alveoli, black bodies are red blood cells (erythrocytes)

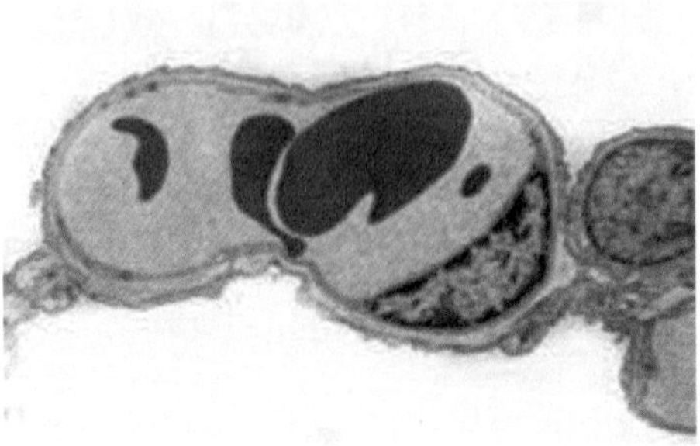

Background

Exercise does not cause asthma. But exercise, especially vigorous endurance training in a (winter) outdoor sport is frequently an asthma trigger. Long-term, intense endurance training and competition over several years, particularly in unfavourable environmental conditions, appear to be associated with an increased risk of developing exercise-induced bronchoconstriction/exercise-induced asthma in elite athletes. Whereas light to moderate endurance training seems to be beneficial for children and adults suffering from asthma.

Exercise induced asthma (EIA) occurs when the airways narrow as a result of exercise. Exercise-induced asthma and exercise-induced bronchoconstriction are synonymously used, the second term explaining the central mechanism of action of the condition. Exercise-induced bronchoconstriction (EIB) occurs after several minutes of intensive aerobic activity. This increased respiration with direct inhalation of air, which has not been warmed and humidified by the nasal passages, generates an irritation of the airways with a water-loss and heat loss, leading to mediator release, airway inflammation, and increased parasympathetic nervous activity in the airways, finally causing a narrowing (bronchial constriction) and inflammation (bronchial hyper responsiveness).

Figure 2: Mechanism of Exercise Induced Asthma

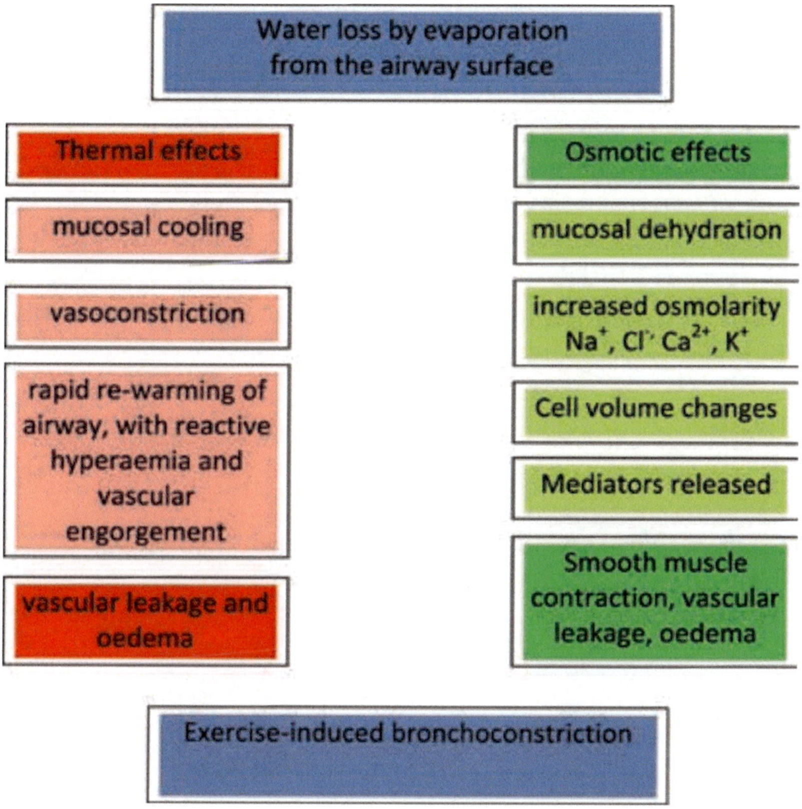

Exercise induced asthma (EIA) clearly impairs performance and athletes affected by it, who have had inadequate treatment, are seriously disadvantaged. EIA is frequent with around 15% of athletes suffering from it, more in endurance and outdoor winter sports (up to 50% in cross country skiing). Because of its sometimes atypical symptomatology, exercise induced asthma may not always be recognised, as the athlete's own perception of respiratory symptoms (like shortness of breath or slight coughing) is an unreliable diagnostic tool. As a result, athletes with EIA sometimes go without any treatment. For these reasons, it is important the diagnosis be either confirmed or rejected, so we know whether treatment is needed.

Good treatment options for EIA are available and with the appropriate treatment the athlete is able to reach his top potential and reach the podium. However, studies show clearly that use of anti-asthmatic medications in otherwise healthy athletes doesn't bring any beneficial effect on performance, but possibly does have side effects.

Use the so-called *'refractory period'*—after a good warm-up with stepwise accelerations up to competitive intensity in the immediate preparation of a race, the bronchial system goes into a protected state for about 4 hours, where it is inert to any bronchoconstriction or inflammatory response and allows further vigorous efforts without being provoked.

Prevention and Treatment Table for Exercise Induced Asthma

Prevention	• Follow the recommendations in chapter 'Prevention of Infectious Diseases in Sports' in order not to catch ongoing respiratory infections, leading to a chronic condition • Look for the 'refractory period' as described above
Treatment by Yourself	Follow your doctor's instructions.
When is a Doctor Needed?	If exercise-induced asthma/bronchoconstriction is suspected. Watch out for the symptoms as described above.
Return to Play/ Sports	Once diagnosis is established, treatment may be started without delay. Discuss and adapt the appropriate treatment plan with your sports medicine physician.

What Does the Doctor Do?

The doctor takes the history, performs a clinical examination, and lung function tests at rest. In exercise-induced asthma/ bronchoconstriction at rest, clinical examinations and lung functions are normal. Therefore, a specific exercise induced asthma test will be a performed in order to confirm or to rule out EIA/EIB. If not yet done, additional allergy testing (e.g. skin prick test) may be helpful to recognise possible allergens (pollen, mite dust, etc.). Therapy consists in a stepwise applied, combined treatment approach with a bronchodilating spray (to open the airways), an inhalative corticosteroid (to prevent the inflammatory response), and a leukotriene antagonist (anti-allergy tablet to prevent airway inflammation)—discuss your individual treatment plan with your doctor.

Good to know: As an add-on (but not replacing the main therapy stream as described above!) possibly fish-oil (n-3 fatty acids), Vitamin C, and Vitamin D could be beneficial in reducing the inflammatory response of the airways. Talk with your doctor about this interesting option

Literature

'Exercise-induced bronchoconstriction' retrieved from Wikipedia website 18.4.2016, https://en.wikipedia.org/wiki/Exercise-induced_bronchoconstriction

Kumar A et al. N-3 Fatty acids and asthma. Nutr Res Rev. 2016 Jan 26:1-16.

Bonini M et al. AIDA and the Italian Unit of the GA2LEN Olympic Study. Asthma, allergy and the Olympics: a 12-year survey in elite athletes. Curr Opin Allergy Clin Immunol. 2015 Apr;15(2):184-92

Khan, DA (Jan–Feb 2012). 'Exercise-induced bronchoconstriction: burden and prevalence '. Allergy and Asthma Proceedings 33 (1): 1–6

Stickland MK et al (March 2012). 'Effect of warm-up exercise on exercise-induced bronchoconstriction '. Med Sci Sports Exerc 44 (3): 383–91

Carlsen KH. Sports in extreme conditions: the impact of exercise in cold temperatures on asthma and bronchial hyper-responsiveness in athletes. Br J Sports Med. 2012 Sep; 46(11):796-9

Tecklenburg-Lund S et al. Randomized controlled trial of fish oil and montelukast and their combination on airway inflammation and hyperpnea-induced bronchoconstriction. PLoS One. 2010 Oct 18;5(10):e13487

Hemilä H. Vitamin C and exercise-induced bronchoconstriction in athltes. J Allergy Clin Immunol. 2009 Jan;123(1)274-5

Lund TK. Asthma in elite athletes: how do we manage asthma-like symptoms and asthma in elite athletes? Clin Respir J. 2009 Apr;3(2):123

Carlsen KH et al. (April 2008). 'Exercise-induced asthma, respiratory and allergic disorders in elite athletes: epidemiology, mechanisms and diagnosis: Part I of the report from the Joint Task Force of the European Respiratory Society (ERS) and the European Academy of Allergy and Clinical Immunology (EAACI) in cooperation with GA2LEN '. Allergy 63 (4): 387–403

Carlsen KH et al. (April 2008). 'Treatment of exercise-induced asthma, respiratory and allergic disorders in sports and the relationship to doping: Part II of the report from the Joint Task Force of European Respiratory Society (ERS) and European Academy of Allergy and Clinical Immunology (EAACI) in cooperation with GA2LEN '. Allergy 63 (4): 492–505.

Fitch KD et al. Asthma and the elite athlete: summary of the International Olympic Committee's consensus conference, Lausanne, Switzerland, January 22-24, 2008. J Allergy Clin Immunol. 2008 Aug;122(2):254-60

Anderson SD, Kippelen P. Airway injury as a mechanism for exercise-induced bronchoconstriction in elite athletes. J Allergy Clin Immunol. 2008 Aug; 122(2):225-35

Fitch KD. Beta2-Agonists at the Olympic Games. Clin Rev Allergy Immunol. 2006 Oct-Dec;31(2-3):259-68.

Asthma in Sports – With Good Treatment Reaching the Podium

Symptoms

Coughing episodes, shortness of breath, difficulties in respiration, in particular difficulties exhaling. Wheezing chest.

Background

Asthma. Greek meaning: shortness of breath. Asthma is a condition in which your airways narrow, swell, and produce extra mucus. This can make breathing difficult and trigger coughing, wheezing, and shortness of breath.

There are different asthma types. Basically asthma has a genetic determinant, so the family history is important. It means one of your closer ancestors or siblings is also suffering from the disease. Asthma almost always shows different clinical pictures at different ages, usually being quite strong and prominent in childhood, getting better in adolescence and in adulthood. Everyone should be a non-smoker, though this even more important for a person with asthma.

Prevention and Treatment Table for Asthma

Prevention	• The predisposition for the illness is mostly genetically determined • If there is an allergic component, reduction of the irritating stimulus (e.g. mite dust, pollen) leads to distinct improvement

Treatment by Yourself	• Stick to the treatment plan of your doctor • Sports, particularly endurance sports, are good for your lungs and help you develop a good feeling about yourself. They keep you in good shape and train not only the cardiovascular system and your working muscles but also the respiratory muscles. This is the reason why even severely asthmatic children profit from moderate regular endurance training, adapted to their level of performance • The other side of the coin is that it is not yet clear, but possible, that high performance endurance training and competition may affect the respiratory system and increase the number of athletes needing anti-asthmatic treatment. It is also unclear whether this treatment for asthma is only temporary, i.e. reversible after stopping high performance sport
When is a Doctor Needed?	• If asthma is suspected • With asthma, follow-up usually about twice a year
Return to Play/Sports	For safety reasons, the coach must know about the illness and be informed about treatment. With a good treatment plan and adherence to it, no pause needs to be taken. From the educational point of view, it's important for the coach treats asthmatic athletes like all the others, i.e. not be over-protective of them. However, consider and regularly check the TUE (therapeutic use exemption) with the anti-doping agency (this is usually done in the annual sportsmed exam).

What Does the Doctor Do?

In case of newly suspected asthma, the doctor takes the history focusing on asthma symptoms, onset of shortness of breath while exercising or at rest, coughing episodes, wheezing, etc. They also look at family history and indications of any allergic predisposition. A clinical examination, lung function tests, and usually a chest x-ray and allergy tests will be performed to either confirm or rule out asthma.

In case of follow-up, the doctor takes the intermediate history focusing on symptoms like coughing episodes, shortness of breath in rest, training or competition, etc. A clinical examination and lung function tests are performed to have objective measures of functional lung values of the asthmatic under treatment.

The treatment is built up stepwise, along the GINA guidelines according to the needs (Global Initiative for Asthma; 'as much therapy as is needed to control the illness, but not more'). The most important treatment (the first and second steps) are the anti-asthmatic cortisone spray (to reduce the allergic, spasm reaction locally). This is often combined with a bronchodilating medication (to open the airways for better airflow) and/or a leukotrienantagonist (montelukast), a tablet acting in an anti-allergic way. This is helpful if spray treatment is not sufficient and is intended to minimise use of cortisone. If asthma control remains insufficient, there are further treatment options (e.g. using higher doses).

With the anti-asthmatic medication you need to check the TUE (therapeutic use exemption) regulations of your country and your international sports federations, sometimes they are different! Remember, you need to check whether you need a TUE (therapeutic use exemption) before starting any treatment.

Literature

'Asthma' retrieved on Wikipedia website 18.4.2016, https://en.wikipedia.org/wiki/Asthma

GINA guidelines for treatment: 'Global Initiative for Asthma' retrieved on GINA website 18.4.2016 http://ginasthma.org/2016-pocket-guide-for-asthma-management-and-prevention/

Bonini M et al. AIDA and the Italian Unit of the GA2LEN Olympic Study. Asthma, allergy and the Olympics: a 12-year survey in elite athletes. Curr Opin Allergy Clin Immunol. 2015 Apr;15(2):184-92

Lund TK. Asthma in elite athletes: how do we manage asthma-like symptoms and asthma in elite athletes? Clin Respir J. 2009 Apr;3(2):123

Fitch KD et al. Asthma and the elite athlete: summary of the International Olympic Committee's consensus conference, Lausanne, Switzerland, January 22-24, 2008. J Allergy Clin Immunol. 2008 Aug;122(2):254-60

Fitch KD. Beta2-Agonists at the Olympic Games. Clin Rev Allergy Immunol. 2006 Oct-Dec;31(2-3):259-68.

Cardiovascular System, Heart, Vessels, Blood

Fainting or Nearly Fainting Due to Hypotension (Low Blood Pressure) – No Real Worries

Symptoms

'Everything is turning black', feeling weak and unsafe on your legs. Getting much better after sitting or lying down.

Background

Many young people and athletes have low blood pressure. Many have experienced to feeling a bit shaky after having tied one's shoes or getting out of bed too quickly in the morning. Some have even experienced a moment when 'everything went black', i.e. (nearly) fainting after standing up.

Blood pressure reflects the blood flowing through our blood vessels to all body organs and to reach all corners of our body—the small and fine capillaries in toes, fingers, and in our brain. Blood pressure is comparable to a fire fighter's water hose; it needs enough water (i.e. circulating blood), a good pump (i.e. our heart), and intact fire hoses (i.e. our arteries/veins) to have a working system and a good enough pressure to reach everywhere required. With a fairly low pressure and a change in position (e.g. from lying to standing or standing after having tied one's shoes), the brain becomes higher than the heart and blood pressure is insufficient to reach and irrigate the brain. This results in the person (nearly) fainting.

Blood pressure is measured with a cuff wrapped around our upper arm using a pressure measuring system. It indicates the pressure with two numbers in millimetres of mercury (i.e. abbreviated as Hg), like 120/80mmHg. The upper shows the current maximal (systolic, here 120mmHg) and the lower, the current minimal pressure (diastolic, here 80mmHg) in the bloodstream.

There is often an additional mechanism to explain a fainting episode—the vaso-vagal mechanism. This is a momentary dysfunction of the vegetative nervous system. In some situations, e.g. in a crowd at a music concert or a sport event, it is hot, busy, everything is tense, and you cannot really move and do what you want to do. What happens is that the vegetative nervous system is not taking over and doing what it should do (i.e. making the heart pump more quickly and contracting the vessels of the legs), so your blood pressure may fall and fainting may occur.

Is this dangerous? No. Having low blood pressure is a sign for longevity. High blood pressure (so the contrary) is one of the main risk factors for many diseases, like heart attack, stroke, etc. Having low blood pressure is therefore an advantage.

Prevention and Treatment Table for Low Blood Pressure

Prevention	• Eat breakfast! This gets you ready for the day • Drink regularly, look for 1.5–2l liquid uptake a day • If you have (fairly) low blood pressure, be careful with rapid movements and changes in body positions: o After tying your shoes, stand up slowly o When getting out of bed, sit for 20sec, then stand up
Treatment by Yourself	If there are bad days, with the feeling of 'everything is getting black', drink ½ l of a sports drink (with carbohydrates and minerals). If this is not available, prepare ½ l of tea, put enough sugar in and a tiny pinch of salt (point of a knife), or drink a bouillon (i.e. salted soup). It's the sodium (Na^+ in the sodium-choride, NaCl) that raises blood pressure.

	For people with high blood pressure it is the opposite, as they should try to reduce salt intake in order NOT to raise blood pressure any further. If you have low pressure, however, you may, as a self-treatment option, use some additional sodium chloride (plain salt; NaCl) in drinks or food, to raise your blood pressure to normal levels.
When is a Doctor Needed?	If you have a real fainting episode, you must see a doctor. This is essential even if you are an adolescent or young adult, in order to rule out other possibly dangerous conditions.
Return to Play/Sports	Once the doctor's check is done and you are managing well with the self-treatment option, no restrictions.

What Does the Doctor Do?

The doctor performs a check-up by taking the history, clinical examination, most probably an ECG (resting 12-lead Electro-CardioGram), more extensive testing of the blood pressure, possibly a blood test. Depending on your history and these findings, if treatment is required, it will be started.

You must inform your doctor that you are an elite athlete, as almost the medications used to raise blood pressure are not allowed, as they are 'stimulants', good for raising blood pressure, but forbidden by the anti-doping code. If a medical treatment is indicated, a TUE (therapeutic use exemption) is required *before* starting treatment.

Literature

O'Connor FG, Levine B. Syncope in athletes of cardiac origin: 2B. From personal history and physical examination sections. Curr Sports Med Rep. 2015 May-Jun;14(3):254-6.

Murrell CJ et al. Syncope is unrelated to supine and postural hypotension following prolonged exercise. Eur J Appl Physiol. 2011 Mar;111(3):469-76.

Williams CC, Bernhardt DT. Syncope in athletes. Sports Med. 1995 Mar;19(3):223-34.

Sudden Cardiac Death vs Why Athletes Live Longer – a Serious Sports Paradox

Symptoms

Sudden death due to a cardiac event on the sport field/pitch.

Background

Sudden cardiac death is an issue in sports and creates enormous media attention. And it's clear: every single sportsman or woman lying dead on a pitch is a catastrophe, and every endeavour must be made to prevent such events.
So what is the reason for these sudden cardiac deaths?

Looking at the data (mainly from big popular running events), we recognise that one cardiac death may occur for every 125,000hours of sport competition. In younger sportsmen and women (<35 years), almost all deaths come from heart abnormalities, which somehow lead to heart rhythm abnormalities and eventually a fatal outcome. The most frequent among these is the hypertrophic obstructive cardiomyopathy (acronym HOCM). The good news is that the vast majority of these conditions can be detected by a sportsmed exam with history taking, clinical examination, and 12-lead ECG. In athletes above 35years of age, the etiology is mainly a non-detected coronary heart disease, causing a fatal myocardial infarction. This condition is more difficult to detect.

On the other hand endurance sports (and also sports in which endurance plays a role) prolong life expectancy by about 8 years, as regular sport activities reduce significantly the risk for many common diseases, like arterial hypertension (high blood pressure), stroke, coronary heart disease, diabetes, etc.

This sports paradox now shows that life expectancy for endurance athletes is distinctly longer, but the risk of having a sudden cardiac event during high performance is elevated. Still, endurance sport is absolutely worthwhile: even taking into account this elevated risk during the hours of training and competition, life expectancy is raised!

Whether we are talking about sport after your career, being in masters category or even later, or for all weekend warriors and recreational sportsmen and women, it's certainly wise to adapt the rhythm and intensity of your participation according to your age.

Prevention and Treatment Table for Sudden Cardiac Death

Prevention	• As an elite or ambitious athlete: stick to the recommendations and have a yearly sportsmed exam done • As many good, international studies show: a thorough clinical exam and a resting 12-lead-ECG (electro-cardio-gram) are the things to be done on an annual basis or every other year
Treatment by Yourself	Not applicable. Many sport fields/pitches are equipped with an AED (automatic external defibrillator). A fantastic thing, which will hopefully save lives, but you can't rely on that. You, as an athlete, need to have the annual check-up. By the way: everybody should be able to deliver first aid and CPR (cardio-pulmonary resuscitation). Have you done your first aid course with basic life support (BLS) including AED?
When is a Doctor Needed?	• In case of chest pain (at rest or under effort), (nearly) fainting under effort, or with any suspicion of a cardiac problem see a doctor or an emergency department immediately! • If you have a family history of cardiac events, talk to your doctor about it. According to your family history you may then take appropriate action

Return to Play/Sports	Out of the regular screening, no limitations for almost all athletes. An athlete suffering a sudden cardiac death-like event is immediately brought into intensive hospital care. Beside treatment and observation on the intensive care unit, further exams are conducted by specialised cardiologists in order to diagnose the underlying cardiac illness and completely understand the event. The further treatment plan will be established including the discussion, how far an RTP may be realistic or not. Finally, there are a very few conditions in which, quite sadly, sport cannot be recommended as the risks arising from vigorous efforts are too high. This decision needs a lot of experience and expertise in the field of sports cardiology and will only be taken after having done serious testing and imaging of this athlete's heart and having carefully considered all treatment options.

What Does the Doctor Do?

Prevention, with the annual sportsmed exam, is the most important thing to do. In case of a sudden cardiac event, emergency treatment is immediately started—advanced cardiac life support (ACLS) including defibrillator.

Later on, close family members of the concerned athlete will undergo further cardiac screening, as there is a genetic predisposition for cardiac events.

Literature

Chatard JC et al. Screening young athletes for prevention of sudden cardiac death: Practical recommendations for sports physicians. Scand J Med Sci Sports. 2016 Apr;26(4):362-74.

Schmied C, Borjesson M. Sudden cardiac death in athletes. J Intern Med. 2014 Feb;275(2):93-103.

Ljungqvist A et al. The International Olympic Committee (IOC) consensus statement on periodic health evaluation of elite athletes.Br J Sports Med 2009; 43:631-43

Maron BJ et al. Cardiovascular preparticipation screening of competitive athletes. A statement from the Sudden Death Committee, American Heart Association. Circulation 2007; 115:1-13

Corrado D et al. Cardiovascular pre-participation screening of young competitive athletes for prevention of sudden death. European Society of Cardiology. Eur Heart J 2005; 26:516-24

Deep Vein Thrombosis, Pulmonary Embolism – Rather Seldom, but Good to Know

Symptoms

Deep vein thrombosis: Swelling of one leg, mostly painful when walking, often red-blue-purple coloured.

Pulmonary embolism: Shortness of breath, possibly painful breathing, possibly coughing with spitting of blood (rare but very specific). Often raised heart rate. Pulmonary embolism occurs as a consequence of deep vein thrombosis.

Both, deep vein thrombosis and pulmonary embolism, occur more often after long range travelling (e.g. flights longer than 4h).

Figure 1: Drawing of Deep Vein Thrombosis and Pulmonary Embolism

1.1 deep vein thrombosis *1.2. pulmonary embolism*

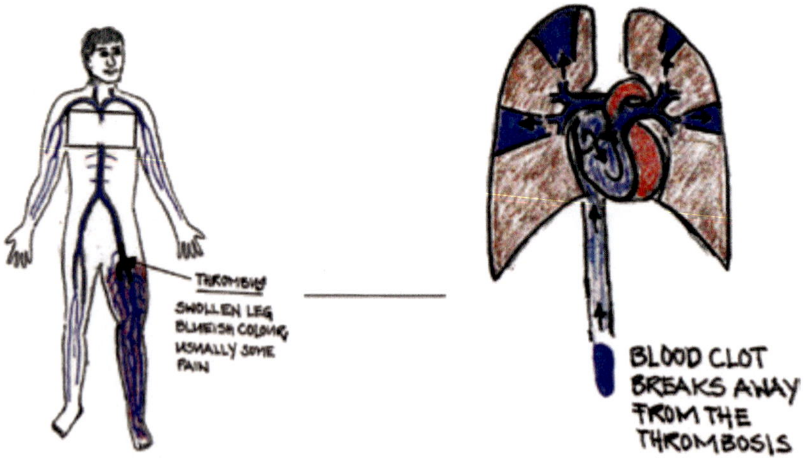

Background

Deep vein thrombosis (Figure 1.1) is the formation of a clot in deeper veins (i.e. thrombus), typically in one lower limb, mostly starting in the calf. As it evolves further, the clotting continues and raises inside the vein system obstructing further the veins higher up the leg, going into the popliteal hollow, thigh, possibly even touching veins in the groin region. As blood flow back to the heart is impaired, the leg becomes more and more swollen and becomes red-blue-purple.

A pulmonary embolism (Figure 1.2) occurs when a *thrombus* breaks away from the whole clotted block inside the obstructed vein and is flushed back to the heart and lungs, now named *embolus,* thus the name pulmonary embolism. This blood clot goes through the right side of the heart and is ejected in one (or often several pieces) into the lungs, and eventually gets stuck within the lungs. Depending on the size of this embolus, the disease is more severe and blocks a bigger (central) or smaller (peripheral) part of lung circulation. This is serious, and in the case of a *central pulmonary embolism, life threatening!*

Sportsmen and women are not more prone to this disease than other people. Having a positive family history (one or several close relatives with the disease) makes you more likely to get it. Further risk factors are: smoking, birth control pills, long distance travelling, dehydration, long period of immobility (e.g. having a cast after an injury), operations, etc. Having two or more of the risk factors does not just double but quadruples your risk.

Prevention and Treatment Table for Deep Vein Thrombosis and Pulmonary Embolism

Prevention	• With long travel, for all, the goal is to keep the circulation going and prevent blood clotting, mostly occurring in a vein of the lower limbs, therefore: o Drink enough (water, tea, coffee, etc.) to be well hydrated o Stand up regularly, walk a few steps and move your legs and feet

	o Move your legs and feet from time to time while sitting in your chair o (Possibly) wear compression stockings (essential if you're prone to have thrombosis by personal history, family history, or other reasons) o **Only with a positive history:** Most people with either a former history of thrombosis or pulmonary embolism or a predisposition need to prevent further events with an anticoagulation medication for the duration of the flight, talk to your doctor about it. Otherwise healthy people don't need that.
Treatment by Yourself	See prevention.
When is a Doctor Needed?	If you suspect one of both diseases, you must see a doctor or an emergency department the same day!
Return to Play/Sports	Depending on the illness and the severity. Needs to be individually planned and put down in a written RTP plan. A return to top level sport is possible for both diagnoses. But you really need to allow enough time and seek experienced professional assistance by a sports medicine physician with a good background in internal medicine.

What Does the Doctor Do?

The doctor wants to see you the same day, taking history, clinical examination, blood tests. With these first basic exams it's often possible to rule out the two diagnoses. If this is not possible, further exams and imaging are needed the same day: ultrasound of the veins, possibly a CT scan of the chest. It's all about confirming, or hopefully, ruling out the diagnosis. If confirmed, an anti-coagulatory treatment is started immediately: for deep vein thrombosis, 3 months; for pulmonary embolism, 6 months. After the treatment period often further blood tests are performed in order to rule out any familiar predisposition or other underlying clotting disorder.

Literature

Sedaghat-Hamedani F et al. Biomarker changes after strenuous exercise can mimic pulmonary embolism and cardiac injury--a metaanalysis of 45 studies. Clin Chem. 2015 Oct;61(10):1246-55.

Casals M et al. Do Basketball Players Have a High Risk of Pulmonary Embolism? A Scoping Review. Med Sci Sports Exerc. 2016 Mar;48(3):466-71.

Grabowski G et al. Venous thrombosis in athletes. J Am Acad Orthop Surg. 2013 Feb;21(2):108-17.

Varicosis – Mainly an Aesthetic Thing

Symptoms

Visible swelling and protruding of superficial veins.

Background

Varicosis: from the Latin word *varix,* meaning enlarged vein knob; and *osis* meaning condition. So, the disease it is about distinctly enlarged veins in the lower limbs. Veins are the vessels carrying blood from the periphery back to the heart. To do this, veins have *valves,* constructed like non-return valves, which are essential in supporting the venous blood flow and, especially in a person standing upright, sustaining the venous blood column and holding the venous blood at the level it has reached. Beside the valves, the *muscle pump,* i.e. the action of the muscles surrounding the veins, pumps the blood inside the veins upwards to the heart. With leaking or missing valves, the whole blood column presses downwards (instead of going upwards) which leads to collection of the venous blood in the legs leading to swelling, formation of varicose veins, oedema (i.e. liquid pressed through the vessel wall and going into the tissues), and impairment of circulation with first purple-blue, later on ochre-brownish skin colouration. The reasons for having varicosis are most often: genetically inherited or as part of a history of deep vein thrombosis (as thrombosis often destroys venous valves or makes them leak).

As you grow older, you may observe a slight enlargement of one or two leg veins. This definitely doesn't mean that you need to see a surgeon. Having tired legs is not a specific symptom and there is no relation between one or two varicose veins and leg tiredness.

Prevention and Treatment Table for Varicosis

Prevention	• As an athlete, you're already doing the best thing you can: you're active! Now, not all sports are the same. As explained, it is the muscle pump of your legs doing the important job. So please keep this in mind • Secondly, be aware that sitting and standing for long periods is really bad for people with varicose veins and venous insufficiency, whereas activating your muscle pump or being in a horizontal position (e.g. lying) is good for your venous system. In German, we use the saying: o 'Sitzen und Stehen sind schlecht' (Sitting and standing bad)! o 'Laufen und Liegen sind gut' (Walking and lying good)!
Treatment by Yourself	Wearing compression socks (medical stockings compression class II are recommended, as soon as a varicosis is established). Sport compression socks are particularly designed for running and athletics and may be particularly helpful in long distance running, but they are not the same as medical compression socks. However, for athletes with vein problems, they are a good option.
When is a Doctor Needed?	As explained above, just slightly visible veins and sometimes tired legs are no reason to see a doctor. But when a number of veins over a larger area, and a greater distance, are really protruding, or when the inner side of your ankles is distinctly swollen and is getting purple-blue to even ochre-brownish, then show them to a doctor.
Return to Play/Sports	No pause necessary.

What Does the Doctor Do?

The doctor takes the history, performs a clinical examination, with a focus on leg veins, blood circulation, and skin condition.

Then it will be decided whether further exams (mostly a duplex ultrasound of the veins of your legs) need to be performed. This exam allows to see, by following your veins, whether both vessel and valves, are working properly or not. Compression stockings (see Treatment by Yourself) are the first treatment step, being regularly active, *no sitting and standing for long periods of time.* Seldom, and only in severe cases, an operation needs to be planned and is usually timed at the end of season.

Anaemia – Clearly Impairs Performance and Recovery

Symptoms

Fatigue, that's the consistent finding, all other symptoms are much less reliable. Possibly: being pale, having higher heart rate at rest, and for a known effort, getting sore legs earlier than usual, hair loss, brittle nails, and burning tongue.

Background

Anaemia is defined as lowered haemoglobin (protein in the blood, binding site of oxygen, gives the blood its red colour) in venous blood. The blood and in particular the erythrocytes (red blood cells) are important for physical performance. The erythrocytes with their haemoglobin are the binding site of oxygen. Oxygen coming through our lungs into our body is attached to the haemoglobin and transported with the red blood cells into the working muscle to deliver oxygen. Beside oxygen transport, blood has other functions in an athlete's performance:

- To buffer (i.e. balance out the acid-base-metabolism) during a resistance effort
- To sustain thermoregulation of the body while performing
- To allow sustainable long lasting effort and good recovery by circulating and transporting basically everything needed for sports performance: nutrients to the muscle and CO_2, acids, etc. away from the working muscle to lungs, kidney, and liver
- To support many reactions of the energy metabolism by keeping up stable steady state conditions (acid-base metabolism, temperature, nutrients, etc.)

In case of iron: to integrate as an essential component many enzymes (i.e. active proteins to facilitate biochemical reactions)—see the following chapter 'Iron Deficiency'

Reasons for anaemia

The most likely etiology for anaemia in athletes is clearly iron deficiency. As iron deficiency is extremely frequent, it is treated in a separate chapter. But there are other quite frequent reasons, like female athlete triad or RED-S (relative energy deficiency-syndrome), Vitamin B12 deficiency, gastro-intestinal blood loss, coeliac disease, hypothyreosis, and more. Your doctor knows more about all this. Blood tests, and if appropriate, further investigations will help find the correct diagnosis.

Good to know: dilutional pseudoanaemia in 10–15% of endurance athletes

The definition of anaemia (see above) neglects that in fact anaemia is the real reduction of the total haemoglobin mass in the body, i.e. absolute anaemia. In contrast, relative or dilutional pseudoanaemia is defined as a lowered haemoglobin and haematocrit due to a distinctly elevated plasma volume, while red cell mass and total haemoglobin mass are normal. Other blood parameters, particularly ferritin, MCV, and MCH are also within the normal range and performance is not affected. This plasma volume increase is considerable and is due to repeated bouts of physical training over the years. The magnitude of the plasma volume depends on the intensity and duration of the effort. In about 10–15% of (mainly endurance) athletes, especially when training time exceeds 10 hours per week, dilutional pseudoanaemia can be observed. The same dilutional effect is found in ultra long endurance distance disciplines or sports events lasting several days (e.g. road cycling tours). As seen in Figure 1.4 in male and female athletes with dilutional pseudoanaemia, the increase in plasma volume causes a slight lowering of the haematocrit while the red cell mass stays high.

Figure 1: Dilutional Pseudoanaemia

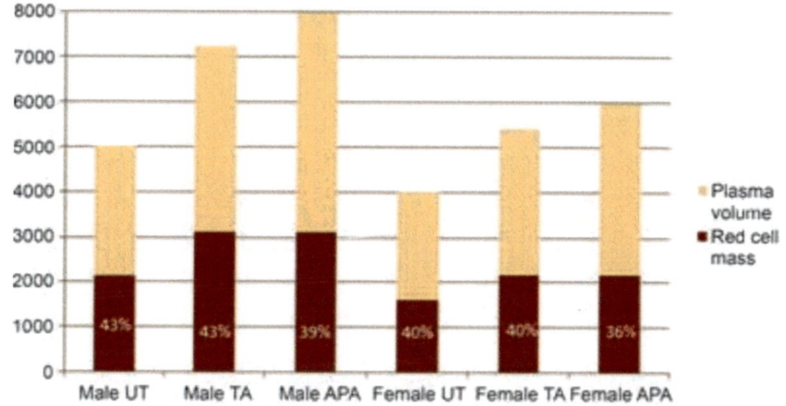

Total blood volume of male and female untrained, top athletes and athletes with dilutional pseudoanaemia in ml.
UT = untrained; TA = top athlete; APA = athlete with dilutional pseudoanaemia.
In the column of the red cell mass the haematocrit in percentage is shown in white letters.

(Clénin et al, Swiss Medical Weekly 2015)

Prevention and Treatment Table for Anaemia

Prevention	As an elite athlete, have an annual sports medicine exam with blood tests (see 'Big Sportslab'). As an endurance athlete go for 2–3 additional 'Small Sportslab per year' to rule out anaemia or iron deficiency.
Treatment by Yourself	Seek professional advice.
When is a Doctor Needed?	If you feel unexplained fatigue or if you have other symptoms of an anaemia.
Return to Play/Sports	After the diagnosis is clear, treatment may be immediately started (see chapter 'Iron Deficiency'). Basically a pause is not needed. But as anaemia leads to a distinct decline in performance discuss with your sports medicine physician when you will be ready for your next competition.

What Does the Doctor Do?

The doctor takes the history, performs a clinical examination, and does a blood test to confirm or rule out anaemia. With your history and the results of the blood tests an initial classification is possible: Anaemia yes/no: if yes, could it be a dilutional pseudoanaemia (relative anaemia, harmless, no further investigations, no treatment) or is it real, absolute anaemia. If absolute anaemia is probable, the etiology needs to be determined. The most frequent reason is iron deficiency. Others as explained above (see background).

Literature

Clénin G, Cordes M, Huber A, Schumacher YO, Noack P, Scales J, Kriemler S. Iron deficiency in sports - definition, influence on performance and therapy. Swiss Med Wkly. 2015;145:w14196.

Steiner, T. & Wehrlin, J. P. Does haemoglobin mass increase from age 16 to 21 and 28 in elite endurance athletes? Med Sci Sports Exerc 2011, 43, 1735–1743.

Heinicke, K. et al. Blood volume and haemoglobin mass in elite athletes of different disciplines. Int J Sports Med 2001, 22, 504–512.

Shaskey, D. J. & Green, G. A. Sports haematology. Sports Med 2000, 29, 27–38 .

Iron Deficiency – Regular Checks Warranted, Have Enough Iron But Not Too Much

Symptoms

Fatigue, general weakness, not ready for optimal performance. Possibly: being pale, having higher heart rate at rest and for a known effort, getting sore legs earlier than usual, hair loss, brittle nails, burning tongue, skin irritation at the corners of the mouth (Perlèche).

Background

Iron deficiency is the most frequent reason for anaemia and impaired oxygen transport in the blood (see chapter 'Anaemia'). But iron is much more than that. Beside its function as an oxygen binding site in *haemoglobin*, it is an essential component of *myoglobin* and *many enzymes. Myoglobin* is the muscle protein binding oxygen and is responsible for oxygen delivery within the muscle cell, as it takes the oxygen brought by haemoglobin and delivers it to the corresponding sites within the muscle. *Enzymes* are active proteins of all kinds facilitating biochemical reactions throughout the body—our focus is on the enzymes involved in energy metabolism, many of which have iron as an integral part. This means not only iron deficiency anaemia (IDA), or lowered haematologic response with less coloured and smaller erythrocytes (IDMH), but also iron deficiency itself (non-anaemic iron deficiency NAID) impairs performance and needs treatment.

You could now argue, just take enough iron. But we definitely need to first look on the other side of the coin: iron has a certain, limited therapeutic range. First, iron overload must be prevented, as abundant iron is falsely stored in organs like the liver and spleen leading to iron storage disease (haemochromatosis with secondary dysfunction of these organs). Second, prevention of any therapeutic iron overload is wise and strongly recommended as it forms *free radicals in the blood* (with intravenous therapy) and an *oxidative reaction in the gut* (with oral therapy) which are in abundance probably harmful. Please find more comprehensive information in articles like 'Iron Deficiency in Sports, Definition, Influence on Performance and Therapy' (Clénin et al 2015).

Prevention and Treatment Table for Iron Deficiency

Prevention	• Enjoy a varied diet, a good reference is the food pyramid for athletes • As meat contains a lot of the preferable haem iron, try to eat meat 5 times a week, and consider iron rich vegetables • If you are vegetarian, iron rich vegetables should be eaten several times daily, like legumes, green leafy vegetables, and cereals • Consider *enhancers* of iron uptake like vitamin C, peptides from partially digested muscle tissue, fermented food, organic acids like malate or citrate, and combine these with your iron rich food and iron tablets (if appropriate). • Think about *inhibitors* of iron uptake, like phytates, oxalates, polyphenols (black tea and coffee), peptides from partially digested vegetable proteins and calcium, and don't consume them together in the same meal with iron rich nutrients especially oral iron
Treatment by Yourself	Don't practice self-treatment with iron, as harmful iron overload may occur. As iron is a vital element and excessive iron probably harms our body through the formation of free radicals and oxidative reactions, we recommend taking iron only under medical supervision and regular blood tests.

When is a Doctor Needed?	With unexplained fatigue, sore legs, or other symptoms mentioned above.
Return to Play/ Sports	Usually no pause needed.

What Does the Doctor Do?

The doctor takes the history, performs a clinical examination, and makes a blood lab test in order to confirm or rule out anaemia and/or iron deficiency. As therapy is usually nutritional (see Prevention), combine with an oral therapy in the form of iron tablets, for about 6–8 weeks. These should contain 40–60mg of elementary iron, as too a high dosage has no further effect, but most probably more side effects (e.g. constipation). Drink fruit juice together with the iron tablet, as Vitamin C enhances the iron uptake, and the fruit juice keeps the bowel movements going. Measure success of treatment with a basic blood test after 8 weeks.

For athletes with repeatedly low iron stores or athletes with a vegetarian diet, a maintenance therapy is an option, either with an intermittent uptake of iron tablets twice a week (40–60mg elementary iron; two days on, five days off) or a daily supplement with a preparation containing 14mg of elementary iron, corresponding to the RDA, recommended daily allowance.

In cases of serious incompatibility with oral therapy, concomitant disease (e.g. depression), or low iron stores before an altitude training camp, IV iron therapy may be considered. However, long-term daily oral iron intake or IV supplementation in the presence of normal or even high ferritin values is not recommended and is most probably harmful.

Literature

Clénin G, Cordes M, Huber A, Schumacher YO, Noack P, Scales J, et al. Iron deficiency in sports - definition, influence on performance and therapy. Swiss Med Wkly. 2015;145:w14196.

Sandström, G et al. Iron deficiency in adolescent female athletes - is iron status affected by regular sporting activity? Clin J Sport Med 2012, 22, 495–500

Latunde-Dada, G. O. Iron metabolism in athletes- achieving a gold standard. Eur. J. Haematol. 2012. doi:10.1111/ejh.12026

Peeling, P. Exercise as a mediator of hepcidin activity in athletes. Eur. J. Appl. Physiol. 2010, 110, 877–883

Clénin, G. E. Eisen im Sport - oft zu wenig, gelegentlich aber auch zu viel! Schweizerische Zeitschrift für Ernährungsmedizin 2006, 21–25.

Hypertension (High Blood Pressure) – No Contraindication for Elite Sports, but Treatment Needed

Symptoms

Mostly little or no symptoms.

Hypertensive crisis: When blood pressure rises dramatically, turning into a hypertensive crisis reaching values of above 200/110mmHg, people describe a severe headache, a feeling of being really unwell, pressure on the chest and whole upper body, and dizziness.

Background

Why worry, when there are nearly no symptoms?

Luckily, slight rises in blood pressure cause no harm in short term. It's a really significant rise, a hypertensive crisis, as described above, which is an emergency and needs immediate treatment within the hour. The problem with blood pressure is the long-term damage: elevated blood pressure, arterial hypertension, is still one of the *major risk factors for coronary heart disease (heart attack)* and *cerebrovascular disease (stroke*). Blood pressure slightly rises with age, and about 25% of the population will, during their life, suffer from arterial hypertension.

What happens when we have higher blood pressure?

Vessels get worn out: smaller fine vessels, e.g. capillaries in the retina of the eye or capillaries of the glomeruli (filters) in the kidney, may be seriously damaged over the years; and larger vessels have the tendency to develop atheromatosis (wall thickening, adhesion of blood fat components with finally significant narrowing or even occlusion of the affected vessel, leading to myocardial infarction or stroke). Therefore blood pressure needs to be kept within the normal range.

What's a normal range?

Blood pressure is measured by indicating two values, the upper (systolic) value indicating the current maximal blood flow and the lower (diastolic) value indicating the current minimal blood flow. The values may vary quite a bit and are normal *under 140/90mmHg.* A single elevated value is not, of itself, hypertension though. It's the time duration you are above these limits, or better still, the percentage of values out of many measurements taken the same day that tells us whether treatment is necessary or not.

Arterial hypertension is very often genetically determined, so if your parents or grandparents have it, you run the risk of having it (or to getting it), too.

Important: Untreated hypertension in athletes seems to measurably decrease exercise capacity (Mazic et al 2015).

Prevention and Treatment Table for Arterial Hypertension

Prevention	• Continue lifelong sports. When older, continue cycling, swimming, jogging, walking, moving, keeping fit • Keep your weight within a good range, as overweight is a risk factor for hypertension
Treatment by Yourself	• There is a bunch of life style interventions that have been effective: o Move regularly—30min a day at a moderate activity level and/or take vigorous exercise 3x/ week 20–60min o Reduce alcohol consumption and stop smoking o Reduce stress o If overweight, try to reduce bodyweight

	o Reduce salt intake, as our salt consumption is generally too high and the sodium in the salt raises blood pressure Most of these recommendations are for people who are not athletes, but keep them in mind anyhow
When is a Doctor Needed?	If your blood pressure is too high, check it regularly to see if it was just a single finding or whether it's a real problem. Blood pressure is tested in the annual sportsmed exam. Luckily, it is not usually an issue among sportsmen and women, but there are a few who need to be concerned. Best to keep it in mind.
Return to Play/Sports	Generally sport is possible at the highest levels. Endurance sports are even beneficial. Under treatment plenty of sport disciplines are possible. When it comes to pure strength sports (e.g. weight lifting) a shift to another sport needs to be considered, as pure strength activity massively increases blood pressure at the moment of action without offering any other beneficial effects for blood pressure regulation.

What Does the Doctor Do?

The doctor takes the history (in particular family history), clinical examination with some blood pressure measurements, takes a resting 12-lead-ECG. You will most probably be instructed to do home measurements (showing BP measurements throughout a whole day). Often a 24h blood pressure measurement will be done, looking systematically at your BP for 24h.

If the diagnosis is confirmed, further exams will be necessary to rule out the secondary arterial hypertension. 80% of people concerned have the primary form (genetically determined, and that's it), however the other 20% have other medical conditions leading to high blood pressure and these must be ruled out. When it comes to treatment, remind your doctor, that you are an elite athlete as a few of the available medications are banned by the anti-doping code or just not appropriate for you as an athlete, but there are enough good treatment options.

Literature

Berge HM et al. Blood pressure and hypertension in athletes: a systematic review. Br J Sports Med. 2015 Jun;49(11):716-23.

Mazic S et al. The impact of elevated blood pressure on exercise capacity in elite athletes. Int J Cardiol. 2015 Feb 1;180:171-7.

Laine MK et al. Former male elite athletes and risk of hypertension in later life. J Hypertens. 2015 Aug;33(8):1549-54.

Leddy JJ, Izzo J. Hypertension in athletes. J Clin Hypertens (Greenwich). 2009 Apr;11(4):226-33.

Gastrointestinal System

Constipation – to be Settled With Good Habits and Natural Self-Treatment Options

Symptoms

Not being able to have normal bowel movements. From a slight unease and feeling full, up to serious and very painful abdominal cramping.

Background

Definition of constipation: problematic obstructed bowel with movements less than three times a week.

Bowel movements *require adequate fluid.* When you don't drink enough—i.e. 1.5–2l a day for a normal person in winter; up to probably 4.5l for a sportsman or woman in training in summer—digestion cannot work properly. The liquid part is missing and stools are very hard, very dry, and you get constipated (see also chapter 'Drinking in Sports').

Fibres in nutrients are essential for passing stools. Quick food like sandwiches, bars, pasta, and rice do not have much fibres. So, close to important events, continue eating fibres: in vegetables, fruits, and wholegrain products.

For keeping a good rhythm going to the loo: as soon as you feel your stomach grumbling, and it's possible to go to the toilet, make the time to do this. A good moment is a few minutes after having eaten, as our body does have what is called a *gastro-colic reflex*, which means, as soon as the stomach (gastro) fills to a certain level, the reflex sends an impulse to the big intestines (colon) to empty.

For good digestion, it is essential to have *enough time,* time for pauses, time to relax. Digestion is well sustained by the parasympathetic part of the vegetative, involuntary nervous system. This *parasympathetic nervous system* starts to act when we relax and when we stop being active. As soon as we become active, have a distinct goal, are trying to achieve, are using adrenalin, the parasympathetic action stops, which means we cannot willingly digest, but we need to allow time to let it happen.

Prevention and Treatment Table for Constipation

Prevention	• Drink regularly and enough. Control your hydration actively by looking at the colour of your urine • Eat vegetables and fruits 5 times a day • Eat enough fibre (wholegrain products, dark bread, also vegetables, fruits) and always combine it with enough liquid, as fibre need fluids to do their swelling and to act on the intestines to produce smooth bowel movements • Skip low fibre edibles and constipating food (e.g. white bread, dark chocolate, bananas, too much pasta, carrots, black and green tea, coke) • Vary your source of carbohydrates: dark and wholegrain bread, rice, potatoes, try occasionally whole grain pasta and always combine pasta with a veggie sauce (tomato, basil, zucchini, etc.)
Treatment by Yourself	• Add natural products to support digestion: o Go back and check, if you're eating vegetables and fruit 5 times a day o Add pure fruit juices (apple or orange juice) or 1:1 diluted o Eat plums or figs, as they act positively on digestion

	• Use a natural fibre product like psyllium husk (e.g. Metamucil) on an intermittent, or if necessary, daily basis. Make sure you follow the instructions of the manufacturer, drink at least the indicated amount of water, as fibre needs liquid to be able to act
When is a Doctor Needed?	In emergencies, with severe abdominal cramping. Secondly, when it doesn't get better in spite of having followed all the recommendations above.
Return to Play/ Sports	There are quite a few young men and women going to hospital emergencies with acute abdominal pain and cramping. Luckily, it turns mostly out to be 'only constipation'. But, if it was you, an athlete, you cannot perform at all in that condition. Digestion needs to be sorted out for athletes to be able to perform. So be prepared, talk to your sports medicine physician or your GP and check whether you are doing all that can be done.

What Does the Doctor Do?

The doctor takes the history, does a clinical examination, and tries to understand where the problem comes from. The checklist above will be very handy to discuss the different problems related with constipation. Possibly counselling with a (sport) nutritionist could be an option.

Other, stronger medications activating bowel movements exist (pharmaceutical laxatives) but they are potentially harmful and should only be used after consulting your doctor.

Diarrhoea – Be Careful While Travelling

Symptoms

Liquid stool, more than 3 times a day.

Background

Acute gastroenteritis, often of viral sometimes of bacterial origin, is an infection of the intestines, with diarrhoea, nausea, and sometimes vomiting. This illness takes you out. And when I say it takes you out, I mean it like this. It's serious to me, because even today and in well developed countries, athletes miss their competitions because of gastroenteritis. You're so weak, you can't even think of performing, and it will take 10–14 days to be back where you were, possibly longer. And all that, possibly, because of eating spoilt food, drinking unclean water, or insufficient hygiene in the kitchen.

On the other hand, looking at the definitions of constipation and diarrhoea, we recognise the range of normal bowel movements is broad:

- constipation: problematic obstructed bowel movements less than three times a week
- diarrhoea: two liquid stools more than 3 times a day

What about Pharaoh's or Montezuma's revenge?

These names refer to traveller's diarrhoea more frequently encountered in hot and possibly less developed countries. But you don't need to go that far. It's possible to catch infectious diarrhoea with bacteria at home, e.g. in Switzerland. Around Christmas 2014, a big outbreak was traced back to badly cooked poultry meat in 'Fondue Chinoise', meals with the bacteria species 'Campylobacter'.

Prevention and Treatment Table for Diarrhoea

Prevention (at home)	• Don't let germs come into your body • Avoid contaminated food (even if less risky, think about it) • Be careful while processing meat, especially poultry, in your own kitchen. Separate it from all the other food (including a separate knife, a separate cutting board, afterwards wash these items thoroughly) and fry or cook the meat until it is well done • Typical traps are: undercooked chicken or turkey—in a restaurant, give it back or don't eat it (see above)—and old sandwiches
Prevention (while travelling, in hot countries)	• Don't let germs come into your body! • Avoid contaminated food • Only drink beverages from sealed containers • Always boil water before use (also for brushing your teeth) or use bottled water • Only use food that can be peeled or cooked—cook it, peel it, or leave it, that's it. Forget about 'wash it', as your water is not clean • Eat only hot and freshly cooked meals—give it back respectfully, don't eat it, if it's not well done • Typical traps are: o salad buffet (eat salad when you're back home again! Cooked vegetables are okay) o Ice-cream o Open drinks o Undercooked meat (especially chicken!) • Possibly get vaccinations. Available only for a few germs like Typhus, Cholera, enterotox E. coli (ETEC). Discuss this with your sports medicine physician or your GP. Vaccinations do not protect you really (you're just a little less likely to catch gastroenteritis). In any case follow all recommendations above

	• To sport officials, coaches, medical team members: while travelling with a sport delegation in a hot country with lower hygiene standards, consider bringing your own cook with you as this may spare you a lot of hassle. In this particular situation, it's additionally recommended that the medical team should be equipped with enough probiotics (e.g. Perenterol), loperamid (Imodium), and some antibiotics (e.g. Azithromycin)
Treatment by Yourself	• *Hydration* is essential—don't worry about eating initially. • Rehydrate by drinking small portions of either coke or well-sweetened black tea. Good re-hydration is possible with a black tea solution, well sweetened (40-60g/l sugar) and a small pinch of salt (a point of a knife). The sugar and the sodium (Na+ in the NaCl) help better absorption in the stomach and the intestines and deliver some energy. Black tea also acts against the diarrhoea. • If hungry, eat small bits of banana, small bits of white bread, eventually a few small pretzels • As you improve, you may eat soup, some rice, some bread. Still drinking enough in small amounts to keep well hydrated. • Getting better, you may have some pasta, cooked carrots and potatoes, a bit of well cooked meat, etc.
When is a Doctor Needed?	If you risk dehydration and if you have high fever (above 38.5° axillary). and if you have serious abdominal pain and bloody stools.
Return to Play/Sports	When you've recovered. After serious diarrhoea you need to allow 7–10 days before usual training. But plan your RTP with your sports medicine physician early: start with some walking in the first couple of days, continue with light extensive aerobic training, some core stability activity, some flexibility training, and creating your individual program for 7–10 days.

What Does the Doctor Do?

The doctor takes the history, makes a clinical examination, and possibly performs blood tests, stool cultures, and microscopic analysis (to detect the responsible germs) and rules out other reasons for the abdominal pain and bloody stools. Treatment wise, rehydration is essential, combined with the goal of supplying you with some energy. Eating is slowly integrated (as above Treatment by Yourself). Probiotics (medication supporting your own intestinal flora) will bring substantial benefit (e.g. Perenterol twice daily, or Carbolevure three times daily for 10 days, possibly longer, according to stool consistency).

With severe illness with fever, it may be decided to start antibiotic treatment before the test results are back (bacterial cultures and microscopic analyses usually take 3–4 days).

Gastroesophageal Reflux Disease (GERD) – Also Common in Athletes and Young People

Symptoms

Burning stomach, acid regurgitation, heartburn. Despite its name, heartburn has nothing to do with the heart. It's an irritation of the oesophagus by stomach acids that cause a burning discomfort in the upper abdomen and behind the breast bone. This may, in some cases, give discomfort suggesting the pain comes from the heart. Possibly unexplained coughing, possibly more severe, sharp pain in the stomach region.

Background

A high percentage of young people suffer from acid regurgitation and possibly accompanying inflammation of the oesophagus and stomach. The oesophagus enters the stomach just after passing the diaphragm. This passage is quite important, as the oesophagus doesn't have a valve or a particular muscle to close its lower end once the food has passed through. So the stomach acid (pH 2-4, so highly acid) may, in some cases, unfortunately regurgitate and provoke burning, inflammation, or even an ulcer. There are a few known risk factors:

- Having a hiatus hernia, which means that the oesophagus passage through the diaphragm is widened up
- Eating heavy and big meals late in the evening
- Alcohol consumption and smoking
- Late consumption of coffee and black or green tea
- Being overweight

Prevention and Treatment Table for Gastroesophageal Reflux Disease

Prevention	• Prevent stress • Don't eat heavy and big meals in the evening, especially not late • Don't smoke • Consume alcohol, if any, only in a modest and reasonable way
Treatment by Yourself	• See Prevention • No black tea or coffee in the evening • Avoid fatty food like sausages, salami, French fries, butter, sweets in your diet, especially in the evening • Avoid very acid fruits (e.g. citrus fruits) and vegetables (e.g. cucumbers or onions in vinegar) in your diet • Raise the top of your bed (not just the pillow, but the whole bed) about 8–10cm • Avoid being heavily overweight and obesity, respectively reduce bodyweight if BMI>30 • Avoid constipation
When is a Doctor Needed?	When heartburn is severe and you feel a precise sharp pain in the stomach region which doesn't get any better.
Return to Play/Sports	Usually no pause needed. In case of an ulcer and more extensive treatment, the RTP needs to be discussed with the gastroenterologist and the sportsmed physician.

What Does the Doctor Do?

The doctor takes the history and performs a clinical exam. The diagnosis may be clear or the doctor may decide on further investigations. If GERD is highly probable, treatment with proton pump-inhibitor (PPI) medication is usually started. This medication blocks the production of stomach acids (gastric acid) within one or two days. A distinct improvement in symptoms may be observed by then, but at the latest within 3–5days. Therapy is usually continued for 14–28days. In case of a sharp local pain in the stomach region without any improvement on PPI-therapy, a gastroscopy may be needed to have a closer internal look.

Literature

Waterman JJ, Kapur R.. Upper gastrointestinal issues in athletes. Curr Sports Med Rep. 2012 Mar-Apr;11(2):99-104

Krey D, Best T. Dyspneic athlete. Curr Rev Musculoskelet Med. 2014 Dec;7(4):373-80.

Coeliac Disease – Gluten Free Diet for Diagnosed Illness, but *Not* for Others

Symptoms

Symptoms may be quite variable and diverse: sore stomach, feeling full, having grumbling intestines. Typically, stool irregularities may be observed, mostly fatty, stinking, loose stools. Possibly loss of weight, possibly frequent mouth ulcers, possibly feeling tired and not recovering well.

Background

Coeliac disease is intolerance to gluten (from the Greek *koiliakos*, meaning abdominal, used for the description of this particular disease).(1) It is also called gluten-sensitive enteropathy or coeliac sprue. *Gluten* is a protein found in most cereals, especially wheat, barley, rye, and oats. In coeliac patients, the intake of gluten is characterised by an abnormal immune response that provokes destruction of the mucosal surface and finally, complete flattening of the otherwise nicely shaped internal surface. This impairs the whole digestive process and severely harms absorption of many essential nutrients, vitamins, and minerals and leads to a severe deficiency situation (e.g. repeatedly low iron stores, low levels of zinc, Vitamin B12, Vitamin D, and others).

Coeliac disease affects men and women of all ages. You must have a genetic predisposition to develop the disease. Environmental factors are associated with the triggering of coeliac disease in childhood or later in life.(2)(3)

Important: Following a gluten free diet without diagnosed coeliac disease or gluten-sensitive enteropathy doesn't make sense, is hard work, and is not bringing any benefit for you as an athlete [5, 6]

Prevention and Treatment Table for Coeliac Disease

Prevention	No prevention known.
Treatment by Yourself	Don't start a gluten free diet by yourself, as it may mask your symptoms and interfere with the diagnosis (antibody testing may be negative and biopsy of the small intestine may be normal after a few weeks avoiding gluten intake). It is essential to have the diagnosis first, and then take the indicated measures as a gluten free diet is not a trivial undertaking.
When is a Doctor Needed?	To confirm or rule out the diagnosis.
Return to Play/ Sports	• Once the diagnosis is made, a *lifelong gluten free diet* is the therapy [4] • Counselling by a sports nutritionist will help you on your way and is highly recommended • Having the disease and respecting the gluten free diet allows you to perform at the highest elite sport levels [4]

What Does the Doctor Do?

The doctor takes the history, performs a clinical exam, and will most probably first do a blood test in order to check the antibodies. Depending on your symptoms and the result of this antibody testing, it will be decided whether a gastroscopy with biopsy of the small intestine needs to be performed. To confirm the diagnosis such a biopsy is necessary.

Literature

(1) Coeliac disease, general information on Wikipedia website, retrieved online 2.3.2016 https://en.wikipedia.org/wiki/Coeliac_disease

(2) Coeliac disease, general information on Coeliac Australia Website, retrieved online 2.3.2016 http://www.coeliac.org.au/
(3) Coeliac disease brochure for patients from Coeliac Australia, retrieved online 2.3.2016 http://www.coeliac.org.au/uploads/65701/ufiles/Brochures/CDBrochureweb.pdf
(4) Mancini LA et al. Celiac disease and the athlete. Curr Sports Med Rep. 2011 Mar-Apr;10(2):105-8.
(5) Coattrenec Y et al. Benefits of gluten-free diet: myth or reality? Rev Med Suisse. 2015 Oct 14;11(490):1878, 1880-2, 1884-5.
(6) Lis D et al. No Effects of a Short-Term Gluten-free Diet on Performance in Nonceliac Athletes. Med Sci Sports Exerc. 2015 Dec;47(12):2563-70.

Irritable Bowel Disease in Sports – How to Cope With It in Elite Sports

Symptoms

Sore stomach, feeling full, blown up, grumbling intestines, clearly getting better after having bowel movement.

Background

The exact etiology of *ITB (irritable bowel disease)* is not yet clear. Sometimes light forms of other gastrointestinal complaints or illnesses may show similar symptoms and may eventually be involved, like:

- *Intolerance to fructose*: fructose is fruit sugar. In people having intolerance, an overload of fruit sugar may cause fermentation and formation of gas, which expands your bowels. Diagnosis may be made by a specific breath test and treatment consists of a reduction of fructose uptake
- *Intolerance to lactose*: lactose is milk sugar. In people having intolerance due to the (often relative) missing of lactase (enzyme, responsible for the lactose breakdown) fermentation of the lactose and an osmotic reaction takes place, leading to grumbling intestines, feeling blown up, diarrhoea, gas, but also abdominal cramping, typically starting half an hour after milk consumption. Diagnosis may be made by a specific breath test. Treatment consists of avoidance of lactose in your diet (e.g. lactose free milk) or simultaneous intake of medication containing lactase when consuming milk or dairy products
- *Long and slow acting colon*: due to its increased length transit time in the colon, big bowel is increased, leading to the symptoms above

Prevention and Treatment Table for Irritable Bowel Disease

Prevention	General recommendations are difficult. However, try the following: • Follow a regular daily rhythm with eating and drinking, and try to integrate into this rhythm, going to the loo for bowel movement (allow time!) • Have a bottle of water or pot of tea on the table (1.5l) and finish it by bed time—this, in addition to, whatever else you drink (sports drinks, water in training, coffee, or tea). Rethink your drinking volume: in hot conditions, you need much more—maybe 4.5l (look at the colour of your urine, see chapter 'Drinking in Sports')
Treatment by Yourself	Once a diagnosis is made, follow the instructions.
When is a Doctor Needed?	If you observe unexplained weight loss of more than 2kg in 2months, weird stool irregularities, eventually even blood in the stool, or if you feel seriously disturbed in your intestines.
Return to Play/ Sports	Usually no pause needed.

What Does the Doctor Do?

The doctor takes a thorough history, performs a clinical exam, and discusses possible further examinations, if indicated. These may be: a blood test (to exclude deficiencies, exclude coeliac disease etc.); other options, like the breathing tests or gastro or colonoscopy, aren't first line investigations for this particular condition. Treatment consists of having a regular daily rhythm with eating, drinking enough (still a reason for many intestinal troubles!), and having regular bowel movements. Depending on the individual symptoms, treatment modalities are discussed and established. Naturally based medications seem to be promising.

Morbus Crohn (Inflammatory Bowel Disease) in Sports – What to Look For

Symptoms

Sore stomach, diarrhoea, weird stool consistency, with often slimy, and from time to time bloody stools, possibly weight loss.

Background

Morbus Crohn (Morbus means 'type of disease'; Crohn is the family name of B.B. Crohn, a specialist in gastroenterology, 1884–1983) is an autoimmune inflammatory bowel disease affecting different sections of the small and great bowel. It affects the wall of the intestines, causes quite severe inflammation of sometimes large areas of the intestines and leads to the above mentioned stool irregularities. Depending on the percentage of bowel involved, it affects digestion and absorption, and leads in particular to impairment of your top performance.

Prevention and Treatment Table for Morbus Crohn (Inflammatory Bowel Disease)

Prevention	There is no prevention for Morbus Crohn known. Follow a good lifestyle, reduce stress.
Treatment by Yourself	Once the diagnosis is established, follow the instructions of your doctor.
When is a Doctor Needed?	If you observe unexplained weight loss of more than 2kg in 2months, weird stool irregularities with slimy, eventually even bloody stools, or if you feel seriously disturbed in your intestines.

Return to Play/ Sports	Depending on the severity of the disease and indicated treatment, the plan for the return to play/sport needs to be made. Nutritional counselling is part of the return to play plan and is helpful. Follow up with specialists in gastroenterology and a sports medicine physician the same time, as preparation for big events needs close observation and a good communication between all involved.

What Does the Doctor Do?

The doctor takes a thorough history, performs a clinical examination, and discusses possible further exams, if indicated. These are: a blood test (to exclude anaemia, deficiencies etc.), stool exams to check if there's inflammation (calprotectin in the stool), and a colonoscopy. The treatment plan needs to be established with the specialists in gastroenterology first to control the inflammatory acute response. Then together with the sports medicine physician, the long term treatment plan needs to be discussed and put in place.

Sports Nutrition

Basics of (Sports) Nutrition – Still a Source for Major Errors and Performance

Nutrition is *fundamental* to athletic performance, as it is about optimising your energy levels in many different ways. Whether you're an elite athlete or a weekend warrior, the right diet will supply you with the energy needed to achieve your goals and being able to reach your potential.

To meet the demands of daily training and competition and to support recovery after the effort, you need to provide your body with enough energy through an adequate uptake. Dietary energy is like fuel to your body. It's obvious that training and competition generally increase the daily energy requirements and, depending on the type, duration, and intensity of your sports discipline, you need to adapt your intake of food and beverages. The three main nutrients from our diet that supply the body with energy are carbohydrate, fat and protein. These three can be obtained by eating food as proposed by the Food Pyramid for Athletes.

Carbohydrate

Carbohydrate, in the form of glucose, is the main fuel used during exercise and is stored in muscle cells and the liver as glycogen. When physically active, you use the stored glygocen. The muscles and liver can usually store enough glycogen for about 60 to 90min (up to max 120min) of high intensity exercise. If you have ever 'hit the wall' while exercising, you know how body glycogen depletion feels. As carbohydrates help the metabolism of fat, and you've just run out of carbohydrate as a fuel, nothing works. The fat metabolism cannot take over, until some carbohydrates are digested and are ready, in the form of glucose, to restart both metabolisms. The glycogen stores need to be continuously replenished between or during exercise sessions by eating and drinking foods high in carbohydrate. This supplying of carbohydrate will significantly delay the depletion of body glycogen, thereby delaying muscle and general fatigue and sustaining high level performance. Because the body requires less oxygen to burn carbohydrate (in comparison to fat and protein), carbohydrate is considered the body's most efficient fuel source.

Table 1: How to Indicate and Measure Energy

Energy is officially measured in joules. However, as it was measured in 'calories' for many, many years, the common expression is still calories.

1 calorie = 4.184 joule*

*This equation is correct. Our food and the common practice however says 'calories' or 'joules' but in fact we are talking about kilocalories (kcal) and kilojoule (kJ), which means nothing else than 1,000 of them.

Protein

Protein is the nutrient whose main function is to build up and repair muscle and body tissues after exercise as well as to synthetise important enzymes and hormones. Under normal circumstances, it hardly contributes as an energy fuel in sports. In some situations, however, especially when we eat too few calories daily, or during latter stages of endurance exercises, glycogen reserves are completely depleted, and skeletal muscle may be broken down and used as fuel. The latter is a possibly necessary sacrifice in competition, the first is undesirable condition in daily training (compare chapter 'Underweight – What to Do' and 'Female Athlete Triad').

A well-balanced diet covers the protein needs of most of athletes: chicken, turkey, beef, lamb, pork, fish, eggs, dairy foods, and plant sources of protein like tofu, nuts, and seeds. Protein is formed by various combinations of little chemical structures called amino acids. Some amino acids are produced in our body by rearranging the structure of other compounds, while other amino acids (called the essential amino acids) can only be obtained by eating food. Protein from animal foods presents a good variety of amino acids, including the essential ones, while protein from vegetable foods show a different pattern: they usually contain one (or more) of the essential acids in abundance but not the variety. This may be a problem if vegetables make up most of your diet, like for vegetarians. However by thoroughly mixing different plant products, it is possible to cover the needs for proteins, including the essential amino acids as different plants contain different proteins and many are complementary.

The usual targeted recommended dietary intake (RDI) of protein for recreational sport activity is 1g/kg bodyweight. For team athletes, strength-training athletes in a maintenance phase and endurance athletes with a moderate maintenance program, the protein requirement is slightly higher (RDI 1.2–1.4g) and it will be covered by basic nutrition alone. During growth and adolescence (RDI 2g), but also in strenuous endurance or strength-training athletes (RDI 1.7g), protein need is further increased, which needs thorough planning to integrate the recommended four portions of protein by alternating one serving of meat, fish, eggs, cheese, or plant source of protein. In these latter situations, a selective additional protein supplementation to meet the RDI may be considered.

Fat

Fat provides the main fuel source for the long term and is essential for the delivery and uptake of fat-soluble vitamins. Fat provides more than twice the potential energy that protein and carbohydrate do (9 calories per gram of fat versus 4 calories per gram carbohydrate or protein) and is a virtually unlimited source of energy for athletes, as there is enough fat stored in muscle fibres and fat cells to supply more than 100hours of sport activity. To fuel exercise, however, fat needs sufficient oxygen to be consumed simultaneously. So fat fuels low or moderate intensity activity and helps endurance by sparing glycogen reserves even in high-intensity exercise. Most of us have sufficient energy stores of body fat, and it is important to know that the body readily converts and stores excess calories from any source (fat, carbohydrate or protein) as body fat.

You should include moderate amounts of healthy fats into your daily diet, such as nuts, plant based oil (e.g. canola or olive oil), one portion of butter or spread (10g). For each additional hour of exercise, a ½ serving should be added. This contradicts the myth that fats are 'bad'. This perception is wrong and recent studies have underlined the importance of a reasonable fat uptake. What it still true, however, is that fat in biscuits, chips, and deep fried food, and abundant fat in animal foods (e.g. salami, sausages) can be enjoyed, but in reasonable amounts.

Frequently asked questions – myths and facts

1) One of the most common questions in consultations is: Why was I on my last legs? Why did I have this weakness? Shouldn't I take some supplements?

A shared observation among many nutritionists and sports medicine physicians is that sportsmen and women quite frequently suffer a break in their energy supply chain and they strongly believe that this must be related to a specific deficiency, possibly treatable with a supplement. Even with extensive lab tests, we very rarely discover a particular deficiency in these situations. But looking at the food and beverage intake of the particular day, and the day before, we mostly observe quite relevant errors in the management of the energy supply in general.

- Inadequate energy intake for the whole day in long competitions
- Missed meals not adequately replaced
- Bad planning ('we just ate a bit, when we had time' or 'there wasn't anything else available on site but hot dogs and French fries')
- Irregular hydration and irregular nutrition the days before competition due to travelling or stressful days

2) Dietary fat and weight: Athletes wanting to reduce body weight and, in particular, body fat levels ask, 'What should I do? I have reduced my fat intake and still my weight is not moving.'

First of all, we need to check the athlete's goals before asking this particular question. This goes with checking if a weight reduction is really needed. Secondly, we need to address the misconception of fat being the only element responsible. All three types of fuel: carbohydrates, proteins, and fats all contribute to energy uptake. If energy uptake is greater than energy expenditure, the remaining calories will independently from their origin, be stored as body fat. So it's about a simultaneous moderate reduction in energy consumption and a moderate rise in energy uptake (see chapter 'Being Overweight – What to Do').

3) Sports nutrition = carbohydrates. There's a strong belief that, for sportsmen or women, concentrating exclusively on carbohydrates is the right thing to do. Very recently, a group of scientists proposed the opposite—to concentrate on mainly fat instead. As carbohydrates (or fat) would be the only source that energy metabolism is grounded in.

It's true that carbohydrate has a central role in energy metabolism for exercise and recovery, and, on a quantity basis, is the most important nutrient in sport. But as outlined above, to believe in this equation would be a misconception and wilful neglect of the importance of fat and protein, as their essential function cannot be replaced. Nutrition in sports is an 'as well as' function, very much like: Sports nutrition = **carbohydrate** + fat + protein.

In conclusion, nutrition in sport is about having balance. For this purpose the Swiss Society of Nutrition, and in particular the Swiss Forum for Sport Nutrition, has created the 'Food Pyramid for Athletes'. This pyramid gives an excellent overview on a well-balanced diet with sport performance in permanent focus. And you don't need to learn percentages by heart, you may if you like, but be conscious about your nutrition and follow these recommendations. It is in my opinion a good idea to work this pyramid through, read it, and apply it. When you have questions, discuss them with your sports medicine physician and a sports nutritionist. Adopt this pyramid as your specific nutritional target, a blueprint of how it needs to be, and you will be rewarded by having your energy intake organised.

Figure 1: Swiss Sport Nutritional Pyramid (courtesy of Swiss Forum for Sport Nutrition)

Please see over page for the Nutritional Pyramid. To access a larger copy in full, visit: www.forumsportnutrition.ch/wp-content/uploads/pdf/Lebensmittelpyramide_Sport_E1.2.pdf

Literature

Burke L, G. Cox. The complete guide to Food for Sports Performance, Allen&Unwin, Crowsnest NSW, Australia, 2010 p.47-52

Sports Nutrition download online 14.11.2015 from http://nutritionaustralia.org/national/resources/sports-nutrition

The body's fuel sources. Suzanne Girard Eberle. Endurance Sports Nutrition, third edition. p.32-34, Human kinetics, 2014

The truth about fats: the good, the bad and the in-between. Harvard Health Publications. 03.02.2015, online download 18.11.2015 http://www.health.harvard.edu/staying-healthy/the-truth-about-fats-bad-and-good

Swiss Sport Nutritional Pyramid Swiss Forum for Sport Nutrition retrieved 7.5.2016

For athletes exercising ≥5 hours per week

Based on the Food Pyramid for healthy adults of the Swiss Society for Nutrition

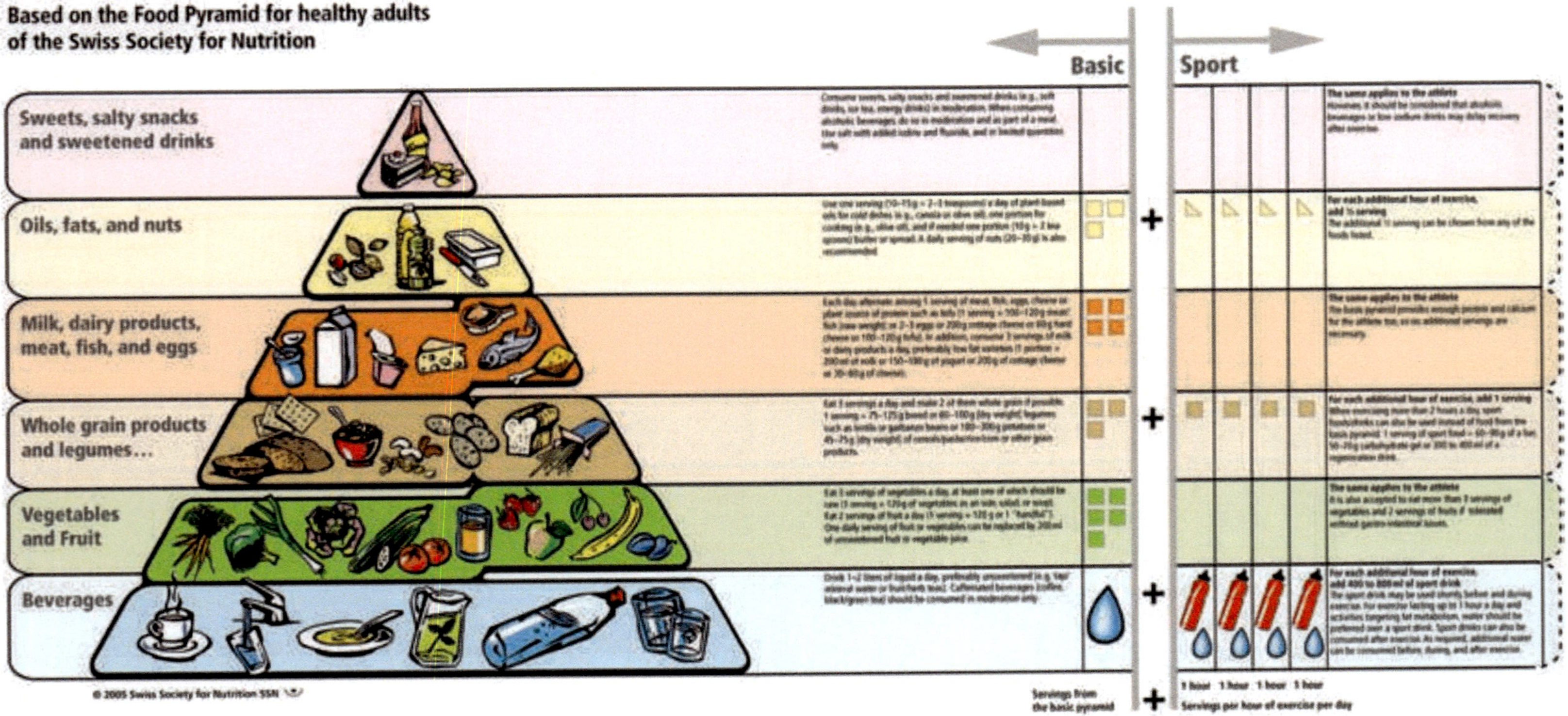

The Food Pyramid for Athletes is based on the Food Pyramid designed and developed by the Swiss Society for Nutrition (Schweizerische Gesellschaft für Ernährung) for healthy adults, which will be referred to as the Basic Food Pyramid. This Basic Food Pyramid has been expanded to cover the energy and nutrient needs for daily exercise typically performed by athletes and active

The Food Pyramid for Athletes is aimed at healthy adults exercising on most days of the week for at least one hour or more per day at moderate intensity, totaling at least 5 hours of exercise per week.

Moderate intensity represents continuous activities such as swimming (2.5 km/h), running (8 km/h) or cycling (2 watts per kg body mass) or the "stop and go" of most intensive match, a soccer game or tennis match. The Basic Food Pyramid reflects balance in food choice, and the same applies to the recommendations for athletes. Both pyramids ensure sufficient energy and nutrient supply for their target population. All foods are allowed, but it is important that a variety of foods are chosen from each section, that produce is chosen seasonally and all foods are prepared and processed with care. The fortified foods and beverages or the use of dietary supplements may exceed the upper tolerable intake level for micronutrients.

Adherence to the Food Pyramid for Athletes offers a solid foundation for longterm, successful performance capability. In contrast to the Basic Food Pyramid, where the recommendations do not have to be followed strictly on a daily basis, it is suggested to ensure optimal regeneration and performance capability. The additional requirement to cover exercise training includes a volume of 1 to 4 hours of moderate intensity exercise per day. For high-intensity exercise and/or greater volumes, the energy and nutrient requirements will be higher. An experienced sports dietitian may help with adjusting food selection and serving size to individual needs.

Serving size selection: From the serving size range given in the pyramid, small athletes of about 50 kg body mass should choose the smallest serving size, whereas the largest serving size applies to athletes weighing about 85 kg, intermediate serving sizes apply to athletes of corresponding intermediate body mass (e.g. medium serving size for 67.5 kg).

Drinking in Sports – Keep Well Hydrated, but We're Not Camels

60% of our body consists of water. Good hydration status is essential for life in general and the maintenance of most of the metabolic processes in a living organism. For an athlete in training and competition, this is even more essential in order to allow a good training regime, to sustain optimal performance and to support ideal regeneration.

Fluid balance is about intake by drinking or eating and about losses, mainly through sweat, evaporation through skin, mucous membranes, respiration (called 'perspiratio insensibilis', as we don't feel these losses), and losses in urine and faeces. Depending on ambient temperature, humidity, type of exercise, its intensity, and duration, sweating and evaporation may vary broadly. Many studies have shown that with a significant percentage loss in body weight (1% during competition), a decline in performance will occur (Goulet 2012, Burke 2010, Coyle 2004). The effect of a 2% loss is clearly more pronounced, and there is an additional deteriorating effect on cognition (Tomporowski 2007, Cian 2001). So, the goal is to replace this loss of body fluid. There are observations that the decline in performance is more pronounced with a higher ambient temperature (Coyle 2004).

Talking about replacing these liquids, and about ongoing effort, it is obvious that it's not only a job to be done by plain water, but it is also about energy uptake of ingested carbohydrates, which are easily digestible and rapidly bring the wanted fuel into circulation. Studies have shown there is 40–60g/hour as optimal amount of carbohydrates in a drink, allowing the best gastrointestinal uptake rate.

Looking at the electrolyte balance with sweating and evaporation, we realise that our body is able to keep blood electrolytes stable for many hours, even during demanding exercises. But we know that the lost electrolytes need to be replaced quickly, for optimal recovery of muscular and cellular function. Therefore, most sports drinks contain a certain amount of electrolytes. Studies about gastrointestinal absorption show sports drinks containing possibly a little lower, but close to the electrolyte concentration of the blood, are best (i.e. slightly hypotonic). Sodium, as one of these electrolytes, seems to assist this absorption additionally (sodium-glucose-water-co-transport).

Among the electrolytes, sodium has a particular place: usually, we have enough sodium in our system through table salt (NaCl) and there's no need to worry about it. But with prolonged training and exercises (>3h), and excessive replacement of fluids by water alone, our body is no longer able to keep the necessary balance and the lack of sodium may turn into a real deficiency, called hyponatremia. This is a serious condition that can, in ongoing long competitions (from 6–12h), result in brain oedema (i.e. accumulation of excessive fluid in the substance of the brain) and death of the athlete. Often these athletes, usually the ones back in the pack, having 4–5 or 6h in a marathon make two mistakes: 1) they drink too much and 2) they drink just plain water and end up with hyponatremia.

What is recommended and how may we proceed?

In the last 15 years, sportsmen and women were told to drink before thirst comes. Is this still correct, or, taking into account these severe cases with hyponatremia, should we return to thirst as a valuable indicator?

Our body is not really good at knowing how well hydrated it is. By far the best (and only) method to judge hydration status is by looking at the colour of your urine (the first sample of the morning is the best indicator) or weighing its specific weight. It should be just slightly yellow (light and pale). If it's fully transparent then you are certainly very well hydrated, if it's yellow, then you should drink more; if it's dark yellow (concentrated), you are dehydrated. If you are consuming a multivitamin or a supplement with Vitamin B2 (Riboflavin) you need to take into account that your urine will be more yellow coloured than usual.

What about thirst now? The answer is clear, you cannot rely on thirst as an indicator in exercise situations. So try to go along with the recommendations, your experiences, and your gut feeling.

If we look at fluid absorption intake recommendations we may keep the following: for a normal person the recommendations propose an intake of 1–2l of liquid a day, preferably unsweetened (e.g. tap/mineral water or fruit/herbal teas). For sportsmen and women, for each additional hour of exercise, add 400–800ml of sports drink, according to ambient temperature, humidity, and training intensity. For exercises lasting up to one hour a day and activities targeting fat metabolism water should be preferred over a sport drink (compare also 'Food Pyramid for Athletes – Beverages').

Table 1: Recommendations for Hydration in Sports

- Begin exercise well-hydrated, aim to drink 200ml (if hot up to 600ml) in the last 45min prior to the event. Do not overhydrate
- Fluid uptake should be regular every 15–20min 150–200ml during exercise
- An optimal sports drink contains carbohydrates (40–50g/l to help delay fatigue by providing glucose to the muscles and improve absorption) and electrolytes (to replace the losses through sweat)
- For long training sessions (>3h) and long and ultra-long events (>2–3h) sodium as an electrolyte is indispensable
- After exercise, replace fluid losses. Weigh yourself before and after exercise. For every 0.5kg body weight lost, drink 500ml fluid, with primarily carbohydrates (and possibly some proteins) to support and facilitate recovery

Literature

Garth AK, Burke LM. What do athletes drink during competitive sporting activities? Sports Med. 2013 Jul;43(7):539-64.

Goulet ED. Dehydration and endurance performance in competitive athletes. Nutr Rev. 2012 Nov;70 Suppl 2:S132-6.

Burke L, G.Cox. The complete guide to Food for Sports Performance, Allen&Unwin, Crowsnest NSW, Australia, 2010

Coyle EF. Fluid and fuel intake during exercise. J Sports Sci. 2004 Jan;22(1):39-55.

Tomporowski PD et al. Effects of dehydration and fluid ingestion on cognition. Int J Sports Med. 2007 Oct;28(10):891-6.

Cian C et al. Effects of fluid ingestion on cognitive function after heat stress or exercise-induced dehydration.Int J Psychophysiol. 2001 Nov;42(3):243-51.

Breakfast, a Good Start to the Day – My Kingdom for a Muesli in a Bowl

Studies show clearly that eating breakfast brings enormous benefits, as it helps improving your cognitive function, boosts energy levels, and is getting you ready for the day. If you look at the glycaemic properties of breakfast, meals with a lower but more sustainable glycaemic load resulted in better cognitive performance and better mood, especially after 3h or later.

This shows quite clearly that, for an athlete, breakfast shouldn't be left out. It further indicates that meals with complex carbohydrates, some proteins, some fat (e.g. wholegrain bread, butter, jam, chocolate milk of milk coffee) are superior to the easy digestible purely refined carbohydrate meal (e.g. toast and honey, orange juice) and also superior to the heavy English breakfast with bacon, eggs, sausages, tea or coffee (mainly fat and some proteins).

Figure 1: A Freshly Prepared Muesli

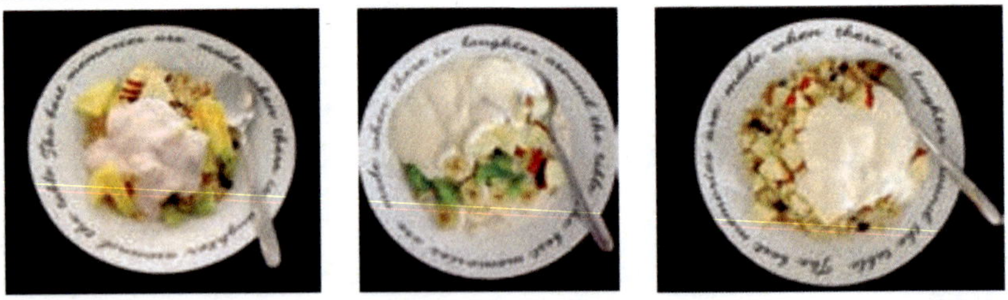

The muesli breakfast is the ideal breakfast meal – my kingdom for a muesli:

- Rolled oats are unsweetened and healthier than refined sugary cereals
- Whole grains deliver sustainable energy over several hours (and do not lead to a high glycaemic peak)

- Rich in fibre to support a good digestion (and as side effect effectively lowering cholesterol)
- Nuts, rolled oats, and other grains are rich in nutrients and unsaturated fatty acids
- Milk is a source of calcium and protein
- Fresh fruits add natural vitamin C and minerals (e.g. potassium, magnesium)
- You stay fuller for longer, don't eat something unhealthy, and avoid a gap before midday

Figure 2: Original Bircher Muesli

Original muesli recipe of Dr Bircher-Benner, Swiss physician, around 1900

- 2 or 3 small apples (or one large one), finely grated (including skin and core)
- 1 tablespoon nuts (either walnuts, almonds, or hazelnuts)
- 1 tablespoon rolled oats (previously soaked in 3 tablespoons water for 12 hours)
- Lemon juice from ½ a lemon.
- 1 tablespoon of either cream and honey or sweetened condensed milk*

*The use of condensed milk was a compromise due to hygiene concerns regarding fresh milk in 1900

It doesn't need to be the traditional Bircher muesli (see Figure 2), create your very own muesli and enjoy – bon appetite!

Literature

Young H, Benton D. The effect of using isomaltulose (Palatinose™) to modulate the glycaemic properties of breakfast on the cognitive performance of children. Eur J Nutr. 2015 Sep;54(6):1013-20.

Adolphus K et al. The effects of breakfast on behavior and academic performance in children and adolescents. Front Hum Neurosci. 2013; 7: 425. Published online 2013 Aug 8. PMCID: PMC3737458

,Hoyland A et al. A systematic review of the effect of breakfast on the cognitive performance of children and adolescents. Nutr Res Rev. 2009 Dec;22(2):220-43.

Artikel über Dr.Bircher-Benner in NZZ (in German) retrieved online 5.6.2016 http://folio.nzz.ch/1997/april/doktor-birchers-neue-weltordnung

Vitamins and Minerals – Good to Know

Athletes (as well as coaches and parents) need a basic knowledge of vitamins and minerals. The following tables give an overview.

Table 1: Vitamins and Their Importance in Sports

Name (medical term)	Importance	Source	Remarks
Vitamin A** (retinol)	Vision: protects eyesight from night blindness, healthy skin and mucous membranes, antioxidant activity, resistance to infection. Protein metabolism	As retinol in: liver, oily fish, egg yolk, full fat dairy product. As beta-caroten in yellow and orange fruits and vegetables (e.g. carrots, pumpkin, apricots, peaches but also cabbage, spinach).	
Vitamin B1* (thiamine)	Nervous system (nerve cell function), energy metabolism from food, especially carbohydrate metabolism.	Fortified and wholegrain breads and cereals, yeast extracts (e.g. vegemite), legumes, potatoes, fish, and poultry.	In case of deficiency: severe neurological disorder, muscle atrophy, heart insufficiency.
Vitamin B2* (riboflavin)	Nervous system, energy metabolism from food, growth.	Milk and dairy foods, yeast extract (e.g. Vegemite), fortified wholegrain breads and cereals, mushrooms	As it is yellow (flavin) it is also used as food colorant (E101). An important component of many multivitamins. Responsible for the yellow urine colour.

Name (medical term)	**Importance**	**Source**	**Remarks**
Vitamin B6* (pyridoxalphosphat)	Red cell formation (haematopoiesis), energy metabolism (formation of amino acids, fat metabolism).	Dairy products, meat and fish, cabbage and legumes, wholegrain bread and cereals, potatoes, bananas.	
Vitamin B12* (cobalamin)	Nervous system (essential for nerve cell function) Formation of all blood cells (haemato-, leuco- and thrombopoiesis), folic acid metabolism.	Meat, fish, dairy products, eggs.	Deficiency leads to a severe pernicious anaemia and funicular myelosis (severe neurological disease).
Vitamin C* (ascorbic acid)	Collagen fibre synthesis, wound healing, antioxidative function (free radical catcher), resistance to infection, absorption of iron	Citrus fruits, peppers, kiwi, cabbage, broccoli, green leafy vegetables, berries	In earlier maritime days, sauerkraut was used to prevent scurvy of the seamen, as it was long-living.
Vitamin D** (1,25-dihydroxy-cholecalciferol)	Bone metabolism, regulation of the calcium/phosporus uptake, muscle metabolism, immune system.	(Oily) fish, butter, eggs, cheese.	Sunlight (20min/d) important for VitD synthesis – but in winter and indoor sports not sufficient. Dietary intake important!
Vitamin E** (alfa-tocopherol)	Antioxidant activity, catcher of free radicals, wound healing.	Wheat germ and wholegrain cereals, vegetable oils, nuts and seeds, egg yolk.	

Name (medical term)	Importance	Source	Remarks
Vitamin K** (phytomenadion)	Blood clotting, bone metabolism, antioxidant activity.	Broccoli, green leafy vegetables, soybean and vegetable oils, poultry.	A certain percentage of these vitamins is synthetised by our own intestinal flora.
Niacin* (Vitamin B3)	Essential in the energy metabolism from food (proteins, carbohydrates, and fats), regeneration of skin, muscles, nerve cells, and DNA.	Poultry, liver, coffee, yeast extracts. mushrooms.	A certain percentage of these vitamins is synthetised by our own intestinal flora.
Pantothenic acid* (Vitamin B5)	Carbohydrate, fat, and protein metabolism, wound healing.	Wholegrain breads and cereals, yeast extract (e.g. Vegemite), fish and meat, eggs, peanuts, soy beans.	A certain percentage of these vitamins is synthetised by our own intestinal flora.
Biotin* (Vitamin B7)	Fat and protein metabolism, growth, mood regulation.	Most vegetables, milk, egg yolk, wholegrain bread and cereals.	A certain percentage of these vitamins is synthetised by our own intestinal flora.
Folic acid* (Vitamin B9)	Formation of red blood cells (hematopoiesis), DNA metabolism.	Green leafy vegetables, broccoli, wholegrain breads and cereals, eggs, legumes, nuts.	Prevention of neural tube defects (in utero), reduction of homocysteine (so folic acid reduces the risk for heart disease).

*water-soluble: all B and vitamin C
** fat-soluble: ADEK

Table 2: A Selection of Minerals and Their Importance in Sports

Name	Importance	Source	Comments
Sodium (Na)	Facilitates the co-transport of glucose and co-transport of fluid in stomach and intestine, major electrolyte outside the cell balances with potassium inside the cell, regulation of blood pressure.	NaCl – our table salt. Our normal nutrition contains usually too much of salt, so there's no need to add additional salt to an athlete's diet. For long ultra-long lasting competitions, sodium is really recommended.	In particular in long lasting endurance sport events (>2-3h), a sodium supply is indispensable. Heavy sweating and abundant drinking of just plain water will otherwise lead to a hyponatremia (lack of sodium) with possibly fatal cerebral oedema.
Potassium (K)	Major electrolyte inside the cell, balances with sodium outside the cell, nerve impulse transmission.	Widely distributed in fruits, especially in bananas and apricots, and vegetables, meat and fish.	
Magnesium (Mg)	Bone structure, muscle contraction and nerve function, enzyme systems.	Dried fruit, wholegrain breads and cereals, fruits, green leafy vegetables, legumes (lentils) and nuts, figs	
Calcium (Ca)	Bone and teeth formation, especially important during growth up to 25yrs of age (age of Peak Bone Mass).	Milk and dairy products, mineral water, nuts.	
Phosphorus (P)	Bone and teeth formation, protein, ATP, and DNA formation.	Widely distributed in foods.	

Name	Importance	Source	Comments
Iron (Fe)	Red cell formation, oxygen transport, enzyme function.	Meat and fish, legumes and cereals, green leafy vegetables.	See separate chapter.
Selenium (Se)	Antioxidant activity.	Lean meat, fish, oysters, chicken. Grains and vegetable oils.	Protection against heavy metal poisoning.
Copper (Cu)	Enzyme function, red blood cell formation, nerve cell function.	Shellfish, liver, tofu, wholegrain bread and cereals, legumes, nuts and seeds, dried fruit.	
Manganese (Mn)	Enzyme function and activation, glucose and fat metabolism.	Rolled oats and other cereals, nuts.	
Zinc	Wound healing, immune system, enzyme component.	Meat and fish, wholegrain bread and cereals, eggs, poultry, legumes and nuts.	
Iodine	Brain function, prevents goitre.	Fish and shellfish, iodised table salt, seaweed	
Fluoride	Healthy bones and teeth.	Fluoridated drinking water.	
Molybdenum	Iron metabolism.	Widely distributed in cereals and vegetables.	

Having gone through this list, you may say, 'That's fascinating, that's real science,' and you are right, it is. Therefore, if you want more details, or have issues to discuss about vitamins and minerals, there are sports nutritionists to help you with all your questions.

If it is about daily life, i.e. what to take home of all of this for your daily training. The 'Food Pyramid for Athletes' is an excellent tool for sportsmen and women. It includes all the above information and use it to influence your diet.

Literature

Food Pyramid for Athletes – Swiss Forum for Sports Nutrition http://www.forumsportnutrition.ch/pyramide/

General information about vitamins and minerals on the Swiss Forum for Sports Nutrition Website; http://www.forumsportnutrition.ch/

Burke L, G.Cox. The complete guide to Food for Sports Performance, Allen&Unwin, Crowsnest NSW, Australia, 2010

Vegetarian or Vegan Diet and High Performance – Is It Worth the Effort?

It's awesome to observe how attentively and carefully people following a vegetarian or vegan diet look after their food. They pay attention to many things to have an all-embracing, complete, and healthy diet. I think all other people, including all athletes, should be respectful towards them and could learn a lesson from them concerning the composition of a carefully chosen diet.

However, food from animal provenance contains some valuable and essential components which food of plant origin completely lacks, or only offers in little amounts, as discussed in earlier chapters of this book ('Basic of Sports Nutrition', 'Vitamins and Minerals', and 'Iron deficiency and Sport') regarding amino acids, in particular essential amino acids (i.e. components of proteins), Vitamin B12, and iron. We need first to clarify the terms. Vegetarian means following a diet of plant origin or from living animals, like honey, milk, eggs, but not meat and no fish. Whereas vegan means following a diet only based on food from plant origin, all foods of animal origin are excluded (no meat, no fish, no eggs, no milk, no honey). Looking at these definitions, we realise the vegan diet makes a serious choice by excluding many valuable sources of protein, calcium, vitamins, and minerals.

I have seen a few vegetarian people and athletes but only a handful following a vegan diet. Vegetarians often, especially kids or adolescents, are not eating meat or fish because they just don't like it. A greater percentage follows this diet for other reasons. In sports medicine consultation, communication is open and we discuss issues frankly and clearly, as the contribution of nutrition to optimal training and performance is quite evident. For people following a vegetarian diet, we need to have a closer look at proteins and essential amino acids, vitamin B12, and iron. Regular blood tests (2 or 3 times/year) to rule out an iron and vitamin B12 deficiency are recommended. If it's about an elite or professional athlete, particularly in endurance sports a controlled substitute with vitamin B12 and iron may be necessary. This needs to be seriously planned and followed by a health professional like a sports medicine physician or a sport nutritionist.

Athletes following a strictly vegan diet have taken on an enormous, even impossible, challenge. On-going professional follow-up in this situation is essential. I must say one very important thing here: growing children on a vegan diet alone, without any vitamin B12 substitute, run the risk of developing pernicious anaemia, impairment of nerve cell function, and severely impaired brain development.

Making your choice towards a thoroughly and carefully executed diet does not necessarily mean it is healthy. In a nut-shell:

- Vegetarian diet and high performance is possible, but adequate planning, focused supplementation, and continuous professional follow up is warranted
- Vegan diet and high performance is an impossible mission and, to be honest, a waste of precious time

Table 1: Practical Recommendations for Vegetarian Athletes in Elite Sports

- Follow the recommendations of the 'Food Pyramid for Athletes'
- Carefully choose. It is very important to vary the 4 servings of protein on a daily basis (egg, milk, cheese, and other dairy products, tofu and other soy products, nuts and seeds) to ideally cover your need in essential amino acids
- Keep an eye on vitamin B12 (dairy products) and iron (legumes, green leafy vegetables, cereals) and eat them regularly on a daily basis
- Regular blood tests to rule out an iron or vitamin B12 deficiency should be performed
- If you are an endurance athlete, discuss with your sportsmed physician or your nutritionist whether an intermittent substitute with oral iron and vitamin B12 is indicated (based on the blood test results)

Literature

Factsheet: Vegetarische Ernährungsweisen im Sport Website of the Swiss Forum for Sport Nutrition, retrieved 5.6.2016, http://www.forumsportnutrition.ch/wp-content/uploads/2015/01/HotTopic_Vegetarische_Ernaehrung_2.0.pdf

Factsheet: Vegetarian eating on the AIS Website retrieved 5.6.2016 http://www.ausport.gov.au/ais/nutrition/factsheets/special_diets/vegetarian_eating

Burke L, G.Cox. The complete guide to Food for Sports Performance, Allen&Unwin, Crowsnest NSW, Australia, 2010

Supplementation – the Cherry on the Cake, But Can't Replace Any Other Thing

Before talking about supplements being the cherry on the cake, we need to address one important thing: contamination of supplements is a big issue and a sad reality. There are numerous personal stories from sportsmen and women of all levels and all over the world to be told. It doesn't necessarily mean the end of a career, but it can and it has. And as many concerned athletes tell, it must be terrible to have worked hard, having given that much of yourself, dedicated that much energy and time, and then be accused of being a cheater. To suffer this false accusation, knowing that you have done nothing wrong, is just beyond our imagination.

The contamination may arise from an unintentional crossover of a little amount of powder of a prescribed medication (e.g. steroid drug) left on a machine and accidentally mixed into your supplement. Or it may be integrated during manufacturing without official declaration. But there is little chance for the athlete to be able to prove it in retrospect, and the law is that the athlete needs to be wise and fully aware of what is getting into his body and to abstain from taking any doubtful product.

What is a supplement?

Is it just about vitamins and minerals? Or is it about all the products you find on the shelves in a health-food store? Or is it only about hardcore body-building products with ingredient names that sound like illegal drugs? Or is also about all drinks, gels, bars, powders, potions, and tailor-made food for athletes? So let's make it clear, and here we can accept the views of former athletes, dieticians, scientists, and sportsmed physicians. For that purpose, the ABCD classification for supplements and sport foods has been developed. It is based on scientific evidence and allows each athlete to integrate sports foods and supplements into their diets so as to reach their performance goals. This information is easily accessible to the sports community and ongoing research projects keep the information and the website up to date.

Table 1: ABCD Classification and Some Examples (According to the AIS Website)

Classification	Scientific Evidence	Subcategory	Examples
A	Supported for use in specific situations to contribute to optimal physical performance.	Sports foods	Sports drinks, sports gels, sports bars, whey protein, electrolyte replacement.
		Medical Supplements	Iron supplement, calcium supplements, multivitamin/vitamin supplement, vitamin D, probiotica (gut/intestinal flora)
		Performance supplements	Beta-alanin, caffeine, beetroot juice, bicarbonate, creatine.
B	Deserving further research.	Polyphenols	Having antioxidative and anti-inflammatory activity like quercetin, tart cherry juice, exotic berries (acai, goji etc.), curcumin.
		Others	Anti-oxidants C and E, carnitine, HMB, glutamine, fish oils, glucosamine
C	Little meaningful proof of beneficial effect.		Categories A and B products outside research protocols, and others (under A-Z of supplements).
D	Banned or at high risk. *Not to be used by athletes.*		Stimulants, prohormones, GH-releasers and peptides, and others.

Ask your nutritionist and sports medicine physician about reasonable prices for supplements (or better still: what is the highest reasonable price) as sale of supplements is about making money. E.g. you should get a really good, well-balanced sports-specific multivitamin for less than $1 per day.

So, it's your decision: balance your very personal pros and cons for taking supplements, discuss it with your coach, your sports medicine physician, and your nutritionist. And don't be too much influenced by such questions as: 'how can I afford to let other athletes get an advantage I don't have?' as still 50% of all athletes are not taking supplements (even not a multivitamin), and are performing very well.

General recommendation about use of supplements:

- If you decide to supplement, choose your product on a rational basis. High quality information is available (see links below)
- Supplementation cannot correct errors in training. So your good training work pays
- Supplements won't correct errors or neglects in basic nutrition. So keep always an eye on your daily nutrition, especially before, during, and after events
- Choose a serious, tested product and stay informed about side and possible negative effects
- Try your product in training before using it in competition

Literature

Supplements retrieved on the AIS Website 5.4.2016 http://www.ausport.gov.au/ais/nutrition/supplements.

Supplementguide Website Antidoping Schweiz retrieved 5.4.2016 http://www.antidoping.ch/de/medizin-substanzen-und-methoden/supplement-guide-nahrungsergaenzungsmittel

Burke L, G.Cox. The complete guide to Food for Sports Performance, Allen&Unwin, Crowsnest NSW, Australia, 2010

Links

For Australian athletes:

http://www.ausport.gov.au/ais/nutrition/supplements.

For Swiss athletes:

http://www.antidoping.ch/de/medizin-substanzen-und-methoden/supplementguide-nahrungsergaenzungsmittel

How About Beetroot Juice, Beta-Alanin, Bicarbonate, Caffeine, and Creatine? – Let's Have a Closer Look

'Nonetheless, in the context of exercise performance, it is clear that carbohydrate (but not fat) still remains king and that carefully chosen ergogenic aids *(e.g. caffeine, creatine, sodium bicarbonate, beta-alanine, nitrates) can all promote performance in the correct exercise setting.'*

(Close GL, Hamilton DL, Philp A, Burke LM, Morton JP 2016)

Ergogenic (i.e. performance enhancing) supplements need to be carefully chosen and I strongly recommend a professional counselling by either an experienced sports nutritionist or sports medicine physician if it comes to a focused use of these products.

I furthermore propose a very conservative approach in the use of performance enhancing supplements with children and adolescents. I'm convinced there's strictly no place for them in kids sport and I recommend restriction in adolescents at least until the age of sixteen. First for safety reasons, as there are no studies on performance enhancing supplements in kids and adolescents and we simply don't know how a growing organism reacts to these substances. Secondly, so much can be achieved in sports performance through the normal training process, without using supplements. And last, but not least, what are we teaching young people if we condition them to believe we still have something up our sleeves and use supplements with the goal to improve performance at this early age?

Beetroot Juice (Cat A)

Active Ingredient	Beetroot juice is a rich source of nitrate (NO_3) which is finally processed into Nitric oxide (NO).
Mechanism of Action	Exact mechanism remains unclear, reducing the oxygen cost of exercise.
Performance Enhancement in	• Reducing oxygen cost of exercise (better economy) in cycling and running events of 4–30min duration, mainly with submaximal and maximal intensity • Better maximal performance in incremental testing without improving the VO2max • Ergogenic during repeated bouts of short-duration maximal intensity exercise with interspersed short recovery periods Chronic (3-15d) as well as acute (single dose prior to exercise) protocols enhance the exercise economy.
Typical Dosages	• 5–8mmol (or 300mg–500mg) consumed 2–2.5h before exercising Average uptake of nitrate 1–2mmol/d out of mainly vegetables (60–120mg/d; as conversion 1mmol = 62mg) Very high nitrate content in green leafy plants and vegetables grown in low light conditions such as: beetroot and beetroot juice, celery, lettuce, rocket, spinach.
Other Effects	• Relaxing the tone of blood vessels (therefore lowering blood pressure) • Regulating platelet aggregation (reducing the risk of atherosclerosis) • Reducing infections in the mouth, gut, and skin • Anti-inflammatory effects (attenuates muscle soreness and sustains jump performance after eccentric exercises)

Side Effects	• Beetroot juice and other vegetable sources of nitrate are unlikely to be harmful. They possibly cause mild gastrointestinal discomfort • Temporary red colouration of urine and stools is common, but this is a harmless side effect • There is not much known about chronic use of nitrate supplements • The use of sodium nitrate or even sodium nitrite, however, can in higher dosages produce toxic effects with a methaemoglobinaemia and possibly fatal consequences

Literature

'Nitrat und Randensaft' Factsheet Antidoping Schweiz retrieved 21.4.2016 http://www.antidoping.ch/sites/default/files/downloads/2014/130326_fb_nitrat_und_randensaft.pdf

'Beetroot juice/Nitrate' AIS website fact sheet – AIS sports supplement program retrieved 20.4.2016 http://beetpower.nl/wp-content/uploads/2015/09/Beetroot_juice_Nitrate_11-_website_fact_sheet-1.pdf

Flueck JL et al. Is beetroot juice more effective than sodium nitrate? The effect of equimolar nitrate dosages of nitrate-rich beetroot juice and sodium nitrate on oxygen consumption during exercise. Appl Physiol Nutr Metab. 2016 Apr;41(4):421-9

Jonvik KL et al. Nitrate-rich vegetables increase plasma nitrate and nitrite concentrations and lower blood pressure in healthy adults. J Nutr. 2016 Apr 13.pii:jn229807.

Wylie LJ et al. Influence of beetroot juice supplementation on intermittent exercise performance. Eur J Appl Physiol. 2016 Feb;116(2):415-25

Clifford T et al. The effects of beetroot juice supplementation on indices of muscle damage following eccentric exercise. Eur J Appl Physiol. 2016 Feb;116(2):353-62

Buck CL et al. Effects of sodium phosphate and beetroot juice supplementation on repeated-sprint ability in females. Eur J Appl Physiol. 2015 Oct;115(10):2205-13

Beta-Alanin (Cat A)

Active Ingredient	Beta-alanin, an amino acid. Carnosin consists of two amino acids: beta-alanin and histidine. Carnosin (in latin, 'carnis' means meat) is nearly exclusively found in meat, in the muscle.
Mechanism of Action	Buffering acids (within the cell).
Performance Enhancement in	• High intensity, lactacid efforts of 1–7min duration (e.g. athletics, rowing, swimming) • Repeated bouts of high intensity efforts (e.g. series of sprints, intervals, isometric force, jump height) • Sprints at the end of an endurance effort (e.g. cross country skiing, cycling)
Typical Dosages	A loading protocol, lasting from 4–10 weeks, may look like this (improves stores of carnosine/ beta-alanin by 40–80%): • 1 week: 4x daily 400mg beta-alanin, pauses of 3h between serves (or twice daily 800mg 'slow-release'/ 'sustained release' formula) • 2–10 week: 4 x 800mg beta-alanin (max 10mg/kg) (or twice 1600mg 'slow-release'/ 'sustained release' formula) • 4 month pause
Other Effects	• Some studies show a better tolerance to training efforts, possibly also due to antioxidative effects of beta-alanin/carnosine
Side Effects	• Tingling sensation of the skin, pins and needles, hot flashes especially with higher dosages, therefore don't go over 800mg or 10mg/kg in one serve • Uptake with meals reduces side effects • Slow release or sustained release formulas cause usually less side effects

Literature

Invernizzi PL et al. Effects of Acute Carnosine and β-Alanine on Isometric Force and Jumping Performance. Int J Sports Physiol Perform. 2016 Apr;11(3):344-9.

Carnosin und beta-Alanin Factsheet Antidoping Schweiz retrieved 21.4.2016

Close GL et al. New strategies in sport nutrition to increase exercise performance. Free Radic Biol Med. 2016 Feb 5. pii: S0891-5849(16)00030-7.

Bellinger PM, Minahan CL. The effect of β-alanine supplementation on cycling time trials of different length. Eur J Sport Sci. 2015 Dec 11:1-8.

Lancha Junior AH et al. Nutritional Strategies to Modulate Intracellular and Extracellular Buffering Capacity During High-Intensity Exercise. Sports Med. 2015 Nov;45 Suppl 1:S71-81.

Sweeney KM et al. The effect of beta-alanine supplementation on power performance during repeated sprint activity. J Strength Cond Res 2010;24:79-87

Stellingwerff T et al. Effect of two beta-alanine dosing protocols on muscle carnosine synthesis and washout. Amino Acids 2011.

Caffeine (Cat A)

Active Ingredient	Caffeine is a natural active ingredient of the coffee bean, the cola nut, mate leaves, guarana berry, and the tea plant (black and green tea).
Mechanism of Action	Caffeine is a stimulating agent. Highest concentration in blood is reached within 30–90min after ingestion. • Reduces perception of fatigue, effort, and pain • Acts directly on the muscle cell (acts on enzymes, enhances effects of adrenalin, enhances cell metabolism) • Improves absorption of carbohydrates in the intestines • Improves fat oxidation (slight effect)
Performance Enhancement in	• Endurance competitions lasting longer than 20min • High intensity efforts from 1–20min duration • High intensity repeated bouts of exercise (team sports)

Typical Dosages	The following three protocols seem to be effective, but focus by choosing one of them (or eventually combine 1 and 3): • 3–6mg per kg bodyweight 1h before the effort • 3–6mg per kg bodyweight in doses of 0.3–1mg/kg spread over the duration of competition • 1–2mg/kg at latest 30min before the end of competition Ingestions above 6mg/kg bodyweight may, because of more frequently upcoming side effects, impair performance. • Coffee (150ml) – 80–150mg • Espresso (30ml) – 30–80mg • Black Tea (1 cup) – 20–40mg • Caffeine gel (1 gel) – 50mg (but may vary) • Coca Cola 250ml – 25mg • Red Bull 250mg – 80mg
Other Effects	• The combination of caffeine and creatine, in case of a concomitant uptake, may reduce the performance enhancing effects of creatine.
Side Effects	• May mainly occur in people not used to caffeine: palpitations, trembling, sleep disturbances, headache, irregular pulse. • Special attention needs to be taken for athletes who are children and younger adolescents. Parents and coaches need to actively decide about the strategy concerning caffeine ingestions for their kids/their team, especially as they are not used to caffeine and do not have the same body weight as adults etc. I propose a conservative strategy, i.e. no caffeine under 16years of age.

Literature

Koffein Factsheet Antidoping Schweiz Retrieved Online 21.4.2016 Http://Www.Antidoping.Ch/Sites/Default/Files/Downloads/2014/110812_Fb_Koffein.Pdf

Higgins S Et Al. The Effects Of Pre-Exercise Caffeinated-Coffee Ingestion On Endurance Performance: An Evidence-Based Review. Int J Sport Nutr Exerc Metab. 2015 Nov 16.

Spriet LL. Exercise And Sport Performance With Low Doses Of Caffeine. Sports Med. 2014 Nov;44 Suppl 2:S175-84.

Owens JA Et Al. Effect Of Energy Drink And Caffeinated Beverage Consumption On Sleep, Mood, And Performance In Children And Adolescents. Nutr Rev. 2014 Oct;72 Suppl 1:65-71

Burke LM, Maughan RJ. The Governor Has A Sweet Tooth - Mouth Sensing Of Nutrients To Enhance Sports Performance. Eur J Sport Sci. 2015;15(1):29-40.

Burke L Et Al: Supplements And Sports Food. In: Burke L, Deakin V (Edit.) Clinical Sports Nutrition. Australia, Mcgraw Hill, P.419-490, 2010

Burke L. Caffeine And Sports Performance. J Appl Physiol Nutr Metab 33:1319-1334, 2008

Bicarbonate (Cat A)

Active Ingredient	Sodium bicarbonate ($NaHCO_3$, HCO_3)
Mechanism of Action	Bicarbonate is an *extracellular buffer substance and facilitates lactic acid removal from contracting muscle*, it keeps the pH (acid-base metabolism) constant. In cases of an accumulation of acids in muscle cells and blood, bicarbonate may buffer these situations. Additional ingestion of sodium bicarbonate temporarily increases the blood concentration of bicarbonate (bicarbonate loading, i.e. enhances the buffer capacity) A *constant pH* secures the activity of enzymes, nerve conduction, energy metabolism, and the functioning of the contractile elements (actin and myosin), whereas acidity impairs all these functions.
Performance Enhancement in	• Lactacid anaerobic efforts of 1–8min, but also in prolonged sports involving intermittent or sustained periods of high intensity work rates (e.g. 60min) • High intensity repeated bouts of exercise

Typical Dosages	Sodium bicarbonate: 300mg/kg bodyweight. Dilute the powder in 1 litre of water or take in capsules with the same amount of water 60–120min before the effort. Uptake over 30–45min, and an increase of the amount of water ingested, reduces side effects.
Other Effects	• Athletes with arterial hypertension or impaired renal function should *not* use bicarbonate • A couple of hours before and after the use of bicarbonate: *no milk, no dairy products, no calcium supplements, no mineral water rich in calcium should be ingested*, as this may lead to hypercalcaemia and a deposit of calcium in organs like the kidney
Side Effects	• Gastrointestinal problems, like nausea and diarrhoea (these symptoms may be controlled by drinking enough water) • Electrolyte disturbances (lowered potassium, increased sodium) • Numbness or pins and needles in hands or feet

Literature

Natrium-Bikarbonat Fact Sheet Antidoping Schweiz retrieved online 21.4.2016 http://www.antidoping.ch/sites/default/files/downloads/2014/110812_fb_natrium_bikarbonat_citrat.pdf

Sahlin K. Muscle energetics during explosive activities and potential effects of nutrition and training. Sports Med. 2014 Nov;44 Suppl 2:S167-73.

Burke LM. Practical considerations for bicarbonate loading and sports performance. Nestle Nutr Inst Workshop Ser. 2013;75:15-26.

Peart DJ et al. Practical recommendations for coaches and athletes: a meta-analysis of sodium bicarbonate use for athletic performance. J Strength Cond Res. 2012 Jul;26(7):1975-83.

McNaughton LR et al. Ergogenic effects of sodium bicarbonate. Curr Sports Med Rep. 2008 Jul-Aug;7(4):230-6.

Creatine (Cat A)

Active Ingredient	• Creatine monohydrate • Our body creates creatine in liver and kidney out of the amino acids glycine, arginine, and methionine. Creatine uptake in the nutrition, mainly found in fish and meat
Mechanism of Action	• Improving energy availability: more creatine phosphate and higher ATP availability (immediate rephosphorylation of ADP to ATP) in the muscle cell • Enhancing muscle mass and strength
Performance Enhancement in	• Better anaerobic lactacid energy availability, improvement in high intensity sprint and strength sports, especially in repeated bouts with short recovery • Enhancing muscle mass In all sports, where absolute strength is the performance enhancing factor (e.g. throwing, bob sled, weight lifting) a supplementation with creatine seems beneficial. Whereas in sports, in which an increase in weight (even if it's muscle mass) may impair performance, possible advantages and disadvantages need to be appraised (e.g. sprint, hurdles, jump, team sports).
Typical Dosages	**Fast load:** 300mg/kg bodyweight daily for 5 days (usually spread in 4–5 serves), then 3g per day as maintenance for 4–12 weeks. Followed by a pause of at least 4 weeks. **Slow load:** 3 (-5)g per day (spread in 1–3 serves) for 4 weeks, then 3g/day as maintenance for 4—12 weeks. Followed by a pause of at least 4 weeks. Uptake is improved after an effort and if ingested together with carbohydrates. Ideally take it round 30min before your regular meal.

Other Effects	• Creatine is *not* recommend in adolescents or children (unclear effects of hormone balance are possible; effect on muscle strength in the growing athlete may provoke serious overuse injuries) • In about 30% of athletes there are no other effects • Creatine may be beneficial and is therefore used in neurological and muscle disorders and in the rehabilitation process • Concomitant uptake of caffeine may reduce the performance enhancing effect of creatine • Yearly blood test recommended (see chapter 'Big Sports Lab'), with particular focus on renal function and liver enzymes
Side Effects	• Athletes with renal function impairment, diabetes or arterial hypertension shouldn't use creatine • Increases bodyweight in the loading phase of about 0.5–1kg (osmotic effect, additional water in the muscle cell) • Possibly further increases in bodyweight in long-term treatments • Anecdotal evidence of more frequent muscle cramps, muscle injuries, and overuse of tendons

Literature

Kreatin Factsheet Antidoping Schweiz retrieved online 21.4.2016

Twycross-Lewis R et al. The effects fof creatine supplementation on thermoregulation and physical (cognitive) performance: a review and future prospects. Amino Acids.2016 Apr 16.

Galvan E et al. Acute and chronic safety and efficacy of dose dependent creatine nitrate supplementation and exercise performance. J Int Soc Sports Nutr. 2016 Mar 31; 13.12

Ramirez-Campillo R et al. Effect of plyometric training and creatine supplementation on maximal-intensity exercise and endurance in female soccer players. J Sci Med Sport.2015 Nov 6.

Kim J et al. Role of creatine supplementation in exercise-induced muscle damage: A mini review. J Exerc Rehabil. 2015 Oct 30;11(5):244-50

Trexler ET, Smith Ryan AE. Creatine and caffeine: considerations for concurrent supplementation. Int J Sport Nutr Exerc Metab. 2015 Jul 28.

Being Underweight, Being Overweight – What to Do

Luckily, most people feel okay with their body and their body image. Regular training helps to form and shape your body a bit, but it is also important to accept your very own body composition to a certain extent, as a fundamental change is neither possible nor healthy.

However, some athletes don't feel okay with their weight and sometimes the coach raises this issue.

How do we measure and judge whether somebody is under- or overweight? For kids and adolescents, we have growth curves for height and weight, and for adults there is the body mass index (BMI). The BMI is calculated by dividing our weight in kilograms by the square of our height in meters.

Table 1: Body Mass Index – Formula and Standard Values

BMI = body weight in kg/ (length in m)^2	
E.g. 72kg / (1.78m x 1.78m) = 22.7kg/m^2	
Underweight	<18.5
Normal body weight	18.5–25
Overweight	25–30
Adiposity	>30

The BMI does have its pitfalls: it does not take into account figure, sex, and body composition, and as mentioned before, the BMI is just a calculated value and norms are a bit arbitrary, using whole numbers. Recent studies indicate that the value of 25, indicating overweight, should probably be raised, as many muscular people with a quite good figure and in good shape reach that value and they are not at any risk. Among athletes that is exactly the problem, as an athlete with a big and well balanced muscle mass but quite lean does have a rather high BMI. Typical example for a muscular-athletic body, with a rather high BMI around 23–26, are male competitive swimmers. So, for adults, the body mass index gives an indication, but nothing more.

To go into more detail, we need to determine the percentage of body fat. The most accurate methods are the dual energy x-ray absorptiometry (DEXA) in lab conditions and, for practical application, skinfold measurement, mostly performed on seven body sites. DEXA, because of its technology and reliability, is considered preferred method. However, its costs, limited availability and the radiation exposure (in fact very low) need to be considered. Skinfold measurement offers a reasonable alternative, and it really measures your subcutaneous fat tissue. If skinfold is repeatedly performed by an experienced investigator it is a valid measurement method. It is not possible, in this book, to give a general interpretation of the requirements of each sport discipline as they vary so much. Each athlete must judge their body fat percentage according to their needs, together with a nutritionist or a sports medicine physician. As a guide, normal values in the general population are: women: 23% +/-5%; men 14% +/-5%. Body fat percentage for sportswomen and men is usually distinctly lower.

Looking at childhood and adolescence, normal values for BMI vary quite a lot and interpretation of the growth curves is recommended instead (see Figure 1). These growth curves indicate the percentages of kids and adolescents within a range. An example: a girl 14 years of age, 45.5kg body weight is at the 25th percentile. This indicates that there are 75% of kids heavier and 25% lighter than her.

Figure 1: Growth Charts Height/Weight for Girls 1–18y and Boys 1–18y

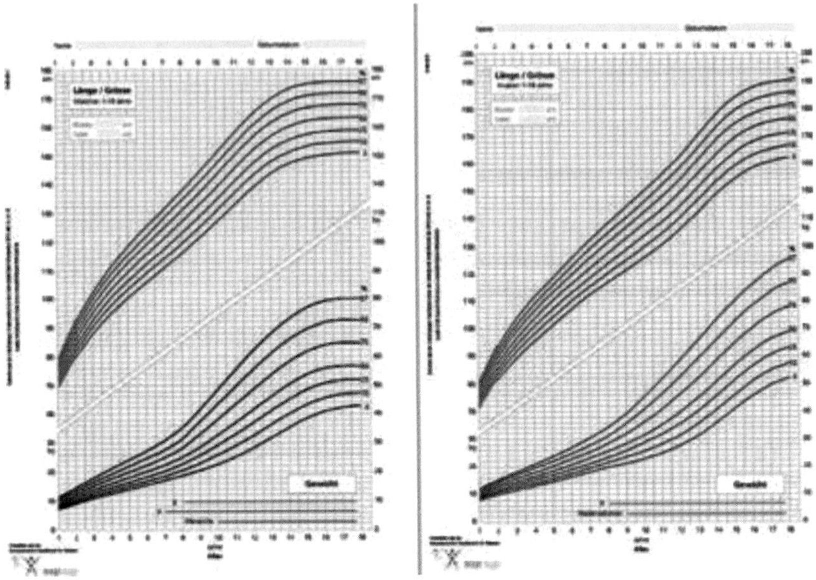

Braegger C, Jenni O, Konrad D, Molinari L (2011) Neue Wachstumskurven für die Schweizerische Paediatrica 22; 1: 9-11.

Looking at these growth charts, it's not only the absolute single value but the longitudinal development and the relation of height and weight (do they correspond? e.g. little and light or tall and heavy?) that help to interpret the situation.

Energy expenditure

It's good to have a basic knowledge about energy expenditure, especially if we talk about a weight issue. Table 2 gives an overview.

Table 2: Estimation of Energy Expenditure in Sports in kcal/h and kj/h
(Adapted from McArdle, Katch, Katch 2009)

Activity	kcal/h	kJ/h	Examples
Rest	60	240	Sleeping, watching TV
Very light activity	150	600	Sitting and standing activities, driving, cooking, desk work
Light activity	250	1000	Walking (slowly), cycling slowly 15km/h, baseball, bowling, horseback riding, gymnastics, moderate strength training*
Moderate activity	450	1800	Jogging 8-10km/h, cycling in a moderate pace 20–28km/h, volleyball, basketball, tennis, brisk walking, intensive strength training*
Strenuous activity	650	2600	Running 12-15km/h, cycling >30km/h, intensive swimming, boxing training, intensive judo training, intensive badminton
Very strenuous activity	900	3600	Running >15km/h; intensive cross country skiing, cycling > 40km/h, ice hockey

*Three general statements about energy expenditure:

1. The table above is a rough estimate, but as it is often better to be 'roughly right, than precisely wrong'; we stick to that. Depending on your exercise intensity, the energy expenditure varies accordingly.
2. Endurance training is about energy expenditure in calories or joule more important than strength training. This means:
   - If it is about *'burning' energy* with the goal of losing weight, because you're an *overweight athlete*, compare the table above to have an idea, what effort is needed
   - If you're an *underweight athlete*, the table above shows you how much energy you need and in your case *must refuel or replace*. For instance, in a training camp with 25 to 30 hours of training/week you need to eat and drink abundantly on any occasion: 30h x 500kcal = 15,000kcal/week of additional energy in kcal to uptake; 2,650 additional kcal per day, so massively more!) in order to keep your weight at least stable.
3. For 'explosive' sports it is best to work with calory restriction combined with short burst of exercise.

Before you seriously start any measures, discuss your issue with a sports medicine physician or a nutritionist. They will help you in your assessment and they will know what to do. Tables 3 and 4 give practical suggestions in case of underweight and overweight athletes respectively.

Table 3: Practical Suggestions in Case of Underweight

- Respect all meals of the day: start with a complete breakfast in the morning sustaining you with energy, have lunch at midday giving you a good break, and enjoy eating dinner in the evening
- Add three snacks according to your training schedule, e.g. at 9am, 4pm, and 9pm
- Don't drink plain water, but have a sports drink with carbohydrates or a diluted fruit juice (1:1 juice and water) or get your own tea ready (sweetened with sugar 40-60g/l)
- Implement the 'Food Pyramid for Athletes' with additional servings in carbohydrates and ½ servings in oils, fats, and nuts per each hour of the sport/day
- And don't forget: Underweight limits your training efforts and decreases your performance.

Table 4: Practical Suggestions in Case of Overweight

- Continue eating normally by keeping your rhythm with three main meals, possibly two light snacks
- Go along with the 'Food Pyramid of Athletes' and follow the basic part, to ensure a healthy and all-embracing diet, skip the additional servings as you need to be a bit mean with calories
- Don't skip entire meals, but use a slightly smaller serving size than before
- Don't use any strict diet rules or products promising to make you thinner shakes or tablets you are getting from any other sources (e.g. internet, word-by-mouth, chemist, etc.), that's all rubbish and not good for you
- Respect the five servings of vegetables and fruits, enlarge the size of the three servings of vegetables and keep the two servings of fruits
- In training just use plain water, don't use a sports drink, as they contain extra energy in form of carbohydrates, which you don't need now
- Have fasting trainings, early in the morning at a slow to moderate pace (e.g. jogging, cycling 3–5x 30min/week). Just drink some water before you start. This will burn a reasonable amount of calories and also train your fat metabolism. After your return, eat a moderate breakfast
- Skip all extra energy sources, in particular soft drinks, alcoholic beverages, sweets

Literature

Aerenhouts D et al. Estimating Body Composition in Adolescent Sprint Athletes: Comparison of Different Methods in a 3 Years Longitudinal Design. PLoS One. 2015 Aug 28;10(8)

McArdle/Katch/Katch. Exercise Physiology: Energy,Nutrition and Human Performance, 3rd ed. Lippincott, Williams&Williams, Philadelphia, USA (2006) and Weineck. Optimales Training, Spitta-Verlag, Balingen, Germany (2009)

Rodriguez-Sanchez N, Galloway SD. Errors in dual energy x-ray absorptiometry estimation of body composition induced by hypohydration. Int J Sport Nutr Exerc Metab. 2015 Feb;25(1):60-8.

De Lorenzo A et al. Body composition measurement in highly trained male athletes. A comparison of three methods. J Sports Med Phys Fitness. 2000 Jun;40(2):178-83..

Stewart AD, Hannan WJ. Prediction of fat and fat-free mass in male athletes using dual X-ray absorptiometry as the reference method. J Sports Sci. 2000 Apr;18(4):263-74.

Urogenital and Endocrinological System

Urinary Tract Infection – When It Burns

Symptoms

Burning sensation when urinating (dysuria), passing frequent small amount of urine (pollakisuria), as strong persistent urge to urinate, a feeling of pressure, sometimes cramping in the lower abdomen, in severe cases, slightly bloody coloured urine (hemorrhagic cystitis). Possibly light fever.

Background

Cystitis is an infection of the bladder. It is frequent and occurs mainly as our own bacteria from the anus region wander up along the urethra into the bladder. This is the reason why women, who have a quite short urethra (about 4cm) and a shorter distance to the anus, have a urinary tract infection more often, while men (urethra >12cm) are seldom touched.

As long as the infection remains in the bladder, it is easily treatable and curable. Signs for an ongoing infection further ascending along the ureter towards the kidneys would be: fever, shivering, ascending pain towards the lumbar region (where the kidney is).

Figure 1: Side View of Male and Female Genitals, Urethra and Bladder

1.1 In males

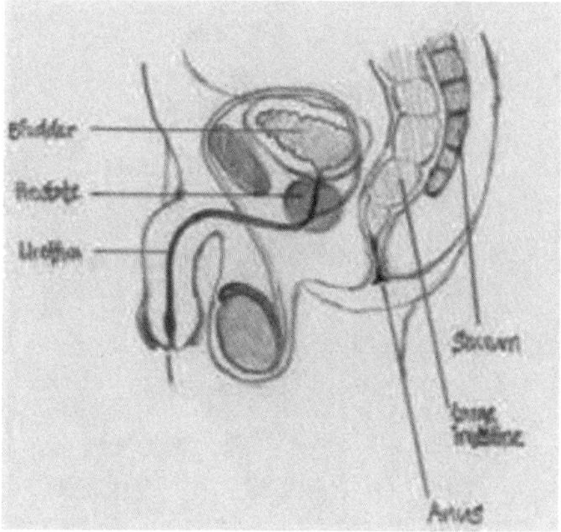

1.2 In females

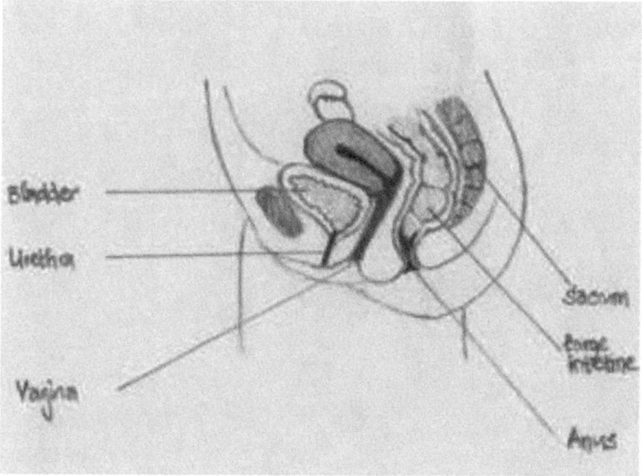

Prevention and Treatment Table for Cystitis

Prevention	• **Hygiene:** don't exaggerate with hygiene measures! Too much scrubbing and lots of soap will even damage your skin around the anus and the genital region. As bacteria thrive better on damaged skin, it is recommended to wash your genital region once daily slightly with a pH neutral soap without scrubbing, and for women: don't douche your vagina*

	• **Wiping your anus:** from front to back after having passed a movement (faeces) is logical advice, as bacteria from the anus will not be pushed towards your urethra • **Drink enough each day:** in order to flush out your bladder frequently • **Underwear:** wear cotton underwear and change daily. If you need to wear tight fitting clothes for training, take a shower, and change clothes soon after training. This avoids warm, moist, airless conditions around your genitals • **Urinate after having sex:** as cystitis may be more frequent one or two days after sex. The movements during sex may transport bacteria close to the urethra and provoke cystitis. Urinating after having sex will hopefully flush them away
Treatment by Yourself	• If cystitis is already established, there is no self-treatment option. • If, in an early stage, you feel bladder irritation or any other early symptom, it may be worthwhile to drink lots to *flush your bladder out.* Once the outbreak is established, drinking a lot is controversial, as it possibly leads only to more pain passing urine. • *Cranberry juice or extract:* cranberry is not an antibiotic and will not usually cure cystitis. But, as it contains a flavonoid substance named proanthocyanidin, it prevents bacteria from attaching to the urogenital cells and may help to prevent urinary tract infections.
When is a Doctor Needed?	When you feel the symptoms as described above. With fever, see a doctor within a few hours.
Return to Play/Sports	Light training is usually possible the next day. If there is a further ascending infection, a longer antibiotic treatment is needed and a few days of rest are indicated.

***Note – for women:**
Exaggerated hygiene in the genital region not only affects skin and the urethra but particularly the vaginal microbioma (i.e. flora in the vagina, microorganisms discovered by A. Doederlein in 1892, therefore also called Doederlein flora or bacteria). The low pH <4.5 in the vagina is the main mechanism controlling the composition of the vaginal flora. Too much soap (usually high pH between 9–11) or a vaginal douche will change this composition and possibly allow the genesis of vaginal infection with yeast or bacteria. The same situation occurs after a therapy with antibiotics for several days, as antibiotics often destroy or impair the vaginal flora. Women prone to vaginal infection after antibiotics may profit from regular application of a suppository containing this vaginal flora (e.g. FloraFemme).

What Does the Doctor Do?

The doctor takes the history, performs a clinical exam, and tests the urine. Normally diagnosis is then obvious and antibiotic treatment is started. There are different antibiotics available, single dose or for three days or longer. The doctor will discuss with you the appropriate treatment for your situation.

Literature

Jepson RG et al. Cranberries for preventing urinary tract infections.Cochrane Database Syst Rev. 2012 Oct 17;10:CD001321. doi: 10.1002/14651858. CD001321.pub5. Review.

Wang CH et al. Cranberry-containing products for prevention of urinary tract infections in susceptible populations: a systematic review and meta-analysis of randomized controlled trials.Arch Intern Med. 2012 Jul 9;172(13):988-96.

Sexually Transmitted Diseases – About Safer Sex, Respect, Enjoyment, and Fun

Why do we need to talk about sexuality? Because this book is about complete athletes' health, and sexuality is one part of healthy, human behaviour, so we need to briefly address this topic. Sexuality is a precious gift two persons may share with each other intimately. Enjoy – have fun – *but be respectful and reasonable!*

Finally, and this concerns all young people as hardcore sex and porn is readily available – sought for or often even not sought for. Please, boys and girls, what's shown in hardcore pornography is not real life, it's mostly disrespectful, often even dangerous and insane, and has nothing to do with sexuality within a respectful and loving relationship.

Symptoms

May vary, often a burning urethra with or without matter (urethritis). Possibly laceration of the genital skin, possibly enlargement of the lymph nodes in the inguinal, possibly fever, possibly pain in the lower abdomen and the pelvis. In females, often a vaginal discharge.

Prevention and Treatment Table for Sexually Transmitted Disease

Prevention	Safer sex! There's no sex without protection with a condom. Short but clear message!
Treatment by Yourself	Be strict with prevention. If you catch a sexually transmitted disease, go to a doctor as it's about serious germs (bacteria and virus) needing professional diagnosis and treatment.

When is a Doctor Needed?	See a doctor if you have a genital infection, don't wait. If you've had unsafe sex and you're catching flu-like symptoms in the following days or weeks, see a doctor. Early HIV infection presents as a flu-like illness.
Return to Play/ Sports	Depending on the diagnosed illness.

What Does the Doctor Do?

The doctor takes the history, clinical exam, and often performs a blood test. If a local infection is visible, swab tests will be taken to diagnose the responsible germs. In bacterial infections, treatment consists of an antibiotic regime for a given number of days (often longer than you expect) to allow good antibiotic penetration to all tissues of the urogenital tract (in order to kill these bacteria). Mostly a partner therapy is indicated. Follow the given instructions to the letter, as you really want to get rid of these germs Ask your doctor how treatment and sport fit together (usually after some days of rest, light and moderate training is possible, but ask).

Amenorrhea, Female Athlete Triad, and Relative Energy Deficiency in Sports (Red-S) – Yes, Red Flag

Symptoms

Missing menstrual cycle for more than six months: primary amenorrhea: no menstrual bleeding at all up to that moment. No menarche (the first occurrence of menstruation) yet.

Or no menstrual cycle after having reached the age of sixteen: secondary amenorrhea: Menarche has taken place. Menstrual cycle was there for a certain time, but has stopped.

Often related to this condition is an underlying eating disorder with underweight and the risk for osteoporosis.

Figure 1: Female Athlete Triad

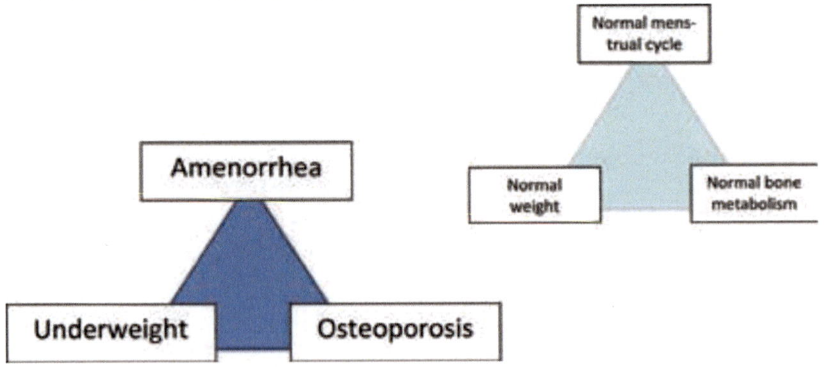

Background

Young girls in adolescence enter puberty and through the hormonal activity of the hypothalamo-hypopituary-ovary axis start having a menstrual cycle. The onset of this first menstrual cycle (i.e. menarche) varies broadly, between 12–16 years of age (or sometimes later). Reasons for delayed onset of the menstrual cycle are: low body weight, familiar predisposition (when did the mother have her first menstruation?), regular sports training with a focus on performance, and other medical reasons.

Do all girls with amenorrhea automatically have a female athlete triad? No, but having a regular menstrual cycle is a sign of normal hormone production in the growing body of a young female. It's oestradiol, the main female hormone and important hormone to sustain the bone metabolism (see following chapter 'Bone Density, Vitamin D3, and Calcium'), which is the last link of the chain responsible for having menstruation or not.

What about RED-S?

Relative energy deficiency syndrome is a slightly new approach to the same topic. It is more comprehensive and includes all situations, where a relative energy deficit may occur.

Prevention and Treatment Table for Amenorrhea, Female Athlete Triad, and Relative Energy Deficiency – syndrome (RED-S)

Prevention (for the coach)	It's the task of every athlete and particularly every coach to keep an eye on this particular issue. As the topic is very sensitive, it needs to be addressed very thoroughly and confidentially. The annual sportsmed exam, offers an ideal opportunity and also the confidentiality to address this topic and also have a regular medical follow-up by keeping either the growth charts in younger adolescents or the longitudinal development of the BMI. **Do:** • Perform in the high level (i.e. high volume of training or ambitious goals) growing adolescent athlete (male and female) an annual sportsmed exam

- Be attentive to an already rather lean female (or male) athlete who tells you, 'I'm fat, I need to lose weight.' Please take a firm stance and reiterate that sport is about performance and stress that anyone who wants to perform needs energy, and energy means eating and drinking
- Be attentive of your young female athletes if they start losing weight
- Be attentive to the eating behaviour of your young athletes, both boys and girls. In trainings camps, eat with them at one table, don't be the police officer, but get an impression of what and how your athletes eat
- If you recognise a possible problem, invite the athlete (possibly together with one of their parents) for a conversation in your office (or another adequate setting) and tell them what you as a coach have observed. In this confidential situation, it's possible to ask whether the menstrual cycle has started and whether it is regular
- If there's a serious problem, you must inform the parents and, together with the athlete and the parents, you should further involve health professionals. Usually it's the team doctor or sports medicine physician who is the next person to contact, but it may also be the GP/family doctor
- If it is a female athlete triad, often a *triangle team of health professionals* is needed: doctor (sports medicine physician or GP), sports nutritionist, and sports psychologist
- If the whole issue is not taken seriously enough, as it is often played down by the athlete, you must insist

Don't:

- I recommend to all coaches: Do not weigh the athletes yourself
- *Never* hang a list of the athletes' weights up in the locker room and *never* communicate it electronically. This may lead to a negative comparison among the athletes

	• Don't think it will be over soon, or it's just something like a mood change. Female athlete triad is a serious illness: in up to 10% of cases, it may have a fatal outcome; and about 60% of athletes with female athlete triad (yes, that many!) will end up in a chronic condition with a lifelong eating disorder. So take your responsibility as indicated above
Treatment by Yourself (for the athlete)	• Take your responsibility as an athlete seriously • Allow sufficient calorie intake to sustain optimal training and recovery, and to reinforce your immune system, e.g. follow the 'Food Pyramid for Athletes' (see chapter 'Being Underweight, Being Overweight – What to Do?') • A healthy, balanced sports diet doesn't contain food bans, everything is permitted (which doesn't automatically mean that everything is good for you) • If you feel something is not okay with your body, talk with your parents, your coach, your sports medicine physician, your GP, or family doctor • If your coach or your parents are concerned about you being underweight, don't trivialise it, don't play it down, follow their suggestions, as it's about your career in sports, about your performance, and about your health
When is a Doctor Needed?	When a secondary amenorrhea persists longer than 6 months, or a primary amenorrhoea occurs. When signs of the female athlete triad are appearing.
Return to Play/ Sports	If the illness is recognised at an early stage, the sport activity may be continued. Almost all athletes having female athlete triad love and adore their sport. Therefore, to prevent them from practicing is a punishment. But in cases of ongoing illness with underweight, a complete ban on sports activities may be needed so as not to take health risks, this is done by the above mentioned team of health professionals.

What Does the Doctor Do?

The doctor takes the history and the clinical exam. Weight and height are determined and the doctor tries to get a more comprehensive overview of the situation. Usually further exams like blood and urine testing are performed. Based to this initial assessment, further measures are then taken.

Literature

Mountjoy M et al. The IOC consensus statement: beyond the Female Athlete Triad--Relative Energy Deficiency in Sport (RED-S). Br J Sports Med. 2014 Apr;48(7):491-7.

Joy E et al. 2014 female athlete triad coalition consensus statement on treatment and return to play of the female athlete triad. Curr Sports Med Rep. 2014 Jul-Aug;13(4):219-32.

Matzkin E et al. Female Athlete Triad: Past, Present, and Future. J Am Acad Orthop Surg. 2015 Jul;23(7):424-32.

Clénin GE et al. Female athlete triad - (k)ein Problem im Kader von Swiss Orienteering, Swiss Orienteering, Olten, Switzerland 2011

Nattiv A et al. American College of Sports Medicine position stand. The female athlete triad. Med Sci Sports Exerc. 2007 Oct;39(10):1867-82.

Bone Density, Vitamin D3, and Calcium – Basic Knowledge for Everyone

Peak bone mass means the maximal bone mineral density and so the highest amount of bone substance we ever reach in our life. In healthy adults—it is the same for both the normal population and very active sport professionals—peak bone mass is reached around the age of 25 years and is, by definition, 100% of our bone mineral density.

Bone is a living tissue, in permanent balance between constitution and degradation of new bone mass. The bone mass is built up during childhood and adolescence, mainly under the influence of sexual hormones, and reaches its peak at age 25. After the age of 40 years, a reduction of about 0.5%/year of bone mass can be observed. So childhood and adolescence are by far the most important times to invest in bone constitution. Therefore it is important to have a closer look at factors impairing the constitution of optimal peak bone mass.

Figure 1: Bone Mineral Density – Constitution of Optimal Peak Bone Mass

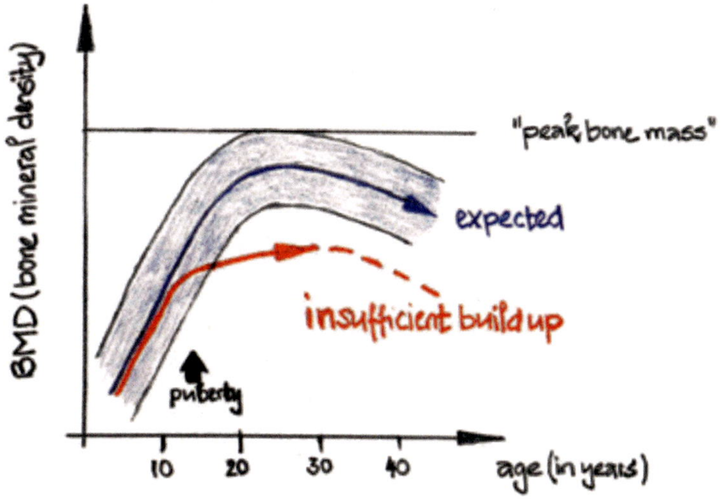

Practical example of an athlete

The subject is a 27y old female long distance runner with a stress fracture of the II.metatarsal bone. Based on a history of a long period of underweight and amenorrhea as an adolescent, a measurement of the bone density using the DEXA method (dual energy X-ray-absorptiometry) was performed. The results (from just one measurement site, normally three or four sites measured: lower back, femur neck, tibia, and forearm) show bone mineral density very low in her femur neck (see Figure 2).

The BMD (i.e. bone mineral density) of this young athlete is far too low for her age and comparable to the lower normal range of BMD of a 60y old woman. This means that she has a serious lack of bone mineral density and suffers from an osteoporosis. Already the athlete has an increased risk of suffering other stress reactions/fractures. Treatment and profound counselling of the athlete are needed.

Figure 2: Example Femur Neck DEXA and Bone Density

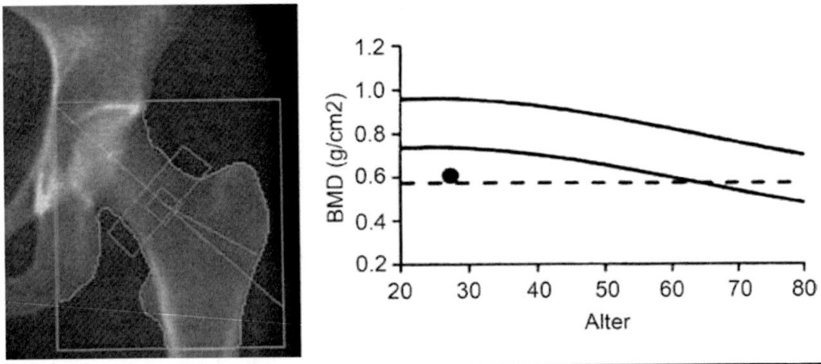

Peak bone mass may be influenced by environmental and lifestyle factors. In men, peak bone mass is 30% higher than in women. In females, the main female hormone estrogen (estradiol) is essential, as it influences BMD in a very positive way. Nutrition also plays a decisive role: calcium, as one of the central bone constitutive minerals, needs to be integrated into daily nutrition as well as vitamin D, which is important in regulating calcium uptake as well as in hardening our bone. There is also a genetic influence on bone mineral density.

Is this just for women?
No, it's not. Boys and men also need to be careful with their calcium and vitamin D intake.

Do I need to have a look at the calcium calculator as a male athlete?
Yes, you should do that.

Looking at the frequency of stress reactions and stress fractures of male and female athletes, we observe that both sexes are about equally affected, so bone health is also an issue for males. Underweight is also an issue in male athletes, as the diet leading to an underweight condition is low in calories, possibly low in dairy products, calcium, and vitamin D (i.e. RED-S, relative energy deficiency syndrome). An underweight athlete is less robust (more prone to infections due to a reduced immune response, less robust locomotor system with more frequent inflammation of anatomical structures like tendons, ligaments, bones leading possibly to stress reaction and stress fracture). It's clear that a stress fracture is not caused by nutrition alone. The main driver will always be the mechanical stress and the impacts, but as an athlete you need to be aware of your risk, so plan to keep your body robust and look for sufficient calcium and vitamin D intake.

Table 1: Prevention of a Low Calcium Intake and a Vitamin D Deficiency

Calcium

- Pay attention to your calcium intake. Your bones need enough calcium to be able to become and stay strong
- Good sources for calcium are: milk and dairy products, some mineral waters (not all, please verify as there are big differences – factor x5), nuts, and green vegetables
- A serving of milk or milk products three times daily is the best foundation for sufficient and successful intake. One serving corresponds to 2dl of milk, one cup of yoghurt, or 40g of cheese
- Distribute your calcium intake throughout the day. This improves the calcium uptake in the intestines
- Try the calcium calculator below to check whether your calcium intake is sufficient or not

Vitamin D

- Vitamin D is, besides calcium, essential for the constitution of healthy and strong bone. Vitamin D additionally promotes the uptake of calcium from food
- Vitamin D is mainly found in food of animal origin. Good sources for Vitamin D are oily fish, dairy products, and eggs. Vitamin D of plant origin is in avocados, mushrooms, dates, and sunflower seeds
- An important contributor to the uptake or generation of vitamin D is the synthesis in our skin. 15–20min of sun exposure to your face and your arms are sufficient, but please without sunscreen (otherwise it is impaired). In some countries in winter (middle and northern Europe, North America), the sun is not strong enough to really help with the synthesis of vitamin D
- Therefore we recommend athletes from these countries check their vitamin D level in the blood (e.g. in the sportsmed exam) and act according to the result (i.e. possibly add a vitamin D supplement)

What do you do for an intolerance or aversion to milk and dairy products?

As milk and dairy products are one of the main calcium sources, it will be difficult to reach the optimal intake without them. But there are possibilities, please discuss it with your sports medicine physician and your nutritionist.

The recommended daily calcium-uptake for adolescents/ young adults should reach **at least 1200mg**.

Table 2: Calculator to Estimate Calcium Uptake (Adapted from Swiss League against Rheumatism 2015)

Products		Consumed Quantity Per Day	X	Content of Calcium	Total Amount of Calcium
Milk and dairy products	Milk	_____dl	x	120mg	_____mg
	Yoghurt	_____g	x	1,2mg	_____mg
		_____x cup of 180g		220mg	_____mg
	Cottage cheese, fresh cheese	_____g	x	1mg	_____mg
Cheese	Soft cheese (e.g. Camembert, Feta)	_____g	x	5mg	_____mg
	Medium hard cheese (e.g. Cheddar, Raclette)	_____g	x	7mg	_____mg
	Hard cheese (e.g.Parmesan, Swiss Emmenthal)	_____g	x	12mg	_____mg
Mineral water	High in calcium (e.g. Contrex, Valser)	_____dl	x	50mg	_____mg
	Medium in calcium (e.g. San Pellegrino, Badoit)	_____dl	x	25mg	_____mg
	Low in calcium (e.g. Evian, Henniez)	_____dl	x	12mg	_____mg
Fresh vegetables and/or nuts	Small serving	_____x		50mg	_____mg
	Big serving	_____x		150mg	_____mg
				TOTAL	_____**mg**

Literature

Walrand S. Effect of vitamin D on skeletal muscle. Geriatr Psychol Neuropsychiatr Vieil. 2016 Apr 21.

Magee PJ et al. Vitamin D status and supplementation in elite Irish athletes. Int J Sport Nutr Exerc Metab. 2013 Oct;23(5):441-8

Bescós García R et al. Low levels of vitamin D in professional basketball players after wintertime: relationship with dietary intake of vitamin D and calcium. Nutr Hosp. 2011 Sep-Oct;26(5):945-51.

Infoblatt Vitamin D Swiss Forum for Sport Nutrition retrieved 5.6.2016 http://www.forumsportnutrition.ch/wp-content/uploads/2015/01/Infoblatt_VitaminD.pdf

Infoblatt Calcium on Website Swiss Forum for Sport Nutrition retrieved 5.6.2016 http://www.forumsportnutrition.ch/wp-content/uploads/2016/01/Infoblatt_Calcium_2.1.pdf

Calcium calculator. Translated and adapted in a new format from the calcium calculator of the Swiss League against Rheumatism 2015 http://www.rheumaliga.ch/Calciumrechner

Hypothyreosis (Underfunction of the Thyroid Gland) in Sports – No Worries Under Treatment

Symptoms

Fatigue, feeling tired and weak, sensation of cold, dry skin, low pulse rate, and exaggerated feeling of sore muscles. Possibly constipation.

*Hyper*thyreosis (*over*function of the thyroid gland) has the contrary symptoms: sensation of heat, frequent sweating, high pulse rate, being nervous and irritated, and passing stool very easily (better than before).

Background

The thyroid gland, a hormone producing organ, works as regulator of many processes in the human body, a bit like an electronic control unit for a car engine. When the thyroid gland works well, the human organism is well balanced.

If it produces *too few hormones (hypothyroidism)* the pulse rate is low, we feel tired, powerless, and experience the sensation of cold, dry skin.

In the opposite condition with the *overproduction of thyroid hormones (hyperthyroidism)* the symptoms are the opposite as described above.

Prevention and Treatment Table for Hypothyroidism

Prevention	No prevention known.
Treatment by Yourself	There is no self-treatment option.

When is a Doctor Needed?	When you think, you have this condition, go and see a doctor.
Return to Play/ Sports	As soon as treatment has started and is well established there's no limitation for sport, including elite and professional level.

What Does the Doctor Do?

The doctor takes the history and performs a clinical examination with palpation of the thyroid gland (which is underneath the skin of our throat, on both side of the trachea, just an inch below the Adam's apple). Blood tests to determine the thyroid hormones and different metabolism parameters are performed. Once the diagnosis is established, treatment is quite simple: you receive the missing hormones in the form of tablets, which need to be taken on a daily basis.

Literature

Kohli S, G.E. Clénin, E. R. Christ «Saure Beine» beim Training auf einen Gigathlon (Sore legs in training for a Gigathlon) Schweiz Med Forum 2005;5:149–152 http://www.medicalforum.ch/docs/smf/archiv/de/2005/2005-05/2005-05-216.pdf

Duhig TJ, McKeag D. Thyroid disorders in athletes. Curr Sports Med Rep. 2009 Jan-Feb;8(1):16-9. doi: 10.1249/JSR.0b013e3181954a12.

Diabetes Mellitus in Sport – a Manageable Challenge

Symptoms

Acute crisis: marked weight loss, being thirsty all the time, heavy drinking (polydipsia; 4 litres per day and more), and frequent letting of urine (polyuria). Vomiting and possibly abdominal pain. Feeling tired and powerless, having troubles with concentration and blurred vision.

Background

Diabetes mellitus roughly translates as the 'honey sweet flow through'. Our pancreas, a large gland in our abdomen, has two major functions: food digestion by the secretion of enzymes and production of hormones, mainly insulin, to regulate blood sugar (in the form of glucose). The insulin produced is carried within the blood stream and acts like a key in a lock: insulin opens the cells to enable the glucose to enter the body cells. In diabetes, insulin is missing through lack of production in the pancreas and glucose rises to enormous levels. This provokes an acute crisis due to these enormous glucose levels with osmotic diuresis. The abundant glucose flows through the kidney taking many litres of water with it, leading to the typical major symptom of an acute onset of diabetes.

In the long run, elevated glucose levels damage the blood vessels leading to early degeneration and destruction of small vessels (e.g. retina, kidney, small capillaries everywhere) and atherosclerosis of larger vessels (e.g. myocardial infarction, stroke). So, it is essential to keep glucose within its normal levels.

Two main forms of diabetes are differentiated:

- **Type I:** almost always *insulin dependent* as the *pancreas fails in its insulin production.* This means treatment with insulin is needed from very early on. As insulin can only be injected, and there are different modalities on how best to connect insulin and meal times, usually several shots of insulin per day are needed. Diabetes type I may occur at any age, but is the more common type in young people
- **Type II:** mostly due to overweight, occurs when the *pancreas is not able to produce enough insulin.* This means other therapeutic strategies may be useful: weight loss, physical activity on a daily basis, medication to improve the insulin effect, medication to produce more insulin, etc. Diabetes type II occurs mainly in middle aged and older people

Physical activity and sport are good for patients with diabetes. With type II diabetes it is even essential. Some patients, by reducing their weight and keeping really active, may actually turn the disease around and they live a normal life again.

Prevention and Treatment Table for Diabetes Mellitus

Prevention	No prevention known for diabetes type I. For diabetes type II keeping fit, keeping body weight in a normal range.
Treatment by Yourself	The treatment of diabetes mellitus needs a professional follow-up, often by a group of specialised people: your doctor, possibly a specialist in endocrinology, a nutritionist
When is a Doctor Needed?	From early on.
Return to Play/ Sports	Physical activity and sports are good and even essential. When an athlete has an acute onset of diabetes, it's the disease that needs to be treated first. Some time (a few weeks) is needed to get everything organised. In this time, discussion about the return to sport takes place. High level sport is possible with diabetes type I, but it requires a highly professional follow-up, a good understanding of the illness, a great effort, and good discipline from the athlete. The coach needs to be informed about the diagnosis and indicated measures in case of hypoglycaemia (i.e. too low blood sugar level).

What Does the Doctor Do?

The doctor takes the history, makes a clinical examination, and takes a blood test and urine sample for analysis. When the diagnosis is confirmed, treatment needs to be started immediately, usually staying in hospital for a few days to get fluid replacement done and the electrolytes and body metabolism well balanced again.

Literature

Ratjen I et al. Type 1 diabetes mellitus and exercise in competitive athletes. Exp Clin Endocrinol Diabetes. 2015 Jul;123(7):419-22. doi: 10.1055/s-0035-1545344. Epub 2015 Apr 8.

Boehncke S et al. [Endurance capabilities of triathlon competitors with type 1 diabetes mellitus]. Dtsch Med Wochenschr. 2009 Apr;134(14):677-82. doi: 10.1055/s-0029-1208104. Epub 2009 Mar 24.

Psychology/Mood Disorders

Sports Psychology – Where is Your Head in It All?

If you go back and have a quick look at the complex figure explaining performance in sports (see chapter 'Training and Performance – the Basics of Success') it explains what you already know: you're doing everything to optimise your performance. The old Olympic principles: *'Citius, altius, fortius'* (Latin for: 'Faster, higher, stronger') just underlines this focus on top performance. You may say: 'I have done it all. What else needs to be done?' Answer: get your head ready, get an adequate mind set. And it is here, where your head should be.

As athlete and coach, you are now at a particular stage of your career. You have experiences and you are giving your best; you are aiming high and you want to achieve more to go to the top (or at least to the podium). This wish, this focus, this goal needs support. You may need to:

- Go for SMART goals: *specific, measurable, assignable, realistic, time-related*
- *Stay positive and be inspired*
- Go for *'realistic expectations and a great performance'* instead of great expectations and a realistic performance
- Learn more and integrate evidence based mental training techniques (e.g. easy to learn visualisation methods, coping methods in nervousness and excitement, etc.)
- Use the *SWOT* analysis: *integrate* your **S**trengths, *address* your **W**eaknesses, *seize* **O**pportunities, and *anticipate* **T**hreats
- Don't fall into the hands (or should I say claws) of an eloquent mental-guru who is not really helping you, but aiming to create dependency, in order to allow them to get the best for them and not for you

- *Train your mind. Be prepared for day X*, waiting for the start, opponent encounter, unfair opponent, wrong umpiring decision, crowd, media, intermediate result
- *Be prepared for the unexpected*

This list is just a short guide to help you to have the necessary mindset for success. You don't need to tick all boxes, but make up your mind and try to work out how you integrate them into your overall plans and your daily training on the way to your top performance. Certainly your experience as athlete and coach allows you to tackle a couple of the boxes, but some of them are extremely challenging, aren't they?

Image 1: Good Communication and Trust Between Athlete and Coach is Essential and a Crucial Aid for Top Performance

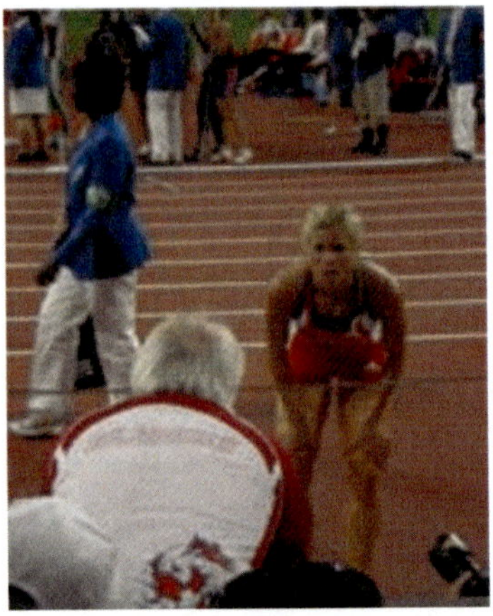

Sports psychology offers answers to that particular need as this evidence based scientific discipline offers tools to manage the above challenges. By addressing these topics, going in depth into strengths, weaknesses, opportunities, threats, setting SMART goals, talking about expectations, training your mind and anticipating many different situations you move closer to being ready for day X, and to face the unexpected. So I encourage you to address the topics in this field and ask for professional support by a sport psychologist.

I'd like to share some personal impressions of three sport movies that I appreciated very much. All three are based on a true story. I hope they may be an inspiration for you on your way as athlete or coach:

- *Team spirit* and *wise decisions:* Invictus (2009) – about the South African Rugby National Team playing the World Cup in South Africa.
- *Passion* and *hard work leading to success:* McFarland (2015) – about runners from a mainly Latino high school in McFarland, California, USA.
- *Having principles, being dedicated,* and *determined:* Chariots of Fire (1981) – about two UK athletes at the Olympics in Paris in 1924.

Literature

Sportpsychology – definition retrieved on the Website of American Psychological Association online on 5.6.2016 http://www.apa.org/ed/graduate/specialize/sports.aspx

Sarkar M, Fletcher D. Psychological resilience in sport performers: a review of stressors and protective factors. J Sports Sci. 2014;32(15);1419-34

Nicholls AR et al. The mediating role of mental toughness in sport. J Sports Med Phys Fitness. 215 Jul-aug;55(7-8):824-34

Collins D MacNamara A. The rocky road to the top: why talent needs trauma. Sports Med. 2012 Nov 1;42(11):907-14

Sleep/Sleep Disorders in Sports – Major Contributor to Recovery

Symptoms

Having difficulty falling asleep (initial insomnia) or having difficulty sleeping through the night (through sleep disorder).

Background

Figure 1: Sleep Pattern – Different Stages of Sleep

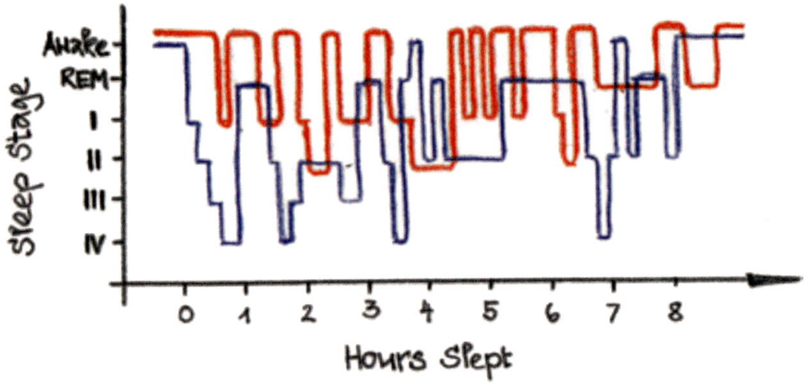

Key:
Blue: ideal sleep pattern, reaching several times deep stages; red: superficial sleep pattern; REM (rapid eye movement)

Our sleep shows different stages of sleeping depths (see Figure 1). To recover, we need to have a nicely undulating sleep with several really deep sleep stages (stage III and IV, as the blue example in Figure 1). If we are tense or under stress, our sleep may show a more superficial pattern (example in red in

Figure 1) and we feel less refreshed and less recovered in the morning. REM (rapid eye movement) sleep is also important and gets its name as our eyes move around rapidly and unconsciously.

Problems with sleep are frequent and common. When we are stressed, tense, or under pressure, sleeplessness may be more frequent. Sleep is essential for our recovery and regeneration. When we are exhausted and lack sleep, one or two nights of good sleep makes the world look better.

Sometimes, sleep disorders may stand alone, but they are often expressions of underlying stress and worry. Talk with someone about it, e.g. your best friend, your partner, your parents, your coach, or your doctor.

Power-nap: studies done in the last decade have shown that sleep behaviours are quite individual and age dependent. Some people seem to profit from a power nap after lunch. But don't go into deep sleep. Have 20min of sleep and wake up again, possibly have a coffee or tea after the power nap, and start refreshed in the afternoon.

There is a valuable list of preventive measures for sleeplessness and a list of *don'ts* for a good sleep quality.

Prevention and Treatment Table for Sleeplessness

Prevention	Preventive measures for a good sleep quality: • Your bedroom's ideal temperature is 16–20°C • Ensure enough oxygen in your bedroom, let fresh air in before going to bed, possibly leave a window open • The bedroom should be calm and quiet; avoid light disturbances (close the shutters/blinds) • The bedroom should be a comfortable place, tidy, clean; a place to enjoy • Have a ritual before going to bed, e.g. brush your teeth, put your pyjamas on, possibly read something (a book, magazine, etc.) • Sleep only as much as necessary to feel rested, then get out of bed

	• Go to bed before midnight, in order to allow enough sleeping time, e.g. at 10 or 11pm • Allow enough sleeping time to be recovered and refreshed, optimal length is individual, as athlete 8h is a reasonable recommendation **Don't:** • Drink caffeinated beverages after 3pm and don't drink alcohol near bedtime • Take your smartphone into your bedroom. Either turn it to silent and keep it out of vision, or it stays outside the bedroom • Take work into your bedroom. If important things come into your mind and you don't want to forget it, write it down on a piece of paper and put the paper away • Take worries into your bedroom. If troubling thoughts come, try to accept them, possibly write them down (as above), but then put them down • Watch thrilling videos of any kind before going to bed, they may excite you too much
Treatment by Yourself	• Go ahead with the recommendations above. Work through them seriously. In sleep disturbances, basic measures are often helpful. • When this doesn't work, if you feel you are worrying about different things or being stressed, possibly causing sleep problems, be courageous and talk with someone about it, e.g. your partner, best friend, parents, coach, or doctor. • Get some tea at your pharmacy, e.g. orange blossom tea (it works!), slightly sweeten it with honey, enjoy it in calm and quiet, go back to bed.
When is a Doctor Needed?	When you feel overly tired and can't overcome it yourself.
Return to Play/Sports	Usually no pause needed.

What Does the Doctor Do?

The doctor takes the history and tries to sort out with you what the problem is. In some situations, when sleep is needed, you may come to the decision that a medication is needed for a short time. Additional methods may be integrated: relaxation therapy, biofeedback, and cognitive behavioural therapy. If there are worries you're dealing with, please share them with your doctor (doctors are bound by confidentiality and it's their job to listen to you and look after your best interests).

Literature

Nédélec M et al. Sleep Hygiene and Recovery Strategies in Elite Soccer Players. Sports Med. 2015 Nov;45(11):1547-59..

Lastella M et al. Sleep/wake behaviours of elite athletes from individual and team sports. Eur J Sport Sci. 2015;15(2):94-100

Juliff LE, Halson SL, Peiffer JJ. Understanding sleep disturbance in athletes prior to important competitions. J Sci Med Sport. 2015 Jan;18(1):13-8.

Depression and Anxiety – How Prone Are Athletes?

Symptoms

Feeling overly sad, feeling tired, and having less interest and pleasure in things that are normally enjoyable. Other characteristics are low self-esteem, anxiety, pessimism, and in worst case, thinking about suicide.

Background

At the outset, we note that, in the 15–30 years age group, roughly 15% of the population suffers from mental disorders. That is exactly the age group most athletes are in. Most of these problems are mood disorders (e.g. depression) and anxiety.

Very recent studies indicate that depression in sport seems to be under-recognised. The prevalence (i.e. proportion of a population to have a condition, e.g. an illness) of depression in young adults is notably high; according to the US Department of Health and Human Services, 8.7% (Rao 2015) of 18–25years olds suffers depression. Studies observing college athletes report prevalence from 5.5% (Uglesic 2014) up to 21% (Trojan 2015). Having lower self-esteem, less social connectedness, and decreased sleep are strong predictors (Trojan 2015). Freshmen and current college athletes seem to be at greater risk of experiencing depressive symptoms than former, graduated college athletes.

Even though sportswomen and men from countries all over the world are telling their stories and publishing books about their life of suffering, the general public and the media still persist in promoting the picture of the 'always-in-a-good-mood, motivated-to-give-their-best' athletes. And that's just not true, and even if this misconception is not intentional and well-meant to support the sportsman and woman, it can make the life of athletes and coaches extremely difficult. It would mean you always have to smile; always be motivated; always be powerful; showing no weaknesses, 24 hours a day, 7 days a week. And that's neither physiologically nor psychologically possible. There is definitely a need for a change!

As members of the general public, as well as being athletes, coaches, and health and sports professionals, we all need to raise the awareness that physiology and performance are very much about recovery and about needing time out and rest. It is essential to allow periods of possibly low motivation, both physically and psychologically. We should imagine our moods having ups and down, like waves - sometimes we will feel really well, on the top, and at other times, we will feel rather dull, possibly even sad. This is physiological and natural and part of a normal modulation of our mood.

Figure 1: Modulation of our mood and examples

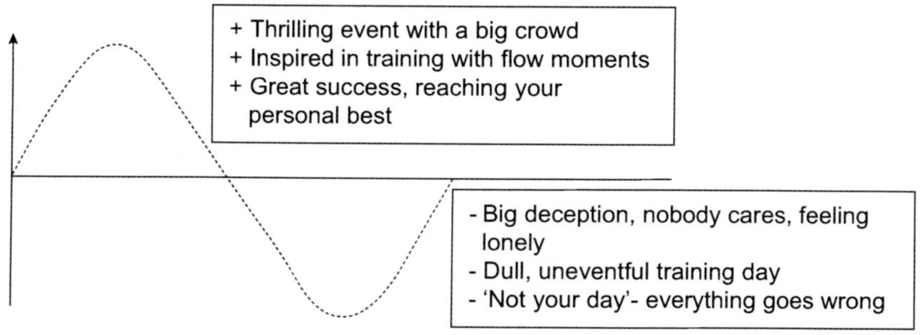

This range is necessary to allow being at the top of the wave again on day X, when it really counts.

Let's spread this word!

If you actually question your mood state, please read the information below. Table 1 presents the self-reporting patient health questionnaire (PHQ-2). These two questions may possibly give you some additional information.

Table 1: The Patient Health Questionnaire-2 (PHQ-2)

Over the past 2 weeks, how often have you been bothered by any of the following problems?	Not at all	Several days	More than half of the days	Nearly every day
1. Little interest or pleasure in doing things	0	1	2	3
2. Feeling down, depressed, or hopeless	0	1	2	3

Total Score:
(in the initial study, a score of ≥3 had a sensitivity of 83% and specificity of 92% for major depression)

Prevention and Treatment Table for Anxiety and Depression Disorder

Prevention	Depression is a highly treatable condition, but some forms of depression are not preventable. The explanation is in a possible malfunctioning of nerve cell connections in the brain circuit. Good health habits may, however, improve mood and possibly prevent depression, as recent studies confirm. Regular exercise, eating a healthy diet, having enough time for fun and relaxation may all contribute to substantial mood improvement and stabilisation.
Treatment by Yourself	Talking to people you are very confident with will help you to sort out, whether it is just a mood change or more. Perhaps the questionnaire above gives additional information, but be careful, it is just a questionnaire, not a diagnosis. **Important:** If you're so down that you're having thoughts about hurting yourself or taking your life, you must be aware of two things: 1. There's always *somebody*, who loves you unconditionally (a family member, a friend, another athlete, a coach, a higher power even), even though you're possibly not conscious of it!

	2. Seek professional advice and give the professionals a chance to work with you (and in case of suicidal thoughts, to save you), it's your own responsibility to seek this professional help Every country has its own emergency system and helping organisations, which are readily available.
When is a Doctor Needed?	As soon as you feel that it is more than just a usual 'downer' or sadness. Don't wait too long.
Return to Play/Sports	Depending on the severity of the illness and according to the treating doctor.

What Does the Doctor Do?

The doctor takes the history and makes a clinical examination. A blood test may be performed to rule out deficiencies or other underlying illnesses (e.g. anaemia, iron, or vit B12 deficiency, hypothyroidism). With the history, specific questionnaires, and by ruling out other illnesses, the diagnosis can be made and treatment options discussed. A regular consultation schedule will be established in order to give assistance to the patient and to treat depression or anxiety (e.g. cognitive behavioural therapy). Treatment options with medications to assure good sleep (often a concomitant problem), to improve and stabilise mood, and possibly to address anxiety are discussed, and if appropriate, started. There are good treatment options available, both naturally (e.g. St. John's wart preparation) or chemically based (e.g. anti-depressants), which allow sports training and performance on a high level. Treatment usually lasts longer to be well balanced and really on track (mostly a couple of months, sometimes more). Talk with your doctor about your profession or your dedication to sports when it comes to treatment and discuss the RTP and if you are ready for competitions. Check if your medication requires a TUE (therapeutic use exemption) according to the WADA anti-doping code.

Literature

Trojian T. Depression is under-recognised in the sport setting: time for primary care sports medicine to be proactive and screen widely for depression symptoms. Br J Sports Med. 2015 Nov 27.

Rao AL, Hong ES. Understanding depression and suicide in college athletes: emerging concepts and future directions. Br J Sports Med. 2015 Nov 27.

Uglesić B et al. Prevalence of depressive symptoms among college students and the influence of sport activity. Coll Antropol. 2014 Mar;38(1):235-9.

Dinas PC et al. Effects of exercise and physical activity on depression. Ir J Med Sci. 2011 Jun;180(2):319-25.

Kroenke K et al. The Patient Health Questionnaire-2: validity of a two-item depression screener. Med Care. 2003 Nov;41(11):1284-92.

Raglin JS. Exercise and mental health. Beneficial and detrimental effects. Sports Med. 1990 Jun;9(6):323-9.

Resilience in Sports – How Do Athletes Cope Best With Exposure to Stress?

Definition

Resilience

- The ability to recover from, or adjust easily to misfortune or change
- The capability of a strained body to recover its size and shape after deformity caused especially by compressive stress

(Merriam-Webster)

To withstand the pressures that athletes experience, they must be able to utilise and optimise a range of mental qualities in order to cope. This internalised know-how, and these psychological capacities, are called resilience. Sarkar and Fletcher outlined very well, in their article (2014), stressors encountered by sport performers as well as protective factors that help them withstand these demands. Figure 1 (courtesy of Sarkar and Fletcher) gives a good overview of the principles of resilience. Stressors can be divided into three main categories: competitive, organisational, and personal, as encountered in the world of ambitious and professional sport. Five psychological factors (positive personality, motivation, confidence, focus, and perceived social support) provide important protection from the potential negative effect of stressors.

Figure 1: Resilience in Sports (adapted from Sarkar und Fletcher 2014)

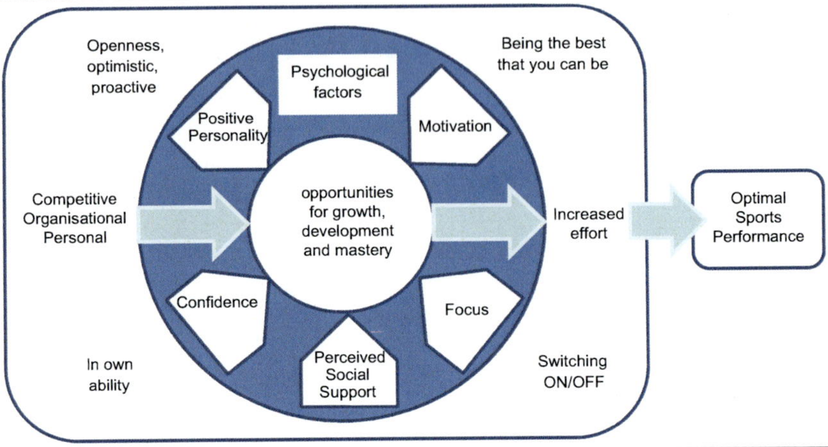

Four particular capacities need to be emphasised, as they can influence resilience:

- *Open, proactive, optimistic* behaviour of an athlete facilitates resilience
- *Be the best you can be*, be determined, and have the will to reach your best. This said, set realistic goals that are accessible to you
- *Know your own ability*, and perform within this ability, not beyond it. In conditions where things are beyond your ability, you become desperate and often struggle in vain
- *Switch ON and OFF*. To be able to switch from the top performing, hardworking athlete to your other life (be it just a normal person, student, husband, father, wife, mother, etc.) requires you to alternate top physical and mental performances with times of perfect relaxation. This is extremely valuable in times of exposure to stress

Why does this topic need to be emphasised that much?

Higher level athletes are persons of public interest. People look up to them. This athlete/crowd relationship is potentially positive and the media, as carrier of news, acts as intermediary. The news may be informative, interesting, and positive for the athlete and coach. It may also be critical, harsh, and possibly even unfair. This is more so when expectations are unrealistic or when the public interest is huge, as in the Olympic Games when the media outnumber athletes by a factor of 3. Stress exposure in events like the Olympics is, for athletes and coaches, extraordinary and unique, and they need to be prepared and ready for it. The following list gives suggestions as to how resilience may be built up:

How to build resilience **(adapted after P.Hassmen 2016)**

- Accept adversity, learn coping strategies
- See possibilities, not obstacles
- Reduce fear of failure
- Learn and grow from setbacks
- Strive for continuous improvement
- Aim for SMART goals (specific, measurable, assignable, realistic, time-related)
- Have positive attitudes and values
- Make an effort at social inclusion
- Assume responsibility (when control is possible)

Literature

Resilience definition by Merriam-Webster retrieved online 3.5.2016 / http://www.merriam-webster.com/dictionary/resilience

Sarkar M, Fletcher D. Psychological resilience in sport performers: a review of stressors and protective factors. J Sports Sci. 2014;32(15);1419-34

Nicholls AR et al. The mediating role of mental toughness in sport. J Sports Med Phys Fitness. 215 Jul-aug;55(7-8):824-34

Collins D MacNamara A. The rocky road to the top: why talent needs trauma. Sports Med. 2012 Nov 1;42(11):907-14

Gustafsson, H., Hassmén, P., & Hassmén, N. (2011). Are athletes burning out with passion? European Journal of Sport Sciences, 1, 1-9. DOI: 10.1080/17461391.2010.536573

Gustafsson, H., Hassmén, P., & Podlog, L. (2010). Exploring the relationship between hope and burnout in competitive sport. Journal of Sport Science, 28, 1495-1504.

Hassmen P. Silent Contributors Symposium 18./19.3.2016, Canberra http://sma.org.au/conferences-events/act-silent-contributors-to-injury-illness-performance-symposium

Addiction/Dependence in Sports– Too Important to Be Ignored

Symptoms

For a better understanding we may look at the definition of addiction and dependence:

Addiction[1]*:* a strong and harmful need to regularly have something (such as a drug) or do something (such as gamble)
Dependence[2]*:* a cluster of physiological, behavioural, and cognitive phenomena in which the use of a substance or a class of substances takes on a much higher priority for a given individual than other behaviours that once had greater value. A central descriptive characteristic of the dependence syndrome is the desire (often strong, sometimes overpowering) to take the psychoactive drugs (which may or may have been medically prescribed), alcohol, or tobacco

Background

Naturally as an athlete, coach, or sports medicine professional, we would like to hear that sport is nothing but protective in the field of addiction, especially dependencies. Scientific data, tell us:

- Athletes *smoke* significantly less, or possibly do not smoke, compared with non-athletes of the same age
- Athletes, especially in ice-hockey, downhill skiing, and floorball consume more *snus (oral smokeless tobacco)* than their non-athletes counterparts do (this is not specific to Nordic countries)
- It is controversial whether *alcohol consumption* is lower or higher in sport. Some studies report a rather beneficial effect

and less consumption, where other studies deliver some evidence for higher and worrisome alcohol consumption particularly in college and team sports in comparison to non-athletes

- There is a mainly positive relationship between *exercise and mental health* with a short term improvement in anxiety and mood. With long term exercise programs, physical activity may be beneficial in healthy individuals as prevention. For people with elevated anxiety or depression, exercise may function as a beneficial means of treatment
- Unfortunately exercise can result in *detrimental changes in mental health.* Some individuals become overly dependent on physical activity and exercise to an excessive degree. This abuse can result in disturbances in mood and worsened physical health

The balance seems to be mixed and that matches my experience. Sport and physical activity has, generally speaking, a rather beneficial effect and may be integrated as part of the therapeutic setting in illnesses like depression, anxiety, and addiction. But there are subgroups among sport performers in which drinking and smokeless tobacco seem to be detrimental. As sport reflects society, there are a certain number of athletes suffering addiction or dependence and needing professional help.

Prevention and Treatment Table for Addiction/ Dependency

Prevention (for athletes[9])	• *Say no. Especially learn how to say no.* If someone is pressuring you to do something that's not right for you, you have the right to say no without giving a reason and the right to just walk away • *Connect with your friends and avoid negative peer pressure.* Pay attention to who you are hanging out with. If you are part of a group in which the majority is drinking alcohol or using drugs to get high, you should definitely think about making new friends

- *Make connections with your parents or other adults.* As you grow up, having people you can rely on and can talk to about life and its challenges and your decisions about alcohol and drugs is very important.
- *Enjoy life and do what you love, don't add alcohol and drugs.* Alcohol and drugs can change who you are, limit your potential, and complicate your life
- *Follow the family rules about alcohol and drugs, if appropriate.* As you grow up and want to assume more control over your life, having the trust and respect of your parents is very important. Don't let alcohol and drugs come between you and your parents. In case your parents are having an alcohol or drug problem, get professional help. Talk to somebody about it, your coach, your doctor or another person you trust.
- *Get educated about alcohol and drugs.* You cannot rely on the myths and misconceptions that are out there among your friends and on the internet
- *Be a role model and set a positive example.* Don't forget, what you do is more important than what you say!
- *Plan ahead.* As you make plans for the party or going out with friends, you need to plan ahead. You need to protect yourself and be smart. Don't become a victim of someone else's alcohol or drug use
- *Speak out, speak up, take control.* Take responsibility for your life, your health, and your safety. Speak up about what alcohol and drugs are doing to your friends, your community, and encourage others to do the same
- *Get help!* If you or someone you know is in trouble with alcohol or drugs, get help. Don't wait. Go talk to your coach, your parents, your sports medicine physician, your family GP, or someone else

Prevention (for coaches and parents)	• *Watch your athletes and children.* You're the coach, you're the parent, so be there for your athletes and your kids. • *Share time and make connections with your athletes and children.* Show your interest for their life, what's going on at school, in further education, what they are interested in, other than sport. Sometimes you may just share time, showing you are there, if needed • *Have clear rules* in your training and in your family about alcohol and drugs. • *Learn how to say no and be consequent.* Follow your rules. Explain them to your athletes and children if it's not clear • *Enjoy life and do what you love*, don't add alcohol and drugs • *Be, as a coach and as a parent, a role model and set a positive example.* Don't forget, what you do is more important than what you say! • *Get yourself educated about alcohol and drugs.* You cannot rely on myths and misconceptions. Learn what's going on • *Get help!* If your athlete or your child or someone you know is in trouble with alcohol or drugs, get help. Don't wait. Go talk to your athletes' parents or your children's sports coach, the sports medicine physician, the family GP, or someone else
Treatment by Yourself	Seek professional help. Your doctor will discuss the topic privately (doctor-patient confidentiality).
When is a Doctor Needed?	ASAP, as soon as the problem is recognised. In many cases, it's recognised but not addressed; it's kept hidden. Often professional help for these serious and harmful illnesses is only sought as a result of external pressure. This pressure may come from somebody around you: athlete, coach, club, doctor, partner, family, or other health or sport professional. *It's this pressure and support at the same time that help the ill person.*

	And don't fall into the trap of co-dependency. In any case, seek professional help. Beware of the trap where people with alcohol problems are sure they are able to manage themselves and they can't!
Return to Play/Sports	If a serious dependency is diagnosed, professional treatment, mostly by an interdisciplinary team (doctor, sports psychology, eventually psychiatry) is needed. For athletes, sport is an essential pillar of their lives and will therefore play an important role in the rehab program.

What Does the Doctor Do?

First of all the doctor takes the history and listens to you. The doctor is a person you can trust and because of the medical secret, what you discuss with your doctor is strictly confident. So that's a good opportunity for a start.

Literature

(1) definition download online 27.11.15 http://www.merriam-webster.com/dictionary/addiction

(2) WHO-definition (world health organization) according to ICD-10; http://www.who.int/substance_abuse/terminology/definition1/en/ download online 27.11.15

(3) Henninger S et al.Physical Activity and Snus: Is There a Link? Int J Environ Res Public Health. 2015 Jul; 12(7): 7185–7198.

(4) Miller BE et al. Alcohol misuse among college athletes: self-medication for psychiatric symptoms? J Drug Educ. 2002;32(1):41-52.

(5) Peck SC, Vida M, Eccles JS. Adolescent pathways to adulthood drinking: sport activity involvement is not necessarily risky or protective. Addiction. 2008 May;103 Suppl 1:69-83.

(6) Veliz P, McCabe SE. Examining Potential Substance Use Disorders Among Former Interscholastic Athletes. Subst Abus. 2015 Oct-Dec;36(4):400-6.

(7) Henchoz Y et al. Video Gaming Disorder and Sport and Exercise in Emerging Adulthood: A Longitudinal Study. Behav Med. 2014 Sep 25:1-7

(8) Martinsen M, Sundgot-Borgen J.Adolescent elite athletes' cigarette smoking, use of snus, and alcohol. Scand J Med Sci Sports. 2014 Apr;24(2):439-46.

(9) 10 Tips National Council on Alcoholism and Drug Dependence.Inc. https://ncadd.org/about-addiction/underage-issues/ten-tips-for-prevention-for-youth

(10) Lichtenstein MB et al.Exercise addiction: a study of eating disorder symptoms, quality of life, personality traits and attachment styles. Psychiatry Res. 2014 Feb 28;215(2)

(11) Reardon CL, Creado S. Drug abuse in athletes. Subst Abuse Rehabil. 2014 Aug 14;5:95-105.

(12) Berczik K et al. Exercise addiction: symptoms, diagnosis, epidemiology, and etiology. Subst Use Misuse. 2012 Mar;47(4):403-17.

(13) Raglin JS. Exercise and mental health. Beneficial and detrimental effects. Sports Med. 1990 Jun;9(6):323-9. Review

New and Classic Therapies in Sports medicine and Sports Physiotherapy – Do They Live Up to Their Promises?

Platelet Rich Plasma (PRP) – shows promising first results

We all know our body has the capacity to fix small injuries itself. With cuts, bleeding will bring platelets and clotting factors to the injury site. These clotting factors, and especially the platelets, stimulate the surrounding tissues to collaborate and close the wound by stopping the bleeding, forming the scar, inducing the surrounding tissues to bring up their own repair mechanisms, and helping the wound to close returning tissues to their former structure and strength. The main active factors in this process are, among others: leukotrien, thromboxan, PDF, VGF.

In PRP (platelet rich plasma) this idea is put into practice; an athlete's venous blood sample is put in a centrifuge to allow separation of the different blood cells. The part of the serum containing a lot of platelets (i.e. platelet rich plasma) is taken, and injected in the injured tendon or close to the tendon origin with the micro-lesions. The platelets and the above named factors are meant to induce a healing response, which helps to cure the injury. Most studies confirm the safety of the procedure and the effect of PRP seems to be equal to other standard therapies, but good quality studies are still missing.

Literature

Guillodo Y et al. Platelet-rich plasma (PRP) treatment of sports-related severe acute hamstring injuries. Muscles Ligaments Tendons J. 2016 Feb 13;5(4):284-8.

Kaux JF et al. Tendinopathies and platelet-rich plasma (PRP): from pre-clinical experiments to therapeutic use. J Stem Cells Regen Med. 2015 May 30;11(1):7-17.

Liddle AD, Rodríguez-Merchán EC. Platelet-Rich Plasma in the Treatment of Patellar Tendinopathy: A Systematic Review. Am J Sports Med. 2015 Oct;43(10):2583-90.

Andia I et al. Platelet-rich plasma in the conservative treatment of painful tendinopathy: a systematic review and meta-analysis of controlled studies. Br Med Bull. 2014 Jun;110(1):99-115.

Stem cells – still a field of research and already quite controversial

Stem cell therapies are an interesting treatment option and a big field of research. Your own body cells (usually taken out of the abdominal subcutaneous tissue, and sometimes combined with venous blood samples and blood cells) are taken to the lab, cultivated, and then re-injected into the injured body site. This procedure could potentially be very promising for cartilage repair and early osteoarthritis, as other treatment options in this field are quite poor. Published studies with quite variable results were almost all working with animal models. Therefore, as mechanisms are still poorly understood, let's wait and see. Stem cell therapy should, if at all, only be performed within clearly defined study conditions.

Literature

Minguell JJ et al. Mesenchymal stem cells and the treatment of conditions and diseases: the less glittering side of a conspicuous stem cell for basic research. Stem Cells Dev. 2013 Jan 15;22(2):193-203.

Verdiyeva G et al. Tendon Reconstruction with Tissue Engineering Approach--A Review. J Biomed Nanotechnol. 2015 Sep;11(9):1495-523.

Valencia Mora M et al. Stem cell therapy in the management of shoulder rotator cuff disorders. World J Stem Cells. 2015 May 26;7(4):691-9.

Shockwave – a therapy that shakes the tissues

Shockwave therapy is a physical therapy with high intensity, high repetition, very low amplitude treatment. It is available as both a radial (i.e. continuous linear waves) and a focused (i.e. targeted convergent waves) application, the latter being much more expensive. The focused shockwave therapy has slightly more literature than the radial, but experience and outcome wise, both modalities are showing similar results. Treatment indications are painful heel (faszitis plantaris) and tendinopathies at various locations.

Literature

Mani-Babu S, The effectiveness of extracorporeal shock wave therapy in lower limb tendinopathy: a systematic review. Am J Sports Med. 2015 Mar;43(3):752-61.

Speed C A systematic review of shockwave therapies in soft tissue conditions: focusing on the evidence. Br J Sports Med. 2014 Nov;48(21):1538-42.

Wang CJ Extracorporeal shockwave therapy in musculoskeletal disorders. J Orthop Surg Res. 2012 Mar 20;7:11.

Eccentric strengthening

Strengthening was always part of the therapy, especially on return from an injury, in the rehabilitation process after an operation. For the last 15 years, evidence has been accumulating that strengthening plays a central role in the therapy of many medical conditions, especially in many overuse injuries especially for tendon healing, but also in muscle imbalance in athletes. It is the therapeutic modality that has immense potential in injury prevention and is an integral part of every training, and most physiotherapeutic, treatment plans.

Eccentric strengthening: strengthening studies have shown eccentric, rather than concentric, strengthening proves to be more efficient, especially in tendon healing, as the tendon becomes stronger, more robust, and more functional.

What is the difference between eccentric and concentric:

- *Eccentric* is the extension movement. In action, the muscle is elongated (the origin and insertion move away from one another). Examples: running downhill, the calf 'lowering' exercises for Achilles tendinopathy

- *Concentric* is the contraction movement. In action, the muscle is shortened (the origin and insertion approach one another) e.g. walking or running uphill.

Literature

Kedia M et al. The effects of conventional physical therapy and eccentric strengthening for insertional achilles tendinopathy. Int J Sports Phys Ther. 2014 Aug;9(4):488-97.

Jensen J et al. Eccentric strengthening effect of hip-adductor training with elastic bands in soccer players: a randomised controlled trial. Br J Sports Med. 2014 Feb;48(4):332-8.

Sussmilch-Leitch SP et al. Physical therapies for Achilles tendinopathy: systematic review and meta-analysis. J Foot Ankle Res. 2012 Jul 2;5(1):15

Brett M et al. Treatment of Tendinopathy: What Works, What Does Not, and What is on the HorizonClin Orthop Relat Res. 2008 Jul; 466(7): 1539–1554.

Cortisone – a blessing or a curse?

To be brief: a cortisone injection is an excellent medication in the doctor's bag, if used conservatively and in particular situations. Usually, cortisone injections are used when to deal with a local inflammatory response which is not responding to conservative treatment. Any cortisone injection needs to be thoroughly evaluated and you, as a patient, need to give informed consent, as there may be side effects related to a cortisone injection (e.g. slightly elevated infection risk at the site of injection, etc.). A few conditions where cortisone is appropriate are:

- Insertional tenosynovitis (i.e. overwhelming inflammatory response of a tendon) which is not responding to conservative treatment. Achilles tendinopathy is an exception and should *not* be treated with a cortisone injection, as cortisone may, in some cases, also lead to a weakening of structures
- Obstinate bursitis (inflammation of a bursa of the elbow, knee, hip)
- Intra-articular synovitis (tenacious inflammation of the inner surface of a joint)

Literature

Leadbetter WB. Anti-inflammatory therapy in sports injury. The role of nonsteroidal drugs and corticosteroid injection. Clin Sports Med. 1995 Apr;14(2):353-410.

Local anti-inflammatory treatment for tenosynovitis

Why am I explaining such a simple treatment? Because, if well done, it is easy, well-tolerated, and amazingly enough, very effective. We don't need to talk about the usual local (i.e. superficially administered as cream, ointment, plaster, spray) anti-inflammatory treatments. They are okay and help to reduce swelling and lead to slight pain reduction. But, we emphasise: *pasta boli*, an easy poultice that does an excellent job, simply my favourite for inflammatory overuse injuries, like a tenosynovitis.

Why is a poultice more powerful than any other cream?

- 8hours (overnight application) of a poultice with an active agent is better than any cream – administered for a week or ten days
- A poultice has an occlusion effect, which means skin penetration is better because of long lasting coverage of the skin by the poultice ingredients
- Salicylic acid, as an active ingredient, is one of the best skin and tissue penetrating agents
- Side effects, like a local skin reaction, are very rare

Literature

Mehallo CJ et al. Practical management: nonsteroidal anti-inflammatory drug (NSAID) use in athletic injuries. Clin J Sport Med. 2006 Mar;16(2):170-4.

Life After Competition Is Over – Start of Lifelong Recreational Sport!

Most end of career decisions are well thought through and based on the fact that the sports career is coming to an end. Other things in life are becoming more important than training and competition. Unfortunately, however, in some cases, a major injury decides when a career ends.

What comes after competition is over?

Quite often, mainly in adolescent athletes, it's about a new challenge in education. In adult elite athletes, after many years of success as a professional athlete, it's mostly about finding another professional life, with a new orientation. The decision that sport is no longer the first priority in your life may take a while to establish itself, but, as in all good decision making, all the pros and cons need to be considered. There is value in writing them down, looking at the positives and negatives of each possibility, and discussing them with your family and your mentor.

What is different?

Simply that all the training time, the many hours of specific training with the team and individually, the special sessions you may have done in the gym, the pool, on the pitch, and all the competitions are disappearing. In addition, all other scheduled appointments, team meetings, travel lasting hours and hours, instructions of the coach, the team manager, sponsor events, and so on are gone. What was a more than 100% job, an activity that gave you back a great deal over many years, is suddenly falling away. And now it's probably no longer your body that is your 'main capital' of being successful and fulfilled. It's now another (mental or practical) ability/qualification that you need at that stage in your life. There will also be a change in not being exposed anymore to the public, a bit less adrenalin and thrill – which will certainly be noticeable.

From the medical point of view, it's the abruptness of stopping these 20–30 hours of sport activity each week. Realising the benefit sport brings to your body, we feel that it can't just be left like that.

What do we need to do?

In many end-of-career-situations, we are often realistically looking at signs of overuse injuries at different locations of the athlete's body arising from many years of training and missing time for complete healing. Now, this is not an excuse for anything, but it does underline the importance of having enough time to recover, as this is the only way to achieve a long lasting successful sports career. And you don't need to hurry: give enough time for complete recovery and slowly get into lifelong recreational sport.

In summary, to gives a good rhythm of a sport activity every other day:

- 3 times a week, an endurance training session of 45–60min
- 1–2 a week, a strengthening session 40–50min focused on core, trunk, and back

Figure 1: Recommendations for Physical Activity (*Training Recommendations UK*)

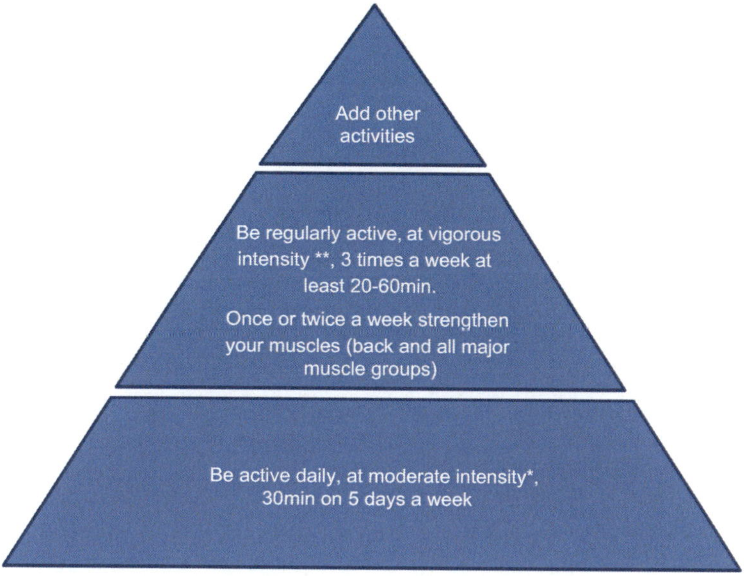

*Moderate intensity physical activities will cause adults to get warmer and breathe slightly harder, but they should be able to carry on a conversation. Examples include: Walking, cycling, light gardening

** Vigorous intensity physical activities will cause adults to start sweating and breathe much harder making it more difficult to carry on a conversation, usually you're able to just finish your sentence before you need to breathe again. Examples include: Running, sports such as swimming and football, heavy gardening, shovelling snow.

Prevention and Treatment Table for End of Career – Lifelong Sport!

Prevention	• *Keep up your good habits.* After a good break away, plan your day, have an agenda, make appointments, have a vision, and put it into practice • *Keep up structure in your life:* but let go the feeling of having to perform at top level. Learn to enjoy movement for its own sake. • *Keep a reasonable level of fitness.* You will not be able to keep your highly trained skills and that's absolutely okay. But try, if possible, even during the long holidays, to take up some recreational sport activity, leisure activity. Continue this leisure sport activity every other day

	• *Fill the gap positively.* It's normal that a certain emptiness will be noticeable. It's normal that without the many hours of training and the thrill and adrenalin of competition, life will feel a bit less tense, possibly a bit boring at times. But plan your life, plan your career after elite sport before retirement, talk to professionals in this field, develop a vision for your professional career after elite sport. Check different options and make your choice • *Don't become overweight.* Get started with the sports activities described above: movement (30min of walking, cycling, etc.) on a daily basis, walk or cycle instead of always using the car. Eat when you are hungry, but respect regular meals: breakfast, lunch, dinner. Skip all sports drinks and sports food, as they were good for you doing 20 and more hours of training, but they contain far too many calories for your reduced training program now • *Try out new hobbies and new sports.* As you now have plenty of time, get started. Start something new, exciting, challenging (e.g. language course, art course, etc.). Try new sport disciplines you've never had the time for (e.g. karate, badminton, mountain biking, kite surfing, etc.) • *Know, who your real friends are.* Look out for the ones who listen, the ones who are there for you, the ones you trust. Remember: social media is a fickle thing.
When is a Doctor Needed?	If you like, your sports medicine physician or your sports physiotherapist are certainly ready to help you with your planning for both, your complete recovery, *and* the new things to try.
Return to Play/Sports	Yes! Go for lifelong sport, not for performance, but for leisure, for fun, and for your health.

Literature

Recommendationforphysicalactivityforadults19-64years,retrievedonline5.6.2016 https://www.gov.uk/government/uploads/system/uploads/attachment_data/file/213740/dh_128145.pdf

Disclaimer/Feedback/Social Media

Important legal advice

The information in this whole manual is general in nature and is only intended to provide a summary of the subject matter covered. It is not a substitute for medical advice and you should always consult a trained professional practising in the area of sports medicine in relation to any injury. You use or rely on the information above at your own risk and no party involved in the production of this resource accepts any responsibility for the information contained within it or your use of that information.

Feedback

Please feel free to give any feedback to this handbook. *Your contribution is highly appreciated and will help improve any further edition.* Thank you!

Please send feedback:
By email: info@smzbi.ch
By post: DrAthletesHealth, Dr.med. German E. Clénin, Sportmed. Centre, House of Sports, 3063 Ittigen, Switzerland

Social Media and Website

If you are interested in receiving recent and regular tweets on Athletes' Health, please follow Dr. German E. Clénin on Twitter under **@DrAthletesHlth**

Visit the website:
www.DrAthletesHealth.ch or **www.DrAthletesHealth.com**

About the Author

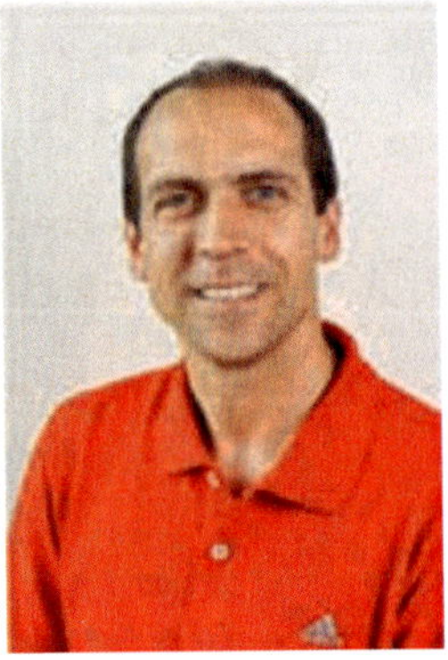

Dr.med. German E. Clénin is a sports medicine physician from Switzerland. After graduating as a physician in 1993 from the University of Berne, he successfully finished his doctoral thesis in sports medicine and exercise physiology at the Federal Office of Sports in Magglingen and the University of Zurich. After training for several years in General Internal Medicine, General and Orthopedic Surgery, Pediatrics, Gynecology, and Dermatology, he headed the Swiss Olympic Medical Center and Human Performance Lab in Magglingen for four years, working with many different sport federations and sportsmen and women of all ages, including many of Switzerland's top performing international athletes. For the last 8 years, he has worked in his own practice in the House of Sport in Ittigen/Berne, Switzerland. He works with athletes at all levels, from top international athletes performing at the Olympic Games and world championships, to weekend warriors and recreational athletes.

He has been and still is Medical Officer for the Swiss National teams of Swiss Orienteering (since 2002), Swiss Athletics (since 2013), and Swiss Ski Freestyle (since 2014). He was Chief Medical Officer for Swiss Cycling for 8 years and supported the Olympic Cross Country, Downhill, and Trial Swiss Mountain Biking teams for numerous European and world championships from 2005 to 2013. He was medical officer for the Swiss delegation at the Beijing 2008 Olympics and Deputy Chief Medical Officer for the London 2012 Olympic Games. He is affiliated with the University of Berne and is actively involved in teaching medical students and junior doctors.

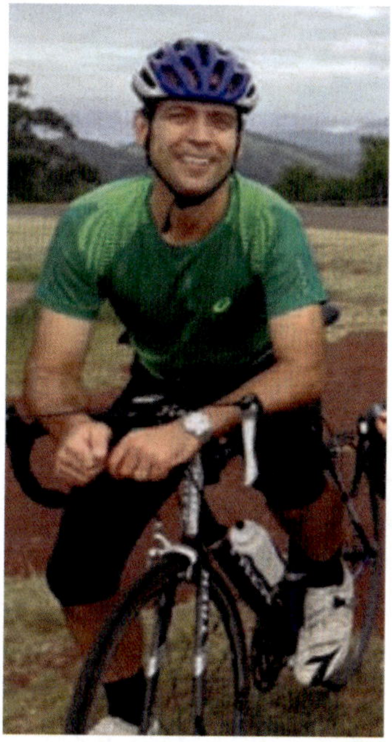

He was Director of the final exams in sports medicine in Switzerland from 2004 until 2014, and is a member of the committee of the Swiss Society of Sports Medicine and, since 2014, Vice-President of that society.

He has particular interests in the fields of athletes' health and performance, iron metabolism and iron deficiency, as well as exercise physiology and teaching. He has a postgraduate Master's degree in Medical Education. He has published in the field of sports medicine, athletes' health, and iron deficiency and lectures nationally and internationally on these topics.

His personal interests in sport are vast and include many different sport disciplines. He keeps fit with a variety of sport activities several times a week (e.g. running, cycling MTB and road, football, swimming, ice hockey, and strength training, etc.). He loves sharing time with his family and is enjoying the privilege of a sabbatical year in Australia (Maleny, QLD), writing this book, visiting friends, and making many good contacts with sports medicine physicians, sports physiotherapists, and other health and sport professionals in Australia and New Zealand.

Testimonials

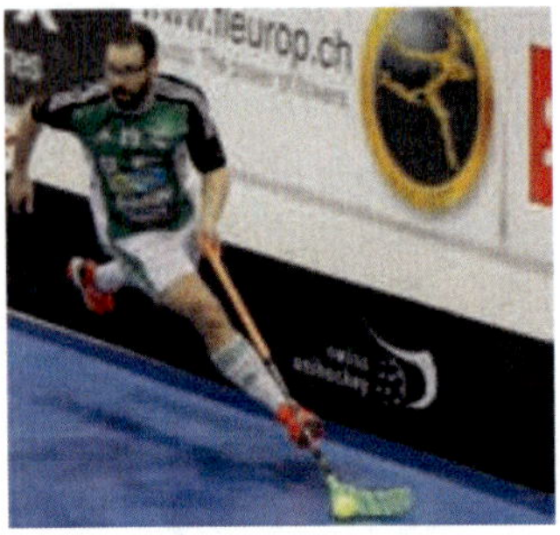

"In order to perform at the top level over several years, you need a high degree of awareness and control of your own body and mind at all times. This book is a perfect advisor which helps you to stay on track!"

Matthias Hofbauer
Captain Swiss Floorball Team
Swiss floorball's record appearance maker with 157 international caps, 5 Bronze medal World Championships, 2 x Top scorer World Championships, 8 x Swiss Champion, 1 x European Cup Champion

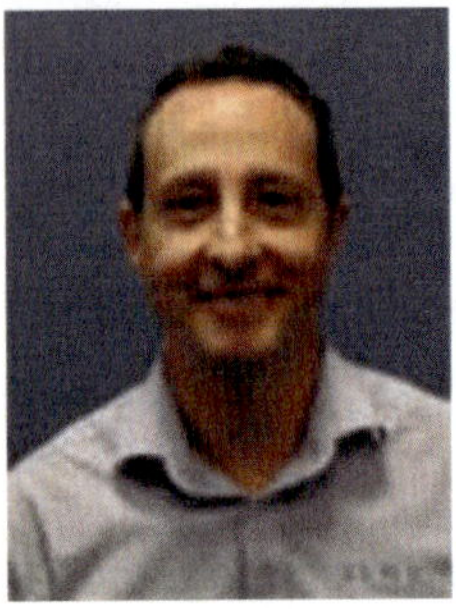

"This is a terrific resource for athletes of all ages and at all levels of sport."

Chris Brady
Sport Physiotherapist
Principal qsmc, Brisbane, Australia

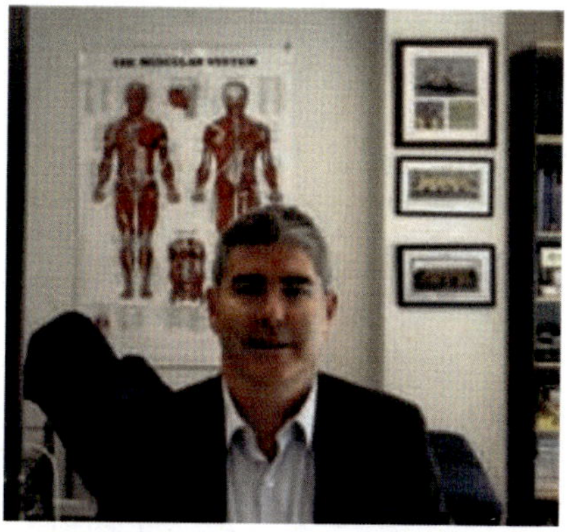

"A great resource for athletes and coaches, covering topics related to performance optimisation, medical illness, injury, rehabilitation and advanced treatment interventions in the broad field of sports medicine.

Valuable tips and practical information, clearly explained and easy to read, from an experienced Sports Physician."

Dr Corey Cunningham
Sport and Exercise Medicine Physician
Chief Medical Officer Australian Paralympic Team
Medical Director, NSW Institute of Sport

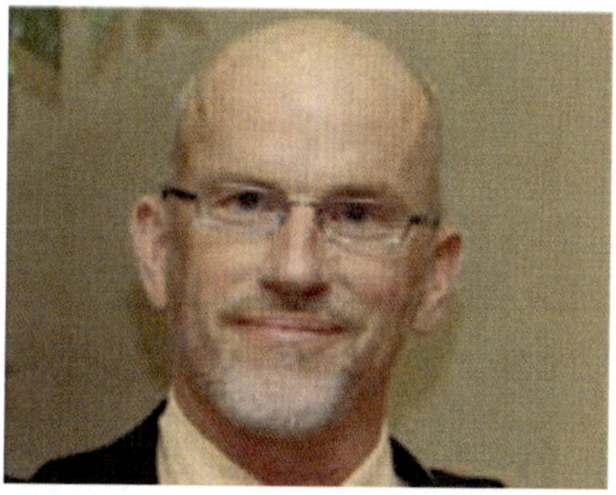

"Written from the perspective of a physician who is also an athlete, 'Athletes' Health and Top Performance?' is an invaluable resource for the elite performer to the weekend warrior.

The book gives advice on when and how to perform self-care as well as signs that indicate when it's time to see a physician.

Athletes of all persuasion will find this book to be an important part of their training regimen."

James MacDonald, MD, MPH
Nationwide Children's Hospital, Division of Sports Medicine
Associate Professor of Pediatrics, Ohio State University, USA
Associate Editor Clinical Journal of Sports Medicine

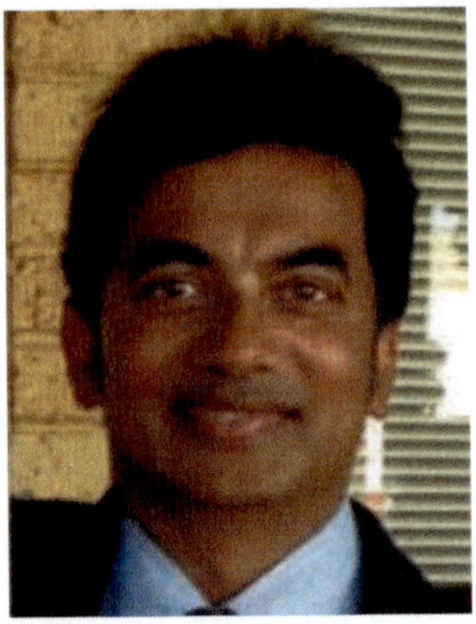

"A very engaging read. I would highly recommend this book!"

Dr Arjun Rao
Consultant Sport and Exercise Medicine Physician FACSP FFSEM (UK)
Specialist Sportscare W.A. Perth, Western Australia.

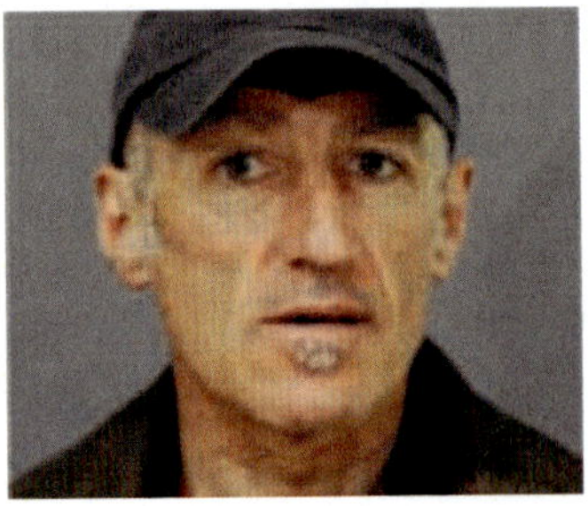

"C'est précisément dans ce genre d'ouvrage qu'émerge la passion. Geri Clénin a toujours été passionné de sport et de santé. Son travail permettra à de nombreux praticiens de ces deux domaines de découvrir de nouveaux champs d'applications. Et ceci avec le soucis du détail et d'une éthique irréprochable, par amour de l'être humain ... et de la vie!

Nicolas Siegenthaler
Teacher, Swiss Olympic Coach
Swiss Olympic Coach of the Year 2012 Elite Category
Swiss Coach of the Year 2006 Junior Category

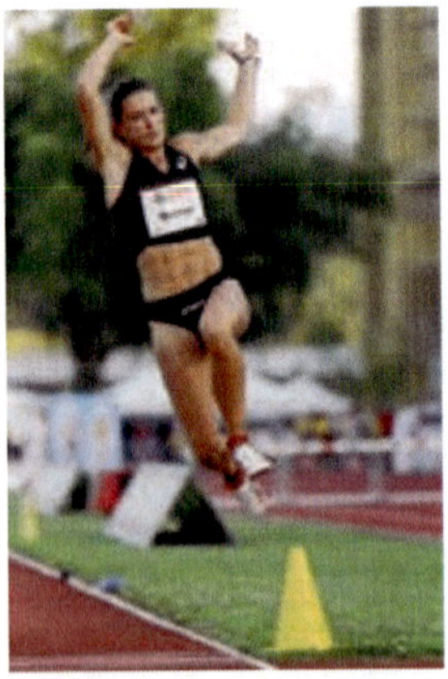

"This book belongs in every competitive athlete's bag. All medical issues of an athlete's everyday life are discussed in a precise, efficient and comprehensive manner."

Ellen Sprunger
Swiss Heptathlete
6124 points 2012, 4th place Universiade 2009, 19th Olympic Games London 2012, member of the Swiss Female Sprint Relay Team

"This book is fantastic; thoughtful and systematic. It informs about the athlete's health on so many beneficial levels and from multiple perspectives.

The competitor's well-being was always vital to me and in this book, Dr. med. German E. Clénin breaks down this complex topic in an easy-to-comprehend way. The chapters are the cumulative result of his profound sports health knowledge and decades of professional experience in this field, from the developing athlete to the accomplished Olympian.

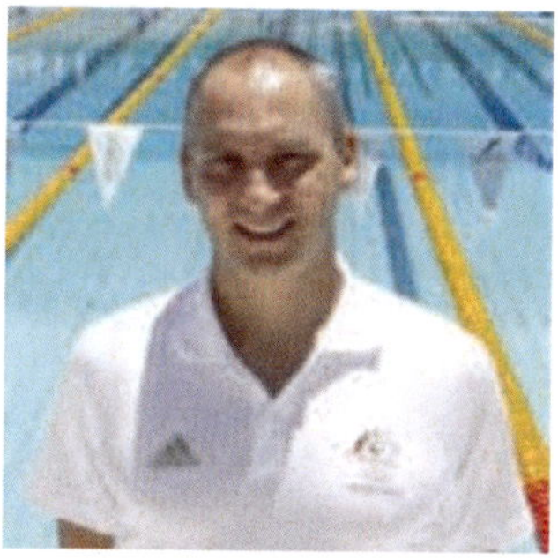

Modern sport is highly complex and today's successful programs undoubtedly recognise the importance of health, stress and performance management. With Dr. Clénin's evidence-based approach, you will gain an insight into many approved contemporary practices across these fields!

Without doubt, you will be a better equipped coach or athlete by reading his book!

A healthy athlete is always a better performing athlete.

Stephan Widmer OAM
Olympic Gold Medal Swimming Coach
2004, 2008, and 2012 Australian Olympic Swim Team Coach,
4 x Swimming Australia Coach of the Year

Made in United States
Orlando, FL
04 November 2026

90205910R00281